An Introduction to Vascular Biology
Second edition

Vascular biology is an exciting and rapidly advancing area of medical research, with many new and emerging pathophysiological links to an increasing number of diseases. This updated and expanded new edition takes full account of these developments and conveys the basic science underlying a wide range of clinical conditions, including atherosclerosis, hypertension, diabetes and pregnancy. As with the first edition, the publication provides an introductory account of vascular biology before leading on to explain mechanisms involved in disease processes. Other emerging topics include the role of nitric oxide and apoptosis in vascular biology. The breadth and range of subjects covered in this new edition do full justice to this increasingly important area of clinical research and medicine. This multidisciplinary approach will suit the needs of all those who are new to the field or working in one small area, with a need to get the wider picture, and also for those seeking to refresh their knowledge with the very latest advances from basic science through to clinical practice.

Features of the new edition

• All chapters fully updated and expanded, including up-to-date references
• Includes several new clinical chapters
• Covers new and emerging areas of research
• Integrates basic science and clinical practice

Reviews of the first edition

'I recommend this book to those seeking an introductory overview into this exciting and rapidly burgeoning area. The authors provide an up-to-date interpretation of vascular biology and how this might relate to disease; the figures are excellent; and the references offer access to further sources of information.' JOURNAL OF THE ROYAL SOCIETY OF MEDICINE

'... it makes excellent reading ... for readers who are interested in gaining fundamental understanding of this critical area. I believe the book offers an excellent pathway towards this goal.' BRITISH JOURNAL OF SURGERY

'It is well written, with the correct balance of figures, tables and text, and also well referenced ... I warmly recommend it.' BIOMEDICAL SCIENCES

An Introduction to Vascular Biology

From basic science to clinical practice

SECOND EDITION

Edited by

Beverley J. Hunt
Departments of Haematology and Rheumatology, Guy's and St Thomas' Trust, London

Lucilla Poston
Department of Obstetrics and Gynaecology, St Thomas' Hospital, London

Michael Schachter
Department of Clinical Pharmacology, Imperial College School of Medicine, London

and

Alison W. Halliday
Department of Vascular Surgery, St George's Hospital, London

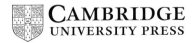
CAMBRIDGE
UNIVERSITY PRESS

PUBLISHED BY THE PRESS SYNDICATE OF THE UNIVERSITY OF CAMBRIDGE
The Pitt Building, Trumpington Street, Cambridge, United Kingdom

CAMBRIDGE UNIVERSITY PRESS
The Edinburgh Building, Cambridge CB2 2RU, UK
40 West 20th Street, New York NY 10011–4211, USA
477 Williamstown Road, Port Melbourne, VIC 3207, Australia
Ruiz de Alarcón 13, 28014 Madrid, Spain
Dock House, The Waterfront, Cape Town 8001, South Africa

http://www.cambridge.org

First published 2002

Printed in the United Kingdom at the University Press, Cambridge

Typeface Minion 10.5/14pt   *System* Poltype® [v n]

A catalogue record for this book is available from the British Library

Library of Congress Cataloguing in Publication data

An introduction to vascular biology : from basic science to clinical practice / edited by
Beverley J. Hunt . . . [et al.]. – 2nd ed.
       p.   cm.
Includes bibliographical references and index.
ISBN 0-521-79652-0 (pbk)
1. Blood-vessels–Diseases.   2. Blood-vessels–Physiology.   I. Hunt, Beverley J.
[DNLM: 1. Blood Vessels–physiology.   2. Blood Vessels–physiology.   3. Vascular
Diseases–physiopathology. WG 500 I635 2001]
RC691.I595   2001
616.1'3–dc21   2001035627

ISBN 0 521 79652 0 paperback

Contents

Contributors

Martin R. Bennett
Unit of Cardiovascular Medicine
Addenbrooke's Centre for Clinical
Investigation
Level 6, Box 110
Addenbrooke's Hospital
Hills Road, Cambridge CB2 2QQ
mrb@mole.bio.cam.ac.uk

Mark Caulfield MD FRCP
The Cardiovascular Genetics Group
Department of Clinical Pharmacology
St Bartholomew's and The Royal London
School of Medicine and Dentistry
Charterhouse Square
London EC1M 6BQ
m.j.caulfield@mds.qmw.ac.uk

Norman Chan MB ChB MRCP DCH
Centre for Clinical Pharmacology
The Rayne Institute
University College London
5 University Street
London
WC1E 6JJ
NNKAChan@aol.com

Philip Chowienczyk
Department of Clinical Pharmacology
Ground Floor
St Thomas' Hospital
London SE1 7EH
Phillip.chowienczyk@gstt.sthames.nhs.uk

Julie T. Daniels
Wound Healing Research Unit
Department of Pathology
Institute of Ophthalmology and
Glaucoma Unit
Moorfields Eye Hospital
London
j.daniels@ucl.ac.uk

Gerard Gardner PhD
The Cardiovascular Genetics Group
Department of Clinical Pharmacology
St Bartholomew's and The Royal London
School of Medicine and Dentistry
Charterhouse Square
London EC1M 6BQ

Kay Lay Goh MRCP
Department of Diabetes and Vascular
Medicine Research Centre
School of Postgraduate Medicine and
Health Sciences
Royal Devon & Exeter Hospital (Wonford)
Barrack Road
Exeter EX2 5AX

Alison W. Halliday
Department of Vascular Surgery
St George's Hospital
Blackshaw Road
London SW17 0RE

Peter Hewins BSc MRCP
Renal Immunology Group
Birmingham Centre for Immune
Regulation
The Medical School
University of Birmingham
Birmingham B15 2TT
P.Hewins@bham.ac.uk

Tim Higenbottam MA MD DSc FRCP
Clinical Sciences
AstraZeneca R&D Charnwood
Bakewell Road
Loughborough
Leicestershire LE11 5RH
tim.higenbottam@astrazeneca.com

Alun D. Hughes
Clinical Pharmacology
NHLI, Imperial College
St Mary's Hospital
London W2 1NY
a.hughes@ic.ac.uk

Beverley J. Hunt MD FRCP FRCPath
Departments of Haematology and
Rheumatology
Guy's and St Thomas' Trust
Lambeth Palace Road
London SE1 7EH
Berverley.Hunt@gstt.sthames.nhs.uk

Karen M. Jurd BSc (Hons) PhD
Principal Scientist, Protection and
Performance Department Centre for
Human Sciences
DERA Alverstoke
Gosport

Brenda A. Kelly
Maternal and Fetal Research Unit/
Centre for Cardiovascular and Vascular
Biology
King's College London
c/o Department of Obstetrics and
Gynaecology
10th Floor North Wing
St Thomas' Hospital
Lambeth Palace Road
London SE1 7EH

Peng T. Khaw
Wound Healing Research Unit
Department of Pathology
Institute of Ophthalmology and Glaucoma
Unit
Moorfields Eye Hospital
London
p.khaw@ucl.ac.uk

Joanne Knight BSc
The Cardiovascular Genetics Group
Department of Clinical Pharmacology
St Bartholomew's and The Royal London
School of Medicine and Dentistry
Charterhouse Square
London EC1M 6BQ

Helen Marriott BSc MSc
Section of Medicine and Pharmacology
Division of Clinical Sciences (South)
Floor F, Medical School
University of Sheffield
Beech Hill Road
Sheffield S10 2RX
h.m.Marriott@sheffield.ac.uk

Nicola J. McCarthy
Unit of Cardiovascular Medicine
Addenbrooke's Centre for Clinical
Investigation
Level 6, Box 110
Addenbrooke's Hospital
Hills Road, Cambridge CB2 2QQ
njm34@mole.bio.cam.ac.uk

Kirsty M. McCulloch
Department of Pharmacology
Quintiles Ltd
Research Avenue South
Heriot-Watt University Research Park
Riccarton, Edinburgh
EH14 4AP
kirsty.mcculloch@quintiles.com

John C. McGrath
Head of Division of Neurosciences and
Biomedical Systems
Institute of Biomedical and Life Sciences
University of Glasgow
West Medical Building
Glasgow G12 8QQ
Jcmcgrath@bio.gla.ac.uk

Alan R. Moody MRCP FRCP
Department of Academic Radiology
Queens Medical Centre
Nottingham NG7 2UH
Alan.Moody@nottingham.ac.uk

Patricia Munroe PhD
The Cardiovascular Genetics Group
Department of Clinical Pharmacology
St Bartholomew's and The Royal London
School of Medicine and Dentistry
Charterhouse Square
London EC1M 6BQ

Nick L. Occleston PhD
Renovo Ltd
Manchester Incubator Building
48 Grafton Street
Manchester M13 9XX
n.occleston@renovo-Ltd.com

Suzanne O'Shea
The Cardiovascular Genetics Group
Department of Clinical Pharmacology
St Bartholomew's and The Royal
London School of Medicine and
Dentistry
Charterhouse Square
London EC1M 6BQ

Lucilla Poston PhD
Maternal and Fetal Health Research Unit
Department of Obstetrics and
Gynaecology
Guy's, King's and St Thomas' School of
Medicine, and Centre for Cardiovascular
Biology and Medicine
St Thomas' Hospital
London SE1 7EH
Lucilla.poston@kcl.ac.uk

Janet T. Powell PhD MD
Professor of Vascular Biology
Department of Vascular Surgery
Imperial College School of Medicine
Charing Cross Hospital
Fulham Palace Road
London W6 8RF
Janet.Powell@wh-tr.wmids.nhs.uk

John W. Quarmby
Department of Vascular Surgery
St George's Hospital
Blackshaw Road
London SW17 0RE

Marlene L. Rose
Professor of Transplant Immunology
National Heart and Lung Institute
Imperial College School of Medicine
Heart Science Centre
Harefield Hospital
Harefield, Middlesex UB9 6JH
Marlene.rose@ic.ac.uk

James H.F. Rudd MRCP
Division of Cardiovascular Medicine
Addenbrooke's Centre for Clinical
Investigation
Addenbrooke's NHS Trust
Hills Road
Cambridge CB2 2QQ
jhfr2@cam.ac.uk

Caroline O.S. Savage MD PhD FRCP
Renal Immunology Group
Birmingham Centre for Immune
Regulation
The Medical School
University of Birmingham
Birmingham B15 2TT
C.O.S.Savage@bham.ac.uk

Michael Schachter BSc MB BS MRCP
Department of Clinical Pharmacology
National Health and Lung Institute
Imperial College School of Medicine
St Mary's Hospital
London W2 1NY
m.schachter@ic.ac.uk

Angela C. Shore PhD
Department of Diabetes and Vascular
Medicine Research Centre
School of Postgraduate Medicine and
Health Sciences
Royal Devon & Exeter Hospital
(Wonford)
Barrack Road
Exeter EX2 5AX
A.C.Shore@exeter.ac.uk

John E. Tooke
Department of Vascular Medicine
Postgraduate Medical School
Barrack Road
Exeter EX2 5AW
J.E.Tooke@exeter.ac.uk

**Patrick Vallance MRCP MD FRCP
FmedSci**
Centre for Clinical Pharmacology
The Rayne Institute
University College London
5 University Street
London WC1E 6JJ
patrick.vallance@ucl.ac.uk

**Peter L. Weissberg MD FRCP FMedSci
FESC**
Division of Cardiovascular Medicine
Addenbrooke's Centre for Clinical
Investigation
Addenbrooke's NHS Trust
Hills Road
Cambridge CB2 2QQ
plw@mole.bio.cam.ac.uk

David Williams MRCP
Department of Obstetrics and
Gynaecology
Imperial College School of Medicine
Chelsea and Westminster Hospital
Fulham Road
London SW10 9NH
david.williams@ic.ac.uk

Preface to Second Edition

The science of vascular biology has emerged and expanded rapidly over the past 25 years. Research in this area has increased understanding of a wide range of clinical conditions. This book provides a broad overview of the field for both specialist and newcomer to the field, and concise resource for the non-specialist. The multidisciplinary team of contributors covers topics ranging from normal and pathological aspects of endothelial cell function to the role of the vasculature in pregnancy, hypertension and atherosclerosis.

The authors have been selected for their ability to provide clear explanations of their area, resulting in an easily readable text with carefully produced illustrations. This second edition has allowed for increased clarity in presentation: the book has been divided into three sections, basic science, pathogenic mechanisms, and clinical practice. There is also inclusion of information on new and advancing areas in vascular biology including chapters on nitric oxide, apoptosis, imaging and pregnancy.

Beverley Hunt

Part I

Basic science

Vascular tone

Alun D. Hughes

Clinical Pharmacology, NHLI, Imperial College, St Mary's Hospital, London

Introduction

This chapter provides an overview of how vascular smooth muscle cells produce force and how this process is regulated. An overview inevitably involves generalizations and this tends to obscure the considerable diversity that exists in vascular smooth muscle. Such diversity is unsurprising if one recalls the variety of functions performed by blood vessels. Large arteries act as elastic conduits, smaller arteries regulate the distribution of blood flow, the microvasculature largely determines vascular resistance and fluid exchange, while the venous system undertakes a capacitive role and governs venous return to the heart. When these differences are compounded with the differences in behaviour required from blood vessels supplying different tissues, one can see that smooth muscle diversity is a positive asset that allows appropriate responses in a particular circumstance.

Owing to space constraints I have not attempted to provide comprehensive source references in this chapter. Instead, recent reviews have been cited and these should be referred to for more detailed information regarding a particular topic and original sources.

Types of stimulus for contraction and relaxation

Under physiological circumstances the primary role of differentiated (as opposed to 'synthetic') smooth muscle is to generate force. Normally, the vascular smooth muscle that makes up the bulk of the blood vessel wall is in a state of continual activation. The amount of force generated by smooth muscle is finely regulated by a variety of extracellular and intrinsic factors. The types of stimuli that act on vascular smooth muscle can be grouped into five categories:

1. Agents acting at G protein-coupled receptors
2. Pressure/tension
3. Agents acting directly on ion channels or signalling systems

4. Extracellular matrix components, cell adhesion molecules and integrins
5. Growth factors

Agents acting at G protein-coupled receptors

This group includes the majority of classical vasoconstrictors, such as α-adreno-ceptor agonists, angiotensin II, serotonin and vasopressin, and vasodilators such as β-adrenoceptor agonists, vasoactive intestinal peptide and calcitonin gene-related peptide. These agents act by binding to receptors that couple to hetero-trimeric G proteins (R_7G: Morris and Malbon, 1999). R_7G form a protein super-family; all possess seven transmembrane domains and in consequence are also known as serpentine receptors (Figure 1.1).

Heterotrimeric G proteins act as signal transducers linking the extracellular ligand to a variety of intracellular signals, such as $[Ca^{2+}]_i$, cyclic nucleotides or ion channels. Heterotrimeric G proteins are membrane-associated proteins composed of α, β and γ subunits with the α subunit possessing guanosine triphosphatase (GTPase) activity (Figure 1.1). In the absence of receptor activation they exist in an inactive guanosine diphosphate (GDP)-bound state. The ligand-receptor complex acts as a GDP/GTP exchange factor promoting formation of a dissociated α subunit–GTP complex and a free $\beta\gamma$ dimer. The α subunit–GTP complex and the $\beta\gamma$ dimer remain associated with the cell membrane and both play signalling roles (Morris and Malbon, 1999). After signalling activation of the intrinsic GTPase of the α subunit catalyses hydrolysis of GTP to GDP which completes the cycle and results in reformation of the inactive $\alpha\beta\gamma$ heterotrimer–GDP complex. The system is regulated at two points. Firstly, downstream targets, including receptor kinases (GRKs) and β-arrestins, can negatively feed back on to receptor–G protein interactions (Lefkowitz, 1998). Secondly, regulators of G-protein signalling (RGS) proteins act to enhance the GTPase activity of α subunits (Dohlman and Thorner, 1997). A number of isoforms of both α and $\beta\gamma$ subunits exist and preferential coupling of the receptor to a specific $\alpha\beta\gamma$ combination probably accounts for the diversity of intracellular events generated by this signalling complex (Hildebrandt, 1997).

Pressure/tension

The ability of vascular smooth muscle to respond to increased transmural pressure by increased tone was first recognized by Bayliss in 1902. The current view is that wall tension or stress, rather than pressure *per se* is the stimulus for contraction. The balance between myogenic tone and endothelium-dependent vasodilatation may coordinate the behaviour of arterial networks (Griffith et al., 1987). While the myogenic response is a very important determinant of tone, perhaps particularly in the microvasculature, the biochemical mechanisms underlying its transduction are still poorly understood; stretch-induced production of vasoconstrictors or

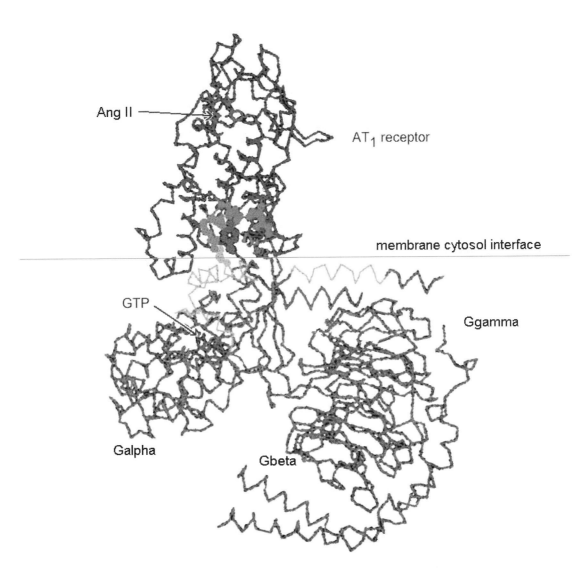

Figure 1.1   Receptor (R₇G) and associated heterotrimeric G protein. Example shown is of an angiotensin II type 1 (AT₁) receptor and a G protein heterotrimer. The image is based on a model constructed by Paiva, A.C.M. Costa-Neto, C.M. & Oliveira, L. Molecular modeling and mutagenesis studies of angiotensin II/AT₁ interaction and signal transduction. On-line Proceedings of the 5th Internet World Congress on Biomedical Sciences '98 at McMaster University, Canada (available from URL:http://www.mcmaster.ca/inabis98/escher/paiva0625/index.html#abstract).

growth factors, stretch sensitivity of ion channels, signalling enzymes and the sensitivity of cell–cell or cell–matrix interactions to tensile stress are all possible candidates for this role.

Agents acting directly on ion channels or signalling systems

A number of agents, such as H^+ ions (intracellular and extracellular pH: Aalkjaer and Peng, 1997), nitric oxide (NO: Ignarro et al., 1999), free radicals and reactive oxygen species (e.g. superoxide anions (O_2^-), hydrogen peroxide: Beckham and Koppenol, 1996; Hancock, 1997), have marked effects on ion channels and intracellular signalling systems. These mechanisms play important roles in physiological and pathological responses in the vasculature.

Extracellular matrix components, cell adhesion molecules and integrins

Cell-to-cell and extracellular matrix-to-cell interactions profoundly affect smooth muscle cell behaviour (Hughes and Schachter, 1994; Braun et al., 1999). Activation of receptors for extracellular matrix proteins (integrins) alters smooth muscle tone. This effect can be mediated by the endothelium (Mogford et al., 1997), or involve direct effects on smooth muscle cells (Mogford et al., 1997; Yip and Marsh, 1997; Wu et al., 1998a).

Growth factors

Vascular growth factors are potent chemoattractants and mitogens. Factors such as platelet-derived growth factor (PDGF) and basic fibroblast growth factor (bFGF) are thought to play an important part in the blood vessel's response to injury (Ross, 1999). Growth factors can also affect vascular tone (Berk and Alexander, 1989; Hughes and Wijetunge, 1998), although the physiological significance of this action is uncertain.

The majority of growth factors act by binding to and inducing dimerization of transmembranous receptors which are intrinsic tyrosine kinases. Dimerization results in transautophosphorylation of tyrosine residues in the intracellular domain of the receptor and leads to recruitment and activation of a range of signalling molecules (Hughes et al., 1996). Increasing evidence suggests an important role for tyrosine kinases in the regulation of smooth muscle tone, even in response to classical vasoconstrictors (Hughes and Wijetunge, 1998).

Regulation of $[Ca^{2+}]_i$ in vascular smooth muscle

The pivotal role of Ca^{2+} in muscle contraction has been recognized for many years. $[Ca^{2+}]_i$ can rise as a consequence of an increase in influx of extracellular Ca^{2+}, alteration in the amount of intracellularly sequestered Ca^{2+} or a decrease in efflux of cellular Ca^{2+}. In general, most contractile stimulants appear to act by altering influx or release of Ca^{2+}. The relative importance of influx or release from stores varies between blood vessels of differing calibre. In the resistance vasculature (i.e. vessels with internal diameters less than 500 μm) and microvasculature (arterioles and precapillary vessels), Ca^{2+} entry through voltage-operated calcium channels appears to predominate (Hughes, 1995).

Ca^{2+} influx

Ion channels, membrane potential and $[Ca^{2+}]_i$

Vascular smooth muscle cells maintain a low $[Ca^{2+}]_i$ ($\sim$ 100 nmol/L) in the face of an immense electrochemical gradient (extracellular Ca^{2+} $\sim$ 1.6 mmol/L, membrane potential (E_m) $\sim$ 60 mV). The smooth muscle cell possesses powerful Ca^{2+}-buffering capacity; $\sim$ 99% of the Ca^{2+} entering the cell is estimated to bind to proteins or to be taken up into stores (Kamishima and McCarron, 1996). Despite this, opening of Ca^{2+} channels causes $[Ca^{2+}]_i$ to rise to micromolar levels. This is sufficient to activate the contractile (and other) processes. There is now substantial evidence that $[Ca^{2+}]_i$ is compartmentalized within the cell and that localized increases in $[Ca^{2+}]_i$ are important to cell function, particularly regulation of ion channel opening (Jaggar et al., 1998a).

The major Ca^{2+}-permeable channel in vascular smooth muscle is the voltage-operated calcium channel (Hughes, 1995). As its name implies, this channel is primarily regulated by E_m and the likelihood of the channel opening (open probability) increases steeply with depolarization. Consequently, E_m is an important determinant of Ca^{2+} influx in vascular smooth muscle cells.

In the main, E_m in vascular smooth muscle is governed by the membrane permeability to four ions, K^+, Cl^-, Na^+ and Ca^{2+}, with K^+ being the major determinant of E_m under resting conditions (Figure 1.2).

Electrogenic pumps such as the Na-K-ATPase or the Na/Ca exchanger also have an influence on E_m and the Na-K-ATPase may contribute up to 10 mV under certain circumstances (Hermsmeyer, 1982).

Most studies of isolated blood vessels carried out under isometric conditions in vitro give values for resting E_m of ~ -60 mV, although more depolarized potentials have been recorded in pressurized arteries (Harder, 1984). In vivo smaller arteries would be expected to be relatively depolarized as a result of 'myogenic' depolarization and prevailing tonic contractile influences such as the sympathetic nervous system and circulating factors. Measurements of E_m in vivo are consistent with this, with E_m being in the range ~ -40 mV (Bryant et al., 1985). This has important consequences for our understanding of the action of some drugs, e.g. dihydropyridine, which act preferentially on depolarized cells.

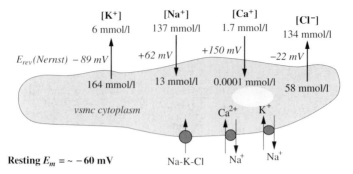

Figure 1.2   Determinants of resting membrane potential (E_m) in vascular smooth muscle. Diagram shows the concentration gradients and equilibrium (reversal) potentials (E_{rev}) of the major ions. The major ion pumps are also indicated.

Unlike most excitable cells, vascular smooth muscle cells rarely display action potentials (for an exception, see Yamaguchi and Jensen, 1993), but show graded depolarization to stimuli. In most cases the vascular muscle cells in the blood vessel wall act as an electrically coupled multiunit. This electrical coupling is due to the existence of intercellular connections (gap junctions) between smooth muscle cells. Gap junctions are formed from the apposition of two hemichannels (connexons), each composed of six transmembrane proteins (connexins). Numerous connexins have been described, but connexin 43 is the most common type in arterial smooth muscle (Brink, 1998; Gustafsson and Holstein-Rathlou, 1999). As a result of the electrical coupling a blood vessel behaves like a three-dimensional electrical cable through which potential changes can propagate (Holman et al., 1990; Tomita, 1990; Gustafsson and Holstein-Rathlou, 1999). Estimates of the cable properties of smooth muscles vary, but values for the length constant of electrical conduction λ are generally in the range 1–2 mm. It has been suggested that smooth muscle cells and endothelial cells may also be electrically coupled via gap junctions in some blood vessels (Gustafsson and Holstein-Rathlou, 1999).

Major ion channel species in vascular smooth muscle

K channels

K channels make up a large family of channels encoded by multiple gene families (Standen and Quayle, 1998). K channels consist of four α subunits that are associated with β subunits to make a hetero-octomer (Figure 1.3). The α subunits form the channel pore while the β subunits modify channel gating properties. Four major types of K channel are present in vascular smooth muscle: voltage-dependent (K_V) channels, Ca^{2+}-activated (K_{Ca}) channels, inward rectifier (K_{IR}) channels and ATP-sensitive (K_{ATP}) channels. The presence of relatively large

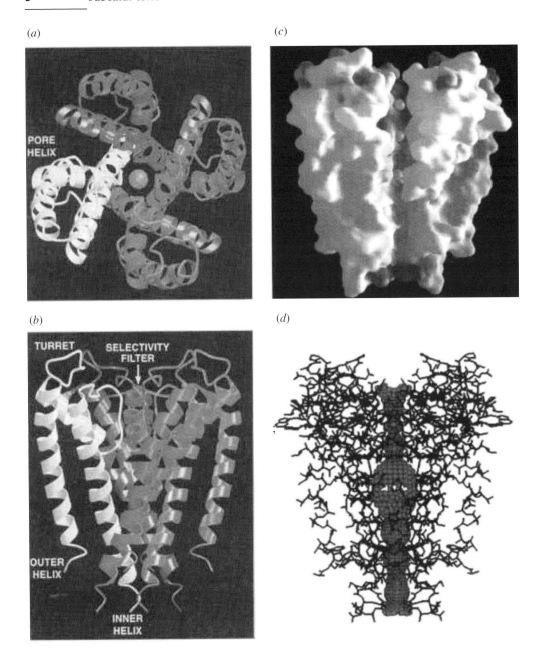

(a)

(c)

(b)

(d)

Figure 1.3   Views of the KcsA channel tetramer, molecular surface of KcsA and contour of the pore. *(a)* Stereoview of a ribbon representation illustrating the three-dimensional fold of the KcsA tetramer viewed from the extracellular side (above). The four subunits are distinguished by colour. *(b)* Stereoview from another (side) perspective, perpendicular to that in *(a)*. Original diagrams were prepared with MOLSCRIPT and RASTER-3D. *(c)* A cutaway stereoview displaying the solvent-accessible surface of the K channel. *(d)* Stereoview of the entire internal pore. This display was created with the program HOLE. Modified from Doyle et al. (1998) with permission.

numbers of K channels (plus the low density of L-type calcium channels and the absence of voltage-operated Na channels) probably accounts for the rarity of action potentials recorded from vascular smooth muscle cells. There is considerable evidence that K channels dominate E_m in vascular smooth muscle under resting conditions. Recent evidence has highlighted the role of K_{Ca} channels in myogenic tone (Jaggar et al., 1998a) and hypoxic vasoconstriction in the lung (Dumas et al., 1999; McCulloch et al., 1999). Many vasoactive agents affect K channel opening. This may account for the ability of these agents to alter E_m (Standen and Quayle, 1998). In some cases (e.g. NO) this may involve direct effects on the channels; in other cases protein kinases, such as protein kinase C, tyrosine kinases or cyclic nucleotide-dependent kinases, appear to mediate this effect. In addition, a num-ber of therapeutic vasodilators act on K channels. Examples include minoxidil and nicorandil which open K_{ATP} channels (Standen and Quayle, 1998), and thiazide diuretics which open K_{Ca} channels (Table 1.1: Calder et al., 1993).

Cl channels

Cl$^-$ ions are actively concentrated inside the vascular smooth muscle cell, probably as a result of the activity of the Na-K-2Cl cotransporter and HCO_3^-/Cl^- exchange. Consequently the equilibrium potential for Cl$^-$ ion (E_{Cl}) is around $-25\,mV$. Opening Cl channels will therefore depolarize smooth muscle cells. Two classes of Cl channels have been identified in vascular smooth muscle – a Ca^{2+}-activated Cl channel (Cl_{Ca}: Large and Wang, 1996) and volume-sensitive Cl channels (Yamakazi et al., 1998; Lamb et al., 1999). Cl_{Ca} has not been identified at the molecular level, but it is a small conductance channel (Klockner, 1993), that opens in response to a rise in $[Ca^{2+}]_i$. Opening of this channel has been implicated in agonist-induced depolarization (Large and Wang, 1996). A number of relatively nonselective blockers of this channel have been described, but in general much remains to be learned about the biophysics, physiological role and regulation of this channel.

Volume-regulated chloride channels form a family currently containing nine members (Jentsch et al., 1999). One of these, CLCN3, has been demonstrated in vascular smooth muscle cells (Yamakazi et al., 1998; Lamb et al., 1999). It has been suggested that this channel contributes to pressure-induced depolarization and plays a role in myogenic responses (Yamakazi et al., 1998).

Voltage-operated sodium channels

There is little evidence that tetrodotoxin-sensitive voltage-operated Na$^+$ channels like those found in neurons or cardiac myocytes contribute to E_m in vascular smooth muscle cells. However, relatively nonselective channels permeable to

Table 1.1 Ion channels in vascular smooth muscle

Channel	Physiological role	Opener	Inhibitor/blocker
Potassium channels			
K_V	Regulation of membrane potential. Hypoxic pulmonary vasoconstriction	Depolarization	4-Aminopyridine, quinidine, phenylcyclidine, tedisamil, tetraethylammonium
K_{IR}	Resting membrane potential K$^+$-induced dilatation	Depolarization	Ba^{2+}
K_{Ca}	Myogenic tone. 'Brake' on agonist-induced depolarization	$[Ca^{2+}]_i$ Depolarization Thiazides NS004	Charybdotoxin, iberiotoxin
K_{ATP}	Metabolic regulation of tone. Reactive hyperaemia. Autoregulation. Endotoxic shock	$[ATP]_I$ Cromakalim, diazoxide, minoxidil, nicorandil, pinacidil, RP-49356	Sulphonylureas, U-37883A, Ba^{2+}
Chloride channels			
Cl_{Ca}	Agonist-induced depolarization in some smooth muscle	$[Ca^{2+}]_i$	Niflumic acids, stilbenes (e.g. DIDS, SITS), furosemide (frusemide)
Cl_v	Pressure-induced depolarization	Increased in cell volume	Stilbenes, 5-nitro-2-(3-phenylpropylamino)-benzoate
Cation channels			
Receptor-operated channels	Agonist-induced depolarization	G protein-linked receptors	Inorganic cations (e.g. Ni^{2+}, Gd^{3+})
Ca^{2+}-activated		$[Ca^{2+}]_i$	
Calcium channels			
L-type	Myogenic tone. Agonist-induced calcium entry	Depolarization, dihydropyridine agonists (e.g. Bay K8644a)	Dihydropyridine antagonists, phenylalkylamines, benzothiazepines
T-type	'Pacemaker' activity?	Depolarization	Mibefradil

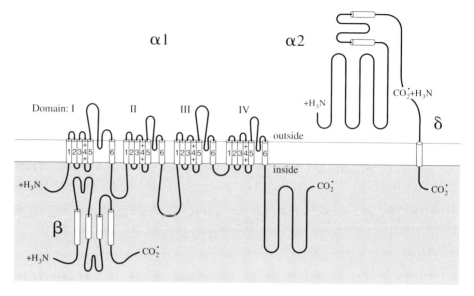

Figure 1.4   Transmembrane organization of voltage-gated Ca^{2+} channels. The primary structures of the subunits of voltage-gated Ca^{2+} are illustrated. Cylinders represent probable α helical transmembrane segments. Bold lines represent the polypeptide chains of each subunit with length approximately proportional to the number of amino acid residues. The α1c subunit (160–273 kDA) consists of four internal repeated domains (I–IV). Each domain contains six α-helical transmembrane regions (S1–S6). Domain I is responsible for channel activation kinetics. S4 is positively charged and forms part of the voltage sensor. The two additional domains between S5 and S6 form pore region of channel. Verapamil and nifedipine bind to helix 5 and 6 regions of domain III. Modified from Hockerman et al. (1997) with permision.

mono- and divalent cations (see below) may contribute to increased Na^+ permeability following agonist activation in some vascular smooth muscle.

Voltage-operated calcium channels

The major calcium channel in vascular smooth muscle is the voltage-operated L-type calcium channel (Ca_v 1.2: Hughes, 1995). T-type channels (Ca_v 3.2) have also been demonstrated in vascular smooth muscle cells, although their physiological significance is uncertain. The molecular characteristics of both L- and T-type channels have now been described (Catterall, 1998). Both channel types consist of α_1, β and $\alpha_2\delta$ components (Figure 1.4). The α_1 subunit forms the pore of the channel, while the β and $\alpha_2\delta$ subunits are involved in membrane targeting (Brice et al., 1997) and modulation of channel opening (Catterall, 1998). The α_1 subunit (α_{1c}) found in smooth muscle is similar to that found in cardiac muscle, though a number of splice variants have been described (Feron et al., 1994; Welling et al., 1997). All classes of calcium antagonists (i.e. dihydropyridines, phenylalkylamines and benzothiazepines) bind to the α_{1c} subunit. Dihydro-pyridines show higher affinity for smooth muscle-type α_{1c} isoforms (Welling et al., 1997). This, in combination with the higher affinity of dihydropyridines for depolarized channels, probably accounts for their selective actions on the vasculature. The L-type channel is also a major target for physiological modulation and many vasoactive agents can modulate its gating properties as well as influencing opening through effects on E_m. Several signalling pathways probably contribute to channel modulation following agonist-induced activation, including tyrosine phosphorylation (Hughes and Wijetunge, 1998) and protein kinase C (PKC: Hughes, 1995). Recently, an endogenous tyrosine kinase (c-*src*) has also been proposed to contribute to L-type channel availability under resting conditions (Hughes and Wijetunge, 1998).

Calcium (cation) channels

Ca^{2+} can also enter the vascular smooth muscle cell through cation channels. Unlike voltage-operated calcium channels which are highly selective for Ca^{2+}, cation channels show limited selectively for divalent cations and also allow Na^+ to enter the cell. Opening cation channels will therefore cause depolarization in addition to Ca^{2+} entry. Three types of cation channel have been described in vascular smooth muscle – those linked to vasoconstrictor agonists, termed receptor-operated channels (ROC: Benham and Tsien, 1987; Wang et al., 1993; Hughes and Bolton, 1995), those opened as a result of a rise in $[Ca^{2+}]_i$–Ca^{2+}-activated cation channels (Loirand et al., 1991) and so-called leak channels which are not known to be regulated (Benham and Tsien, 1987). No physiological role has been assigned to Ca^{2+}-activated cation channels, but opening of ROCs is an important mechanism by which vasoconstrictors induce Ca^{2+} entry and depolarization in some vascular smooth muscle.

Intracellular calcium stores

All muscle types possess intracellular storage sites for Ca^{2+}. In the cytoplasm Ca^{2+} is largely found associated with the endoplasmic (sarcoplasmic) reticulum (SR) and mitochondria. The SR is generally considered to be the site from which Ca^{2+} is released upon activation, although mitochondria may contribute to Ca^{2+} removal.

Ultrastructural studies indicate that the SR is less well organized in smooth muscle than in cardiac or skeletal muscle (Nixon et al., 1994). In keeping with this, Ca^{2+} release from the SR appears to be of lesser importance to the contractile process in smooth muscle. It is most important in large arteries or vessels that show phasic contractions (Ashida et al., 1988; Karaki et al., 1997). However, even in small arteries, release of Ca^{2+} from the stores is important for some responses, e.g. those evoked by brief neural activation (Garcha and Hughes, 1997). Release from Ca^{2+} stores is also believed to be involved in the generation of intense localized rises in $[Ca^{2+}]_i$ (Ca^{2+} sparks). Such sparks are generally seen in the vicinity of the plasma membrane and it has been proposed that they regulate K_{Ca} and other Ca^{2+}-sensitive ion channel activity and may contribute to myogenic responses (Jaggar et al., 1998a,b).

The importance of the SR to Ca^{2+} removal varies depending on the tissue studied (Baro and Eisner, 1995; Kamishima and McCarron, 1998). However, uptake by the SR may also modulate the consequences of Ca^{2+} entry by influencing local $[Ca^{2+}]_i$. In this model (the superficial buffer model: Van Breemen et al., 1995) the SR prevents rises in $[Ca^{2+}]_i$ in the vicinity of the cell membrane spreading to the contractile machinery located nearer the cell interior. The permeability of the store therefore modulates the extent to which Ca^{2+} entering the cell causes contraction. Evidence regarding the importance of this mechanism is equivocal, although it seems likely that the activity of the SR can account for considerable spatial variation in $[Ca^{2+}]_i$.

The net permeability of the intracellular Ca^{2+} store is determined by uptake into and efflux from the SR. Uptake is via a Ca^{2+}-ATPase, probably the SERCA 2b subtype. Activity of this pump is regulated by phospholamban (PLB). PLB is a 24–27 kDa protein which inhibits the SR Ca^{2+}-ATPase when it is dephosphorylated (Kadambi and Kranias, 1997). In vitro PLB can be phosphorylated by cyclic adenosine 3,5-monophosphate(cAMP)-dependent protein kinase, cyclic guanosine 3,5-monophosphate (cGMP)-dependent protein kinase, Ca^{2+}-calmodulin-dependent protein kinase II or PKC. Phosphorylation by cyclic nucleotide-dependent kinases may account for the ability of cAMP and cGMP to stimulate Ca^{2+}-ATPase in smooth muscle (Raeymaekers and Wuytack, 1993). The endoplasmic reticulum Ca^{2+}-ATPase can also be blocked irreversibly by thapsigargin and reversibly by cyclopiazonic acid. The agents have proved to be useful tools for examining the function of the SR in smooth muscle.

Ca^{2+} release from the SR occurs through Ca^{2+}-selective ion channels. Two related types of channel have been described in smooth muscle: inositol 1,4,5-triphosphate (IP_3)-sensitive channels (IP_3R) and ryanodine-sensitive channels (RyR). In some tissues these channels may occupy spatially distinct regions within the cell (Tribe et al., 1994). IP_3R has been isolated from aortic smooth muscle and opens following binding of IP_3. The IP_3R has been reported to be phosphorylated by cGMP-dependent protein kinase. Phosphorylation of the channel results in channel inactivation in vitro, but the physiological significance of this is uncertain (Hofmann et al., 2000). In smooth muscle the IP_3R coprecipitates with cGMP-dependent kinase and another protein IP_3R-associated cGMP-dependent kinase substrate (IRAG). IRAG is a target for cGMP-dependent kinase phosphorylation and phosphorylation of IRAG can inhibit IP_3-dependent Ca^{2+} release (Hofmann et al., 2000). IP_3 is produced as a result of agonist activation of phospholipase C (PLC) which hydrolyses the minor membrane lipid phosphatidylinositol 4,5-bisphosphate (PIP_2) to IP_3 and diacylglycerol (DAG). A number of isoforms of PLC have been described, but the identity of the isoform mediating agonist-induced effects in vascular smooth muscle is uncertain. In the majority of cell types PLC-β is responsible for IP_3 generation following agonist activation; however, a number of recent studies have failed to demonstrate PLC-β in vascular smooth muscle. It has therefore been suggested that PLC-γ or PLC-δ may also play a functional role (Marrero et al., 1994; Lymn and Hughes, 2000).

The physiological role of the RyR in vascular smooth muscle is undetermined. This channel is sensitive to Ca^{2+}, adenine nucleotides, Mg^{2+} and pH and blocked by ryanodine and ruthenium red. Opening of this channel accounts for the ability of caffeine to increase $[Ca^{2+}]_i$. In other tissues (e.g. intestinal smooth muscle and myocardium) the RyR accounts for Ca^{2+}-induced Ca^{2+} release from the intracellular store. In vascular smooth muscle the overall importance of this mechanism is disputed (Ganitkevich and Isenberg, 1995; Kamishima and McCarron, 1997). Nevertheless, the RyR may be involved in Ca^{2+} spark generation (Jaggar et al., 1998b; Coussin et al., 2000) or underlie the establishment of Ca^{2+} waves within the cell (Collier et al., 2000).

Calcium efflux: Ca-ATPase, Na/Ca exchange

Vascular smooth muscle can also extrude Ca^{2+} into the extracellular medium through the action of Ca^{2+} pumps in the cell membrane. Both the plasma membrane Ca-ATPase(PMCA) and the Na^+/Ca^{2+} exchanger contribute to this process. The affinity of PMCA for Ca^{2+} is increased by calmodulin (CaM) and by cAMP-or cGMP-dependent kinases. In general, this is the major efflux pathway for Ca^{2+} in vascular smooth muscle cells. In most blood vessels the Na^+/Ca^{2+} exchanger is probably of minor importance to overall Ca^{2+} homeostasis (Mulvany et al., 1991; Kamishima and McCarron, 1998). Nevertheless, a close association between the SR, the Na^+/Ca^{2+} exchanger and the Na-K-ATPase has been reported in smooth muscle (Moore et al., 1993). If such coupling is a general feature of smooth muscle it is likely to be of functional significance.

This completes the discussion of how $[Ca^{2+}]_i$ is regulated in vascular smooth muscle, but before going on to how a rise in $[Ca^{2+}]_i$ causes force generation, the structural elements of the differentiated smooth muscle cell need to be considered.

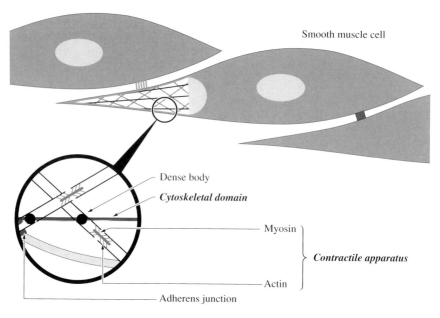

Figure 1.5   The structural organization of the smooth muscle cell. Schematic depiction of the organization of filaments in a vascular smooth muscle cell. Filaments are organized into distinct structural (cytoskeletal) and contractile domains which interconnect via dense bodies. After Small (1995).

The ultrastructure of the contractile apparatus in smooth muscle

The structural elements of the vascular smooth muscle cell can be divided into those common structural elements present in all cells – the cytoskeleton and membrane skeleton – and the specialized arrangement of force-generating components – the contractile apparatus. The major components of the cytoskeleton, membrane skeleton and contractile apparatus are shown in Table 1.2. Unlike cardiac and skeletal muscle, the ultrastructural organization of the contractile apparatus is irregular in smooth muscle (Small, 1995; Small and Gimona, 1998). Studies show filamentous structures in the cytoplasm of smooth muscle cells, but these lack the characteristic geometric arrangement seen in striated muscle, hence the smooth appearance of the cell when viewed by light microscopy. This should not be taken to mean that the contractile machinery is disorganized, as it could equally imply that the three-dimensional pattern is spatially more complex than in striated muscle (Figure 1.5). The contractile machinery in vascular smooth muscle cells is largely made up of actin (thin filaments) and myosin (thick filaments; Table 1.2). Actin-associated proteins (e.g. caldesmon, calponin) are also present and may play a modulatory role in the contractile process.

When actin and myosin are removed from the cell a cytoskeletal network of

Table 1.2 Components of the contractile apparatus and cytoskeleton in smooth muscle

Contractile apparatus	Cytoskeleton		Membrane skeleton	
	Dense bodies	Cytoskeletal domain	Adherens junction	Caveolar domain
Actin (smooth muscle)	Actin (nonmuscle)	Actin (nonmuscle)	Actin (nonmuscle)	Actin (nonmuscle)?
Myosin (type II)	α-actinin	Desmin	Filamin	Dystrophin
Tropomyosin	Calponin	(or vimentin)	Calponin	Caveolin
Caldesmon		Filamin	Vinculin	
Calponin		Calponin	Metavinculin	
		Smoothelin	Talin	
		Synamin	Paxillin	
		Paranemin	Tensin	
			α-actinin	
			Integrins	
			Plectrin	

After Small and Gimona (1998).

intermediate filaments remains. The major component of these intermediate filaments is desmin, though they also contain many other proteins (Table 1.2). The cytoskeleton probably couples the contractile machinery to the cell membrane (and hence to other cells and the extracellular matrix), but is not believed to be otherwise involved in contraction, except to limit overextension or excessive shortening of the cell. The connection between the contractile machinery and the cytoskeleton occurs at cytoplasmic dense bodies, α-actinin-rich structures which are distributed throughout the cytoplasm. It has been speculated that filamin, an actin-associated protein involved in actin polymerization, may be an important regulator of the linkage between the cytoskeleton and the contractile machinery. The cytoskeleton also attaches to the cell membrane and makes connection with the extracellular matrix or other cells via specialized junctional regions known as adherens junctions or membrane-dense plaques. In chicken gizzard smooth muscle these attachment regions appear as submembraneous dense plaques around 0.2 mm thick and 0.05 wide, separated by similar-sized caveolae running along the cell's long axis, giving the appearance of longitudinal ribs. Adherens junctions contain a number of specialized proteins, including vinculin, paxillin and tensin (Table 1.2), which are also present in focal adhesions seen in cultured cells. These proteins are involved in attaching the cytoskeleton to other transmembraneous proteins which couple the cells to other cells (cadherins) or to extracellular matrix proteins (integrins). It is particularly interesting that these points of contact are not merely structural. They are also foci of signalling activity. A discussion of the importance of spatial localization in signalling is beyond the scope of this review; however this topic has been reviewed recently (Bray, 1998).

How increased $[Ca^{2+}]_i$ initiates contraction

The rise in $[Ca^{2+}]_i$ brings about contraction through activation of a signal cascade. The first step in this pathway is activation of CaM. CaM is a widely distributed intracellular protein (17 kDa) that possesses high affinity for Ca^{2+} ions. One molecule of calmodulin binds four molecules of Ca^{2+} via a domain known as the *Escherichia coli* fragment (EF) hand domain, a domain common in a number of Ca^{2+}-binding proteins. This results in a conformational change in CaM-exposing hydrophobic sites which interact with target molecules (Figure 1.5). $(Ca^{2+})_4CaM$ activates a number of cellular enzymes, notably myosin light chain kinase (MLCK). MLCK is a 130–150 kDa serine/threonine kinase which shows a number of structural similarities to other serine/threonine kinases, e.g. cAMP-dependent kinase, CaM (Stull et al., 1998). There are multiple isoforms of MLCK which can be broadly classified into two groups: skeletal muscle and smooth muscle isoforms, the latter group being more substrate-specific. In smooth muscle Ca^{2+}

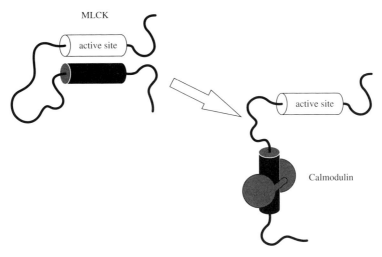

Figure 1.6   Activation of myosin light chain kinase (MLCK). In the absence of active calmodulin
($(Ca^{2+})_4$CaM) MLCK is inactive due to an inhibitory interaction between a myosin-like
pseudosubstrate region of MLCK and the active site. $(Ca^{2+})_4$CaM releases this
autoinhibition, probably by binding to a site near the pseudosubstrate-inhibitory region.

cannot directly activate the actin–myosin interaction, and MLCK is required. Consequently the response to activation in smooth muscle is slow ($\cong 500$ ms) and graded. In the absence of $(Ca^{2+})_4$CaM, MLCK is inactive. This may be because part of MLCK has considerable homology with myosin and effectively acts as pseudosubstrate inhibitor. $(Ca^{2+})_4$CaM releases this inhibition and allows MLCK to interact with myosin (Figure 1.6). The $(Ca^{2+})_4$CaM–MLCK ternary complex catalyses the phosphorylation of myosin at serine 19 on each of the two 20 kDa myosin light chains (MLC_{20}). This allows the actin–myosin interaction to occur, resulting in force production.

Force generation in smooth muscle: actin–myosin interaction

The process of contraction is essentially similar in smooth, cardiac and skeletal muscle. Actin and myosin are the motor proteins (Table 1.2) and contraction occurs by a sliding filament action (Figure 1.7). However, the contractile process in smooth muscle differs in a number of important ways from that in cardiac and skeletal muscle (Table 1.3).

Sensitization and desensitization of the contractile machinery to $[Ca^{2+}]_i$

While $[Ca^{2+}]_i$ is the primary signal for contraction, the amount of force generated can also be altered by changing the sensitivity of the contractile machinery to

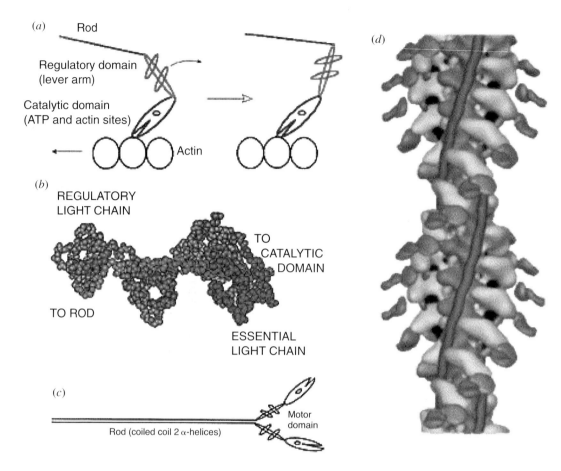

Figure 1.7   Diagram representing lever arm mechanics generating force as a result of the actin–myosin interaction. (*a*) A schematic representation of lever arm rotation as it is thought to occur during force production by a single myosin motor domain bound to actin. The myosin motor domain comprises a catalytic domain and a regulatory domain. The catalytic domain contains an ATP site and an actin-binding site, which has two parts separated by a cleft. The lever arm is the regulatory domain, which is a stretch of myosin heavy chain bound by two light chains, an essential light chain near the catalytic domain and a regulatory light chain. The lever arm rotates about a fulcrum site near the centre of the motor domain, as the ATP hydrolysis products (not shown) are released. The average orientation of the actin-bound catalytic domain does not change during lever arm rotation. The flexibly attached rod portion of myosin connects the motor domain to the thick filament. Rotation of the lever arm slides the actin filament to the left, relative to the thick filament position. (*b*) The regulatory domain, called the lever arm, the scallop muscle myosin consists of essential and regulatory light chains bound to an ~ 8 nm α-helical segment of the heavy chain. Other muscle myosin regulatory domains have similar structures. The figure, with the backbone structure rendered as van der Waals surfaces, was derived from Brookhaven Protein Data

Table 1.3 Comparison of smooth and skeletal muscle

Smooth	Skeletal (striated)
Coordinate activity	Individual recruitment of cells
Inefficient	Highly efficient
Direct activation by Ca^{2+} plays no physiological role	Direct activation by Ca^{2+}
Regulator/graded mechanism	On–off mechanism
Low energy (1% skeletal muscle) requirement for sustained force	High energy requirement for sustained force

$[Ca^{2+}]_i$. Such sensitization is likely to play a significant part in regulating tonic vascular smooth muscle activity and may account for agonist-induced modulation of myogenic tone. Early studies showing that stimulants such as noradrenaline (norepinephrine) increased tone following depolarization with potassium were originally interpreted as indicating receptor-linked influx of Ca^{2+}, over and above that induced by depolarization. However, since the advent of photometric and fluorescent techniques for the measurement of intracellular Ca^{2+} it has become evident that increases in tone following addition of a contractile agonist to depolarized vessels can occur without any detectable increase in $[Ca^{2+}]_i$ (Nilsson, 1998). More detailed studies of intact arteries have shown that in general the ratio of force $[Ca^{2+}]_i$ is higher during contractions induced by receptor agonists than in those induced by depolarization by high potassium. Work by Rembold and Murphy (1993) has also shown that such agonists induce a greater degree of myosin light chain phosphorylation for a given Ca^{2+} level than potassium depolarization, indicating that this effect of agonists involves an increase in effective Ca^{2+}-sensitivity of MLC_{20} phosphorylation.

Caption for fig. 1.7 (*cont.*)

Bank file 1scm (2). (c) A schematic representation of a myosin molecule. There are two motor domains attached to a coiled α-helical rod domain. Each catalytic domain (on the right side) has an ATP site (the circle) and an actin-binding site, which includes a cleft (the v shape). The lever arm is attached flexibly to the catalytic domain and to the rod domain. In muscle, the rod segments aggregate to form the thick filament. Images modified from (*d*). Three-dimensional maps of decorated filaments calculated by cryo-EM and image analysis at a resolution of 2.5–3 nm show the overall shape of the myosin head and its geometry of attachment to actin. Image modified from Cryo-Electron Microscopy of Actomyosin Complexes by Ron Milligan, Scripps Institute, on the Myosin home page (http://www.mrc.lmb.cam.ac.uk/myosin/structure/cryoEM.html).

Biochemical mechanisms of sensitization and desensitization

Recently, our understanding of the biochemistry of Ca^{2+}-sensitization has improved considerably. Work in skinned smooth muscle using techniques which irreversibly permeabilize the smooth muscle cell but preserve receptor coupling has been able to replicate the increases in Ca^{2+}-sensitivity seen with contractile agonists (Pfitzer and Arner, 1998). Studies have shown that this effect can be mimicked by application of GTP-γ-S or AlF_4^-, and blocked by GDP-β-S – non-hydrolysable analogues of GTP and GDP respectively. Such findings were interpreted as indicating that agonist-induced sensitization of vascular smooth muscle occurs by a mechanism involving heterotrimeric G proteins. More recently, the possibility that other GTPases also participate in the contractile process has received increased attention.

At present there are several hypotheses regarding which second messenger(s) are responsible for agonist-induced sensitization of contraction.

Phospholipase C, protein kinase C and lipid-derived signals

The principal phospholipids involved in cell signalling in vascular smooth muscle are phosphatidylinositol (PI) and phosphatidylcholine (PC: Ohanian et al., 1998). Two classes of enzymes hydrolase these lipids to give rise to signalling molecules PLC and phospholipase D (PLD). PLC can utilize PI to give rise to IP_3 and DAG, or PC to generate DAG. PLD preferentially hydrolyses PC to produce phosphatidic acid (PA) and choline. DAG and PA can be interconverted by DAG kinase and PA phosphohydrolase respectively and both molecules have signalling roles. In addition both are substrates for PLA_2 which forms arachidonate and, in the case of PA, lysophosphatidic acid (LPA). Arachidonate may act as an intracellular signal (Somlyo and Somlyo, 2000), while its derivatives (e.g. prostaglandins, thromboxanes, leukotrienes) and LPA act as intercellular signals. The primary role of DAG is as the physiological activator of PKC. PKC is a serine/threonine kinase and numerous isoforms have been identified. DAG binds to PKC, activates it and causes it to translocate from the cytoplasm to the membrane, where it can phosphorylate numerous substrates.

Phorbol esters are powerful activators of PKC that act in a similar manner to DAG. These compounds cause an increase in the Ca^{2+}-sensitivity of vascular smooth muscle. This was therefore widely considered to be the mechanism by which vasoconstrictors increased Ca^{2+}-sensitivity (Lee and Severson, 1994). However, this view has been questioned recently. Phorbol esters are relatively unphysiological activators of PKC and there is increasing doubt about the relevance of their action to physiological activation of the enzyme (Wilkinson and Hallam, 1994). Although phorbol esters do increase Ca^{2+}-sensitivity, their effects are slow (~ 30 min), whereas the effects of agonists are rapid (~ 2 min). Similarly, measurements of PKC translocation have not shown close relationships between the degree of translocation and force production for some agonists. Other studies also indicate that the temporal relationship between agonist-induced rises in tension and the physiologically produced DAG is poor. Indeed, some agonists cause sensitization despite failing to induce detectable rises in DAG (Ohanian et al., 1998). Furthermore, although myosin can be phosphorylated by PKC, the effect of this is inhibitory. PKC can also induce phosphorylation of MLCK in vitro, but there is little evidence that this process is of physiological significance. In permeabilized preparations the effects of agonists and GTP-γ-S on Ca^{2+} release and increased Ca^{2+}-sensitivity can be dissociated, suggesting that PLC activation is not necessary for sensitization to occur. Other problems centre on the putative antagonists of PKC. Many of these agents are now known to be nonselective and inhibit a range of important signal transduction systems. The results of many early studies which interpreted findings with these agents relatively uncritically therefore require reappraisal. More recent studies with more selective PKC inhibitors have been less consistent (Shimamoto et al., 1992; Ohanian et al., 1996; Buus et al., 1998). This is not to exclude PKC from playing a role in agonist-induced sensitization (see below), and the ever-increasing number of isoforms of PKC being discovered certainly opens new possibilities within this field (Morgan and Leinweber, 1998). Nevertheless, the importance of PKC in agonist-induced sensitization remains an unresolved question at present.

Protein phosphatases

Protein phosphatases catalyse the dephosphorylation of cellular proteins. Despite the evidence that cellular phosphatase activity generally exceeds kinase activity, most work has focused on the modulation of MLCK, or other kinases in the contractile process. More recently, control of phosphatases has gained increasing attention as a potential regulatory mechanism.

There are four classes of serine/threonine phosphatases in eukaryotic cells; type 1, 2A, 2B and 2C. The identity of the major myosin light chain phosphatase (MLCP) has only recently been determined (Hartshorne, 1998). It belongs to the type 1 class of phosphatases and consists of a 110–130 kDa regulatory subunit, a 39 kDa catalytic subunit and a 20 kDa subunit of unknown function.

Regulation of MLCP

Somlyo and colleagues were the first to suggest that MLCP might be important in the contractile process (Somlyo and Somlyo, 2000). Originally it was suggested that arachidonate might regulate MLCP. More recent studies implicate monomeric or small G proteins in the regulation of MLCP and smooth muscle tone.

Heterotrimeric G proteins are not the only GTPases present in smooth muscle that participate in signal transduction. Smooth muscle also contains abundant small G proteins ~ 21 kDa belonging to the *ras* superfamily (Somlyo and Somlyo, 2000). Of these, smg p21/rap and rho appear to be the dominant forms in vascular smooth muscle (Kawahara et al., 1991). These GTPases exist in GDP-bound (inactive) or GTP-bound (active) states. Interconversion of these states is controlled by three types of regulatory proteins: guanine nucleotide exchange factors (GEF), guanine nucleotide dissociation inhibitors (GDI) and GTPase-activating proteins (GAPs).

Under resting conditions small G proteins such as rhoA exist mainly as a cytoplasmic complex with a GDI. Following stimulation, a GEF promotes replacement of GDP by GTP, rhoA dissociates from the GDI and translocates to a lipid membrane. The rhoA–GTP complex is the active signalling molecule. After it interacts with its target(s), GAPs stimulate hydrolysis of GTP to GDP. The resulting rhoA–GDP complex then rebinds to a cytosolic GDI, completing the cycle.

Many vasoconstrictors appear to be able to activate rhoA. Exactly how heterotrimeric G proteins signal to small G proteins remains somewhat obscure. p115rho GEF has been reported to associate with some heterotrimeric G proteins ($G_{\alpha 12}$, $G_{\alpha 13}$: Kozasa et al., 1998) and this may account for the ability of some agonists to activate rhoA. Another possibility is that production of phosphatidylinositol-3,4,5-triphosphate by phosphoinositide 3-kinase (PI_3 kinase) is reponsible for the activation of small G proteins. PI_3 kinase is stimulated by some G proteins (Hawes et al., 1996) and is able to activate a GEF (Han et al., 1998).

At present rhoA is considered to be the major regulator of MLCP in smooth muscle (Somlyo and Somlyo, 2000). Work in nonmuscle cells had suggested that rhoA was an important regulator of the cytoskeleton and actin polymerization (Hall, 1999). This effect was demonstrated to involve activation of a rho-dependent kinase (ROK) that phosphorylated the regulatory subunit of MLCP (Kimura et al., 1996).

Numerous studies in smooth muscle have shown that inhibition of rhoA (e.g. by botulinum ADP-ribosyltransferase C_3 (C_3), exoenzyme of *Staphylococcus aureus* (EDIN), or a chimeric protein formed from diphtheria toxin and C_3) can diminish contraction in response to agonists, or GTP-γ-S in permeabilized preparations (Somlyo and Somlyo, 2000). More recently, a cell-permeable inhibitor of ROK (Y-27632) has been described that also inhibits agonist-induced contraction of vascular smooth muscle (Uehata et al., 1997). Together these data strongly suggest that rhoA has a major role in mediating agonist-induced Ca^{2+} sensitization in vascular smooth muscle.

Although rhoA is undoubtedly important, it is not likely to be the sole regulator of MLCP activity. PKC can also affect MLCP (Walker et al., 1998), either by inhibiting MLCP directly, or by phosphorylating an inhibitory protein CPI-17 (Senba et al., 1999). PKC and rhoA may therefore cooperate to regulate MLCP, although current data suggest that rhoA is more important (Somlyo and Somlyo, 2000).

Cyclic nucleotides

In addition to their effects on E_m and $[Ca^{2+}]_i$ homeostasis, cyclic nucleotides affect Ca^{2+} sensitization. cAMP- and cGMP-dependent kinases have been shown to accelerate dephosphorylation of MLC_{20} (Wu et al., 1996, 1998b), but the mechanism of this effect remains uncertain. Indeed, it has been suggested that cAMP may exert many of its effects through cross-stimulation of cGMP-dependent kinase (Francis and Corbin, 1994). Recent data indicate that cGMP-dependent kinase (α isoform) binds to the C-terminal region of the regulatory subunit of MLCP and that abolition of this binding prevents cGMP-dependent activation of MLCP (Surks et al., 1999). cGMP-dependent kinase has been shown to phosphorylate the 130 kDa (regulatory) and 20 kDa subunits of MLCP Nakamura M, as well as several other associated proteins (Surks et al., 1999). However, phosphorylation of the regulatory subunit has not been shown to affect phosphatase activity in vitro (Nakamura et al., 1999).

It is possible therefore that the effects of cGMP-dependent kinase on MLCP activity involve phosphorylation of an associated protein. It has been proposed that telokin, a 17 kDa protein that is identical to the C-terminal sequence of MLCK, could be a target for cyclic nucleotide-dependent kinases in smooth muscle (Somlyo et al., 1998). In vitro telokin can be phosphorylated by cAMP- and cGMP-dependent kinases as well as by p42/44 mitogen-activated protein (MAP) kinases. Telokin has been shown to induce relaxation and dephosphorylation of MLC_{20} in permeabilized ileal muscle and removal of telokin abolished cGMP-induced relaxation. Although these are intriguing data, as telokin is only present in large amounts in some smooth muscles (Somlyo et al., 1998), it seems unlikely that it can be the complete explanation of how cyclic nucleotides affect Ca^{2+}-sensitivity. Perhaps a related molecule or a completely unrelated mechanism remains to be discovered.

Actin-associated proteins: caldesmon and calponin

Two actin-associated proteins, caldesmon and calponin, are possible regulators of the actin–myosin interaction and could contribute to sensitization in vascular smooth muscle. Caldesmon is a 87 kDa protein which binds to actin and inhibits actin–myosin ATPase activity (Marston et al., 1998). In skinned smooth muscle caldesmon has been reported to shift the relationship between MLC_{20}

phosphorylation and force in a rightward direction (desensitization) and in permeabilized vascular smooth muscle cells displacement of caldesmon from actin by a peptide analogue caused contraction. The interaction between caldesmon and actin may be regulated by phosphorylation and p42/44 MAP kinase has been reported to phosphorylate caldesmon in vitro. MAP kinase is known to be activated in response to some contractile agonists (Khalil et al., 1995; Watts, 1996) and could provide a mechanism linking agonist stimulation to phosphorylation of caldesmon. Calponin is another putative modulator of actin–myosin activity. Calponin is a 34 kDa protein specifically found in smooth muscle in association with actin and tropomyosin (Winder et al., 1998). It also blocks actin-stimulated myosin ATPase activity and this action is inhibited by phosphorylation of calponin. CaM kinase and PKC can phosphorylate calponin in vitro (Horowitz et al., 1996), though whether these represent physiological actions of these enzymes remains uncertain.

Latch state

A novel state of actin–myosin cross-bridges, latch state was originally proposed on kinetic grounds by Hai and Murphy (1998) to account for sustained force production in tonic smooth muscles. It is thought to be analogous to the 'catch' state of mollusc muscle which allows force to be maintained for long periods with minimal ATP hydrolysis. A complete biochemical basis for latch state remains to be elaborated, but it is associated with dephosphorylation of MLC_{20} (Arner and Malmqvist, 1998). It is proposed that a specific form of dephosphorylated cross-bridge is generated that remains attached. Whether actin-associated proteins such as caldesmon or calponin contribute to the formation of this state remains speculative.

Conclusions

The generation of arterial tone is a complex and highly regulated process. Many of the basic features and regulators of the contractile process in vascular smooth muscle are now well understood, yet there are deficits in our knowledge. These include the importance of spatial restriction of Ca^{2+} and other messengers to signalling in smooth muscle, the regulation of MLCP and the relationship between ultrastructural structure and function. The recent recognition that unconventional signalling pathways such as tyrosine phosphorylation, small G proteins and the MAP kinase pathway play significant, if as yet ill-defined, roles in contraction will ensure that there will be many new developments in this field in the future.

REFERENCES

Aalkjaer, C. & Peng, H.L. (1997). pH and smooth muscle. *Acta Physiol. Scand.*, **161**, 557–66.

Arner, A. & Malmqvist, U. (1998). Cross-bridge cycling in smooth muscle: a short review. *Acta Physiol. Scand.*, **164**, 363–72.

Ashida, T., Schaeffer, J., Goldman, W.F., Wade, J.D. & Blaustein, M.P. (1988). Role of sarcoplasmic reticulum in arterial contraction. Comparison of ryanodines effect in a conduit and a muscular artery. *Circ. Res.*, **62**, 854–63.

Baro, I. & Eisner, D.A. (1995). Factors controlling changes in intracellular Ca^{2+} concentration produced by noradrenaline in rat mesenteric artery smooth muscle cells. *J. Physiol. Lond.*, **482**, 247–58.

Bayliss, W.M. (1902). On the local reactions of the arterial wall to changes in internal pressure. *J. Physiol. (Lond.)*, **28**, 220–31.

Beckman, J.S. & Koppenol, W.H. (1996). Nitric oxide, superoxide, and peroxynitrite: the good, the bad, and ugly. *Am. J. Physiol.*, **271**, C1424–37.

Benham, C.D. & Tsien, R.W. (1987). Calcium-permeable channels in vascular smooth muscle: voltage-activated, receptor-operated, and leak channels. *Soc. Gen. Physiol. Ser.*, **42**, 45–64.

Berk, B.C. & Alexander, R.W. (1989). Vasoactive effects of growth factors. *Biochem. Pharmacol.*, **38**, 219–25.

Braun, M., Pietsch, P., Schror, K., Baumann, G. & Felix, S.B. (1999). Cellular adhesion molecules on vascular smooth muscle cells. *Cardiovasc. Res.*, **41**, 395–401.

Bray, D. (1998). Signaling complexes: biophysical constraints on intracellular communication. *Annu. Rev. Biophys. Biomol. Struct.*, **27**, 59–75.

Brice, N.L., Berrows, N.S., Campbell, V. et al. (1997). Importance of the different beta subunits in the membrane expression of the alpha1A and alpha2 calcium channel subunits: studies using a depolarization-sensitive alpha1A antibody. *Eur. J. Neurosci.*, **9**, 749–59.

Brink, P.R. (1998). Gap junctions in vascular smooth muscle. *Acta Physiol. Scand.*, **164**, 349–56.

Bryant, H.J., Harder, D.R., Pamnani, M.B. & Haddy, F.J. (1985). In vivo membrane potentials of smooth muscle cells in the caudal artery of the rat. *Am. J. Physiol.*, **249**, C78–83.

Buus, C.L., Aalkjaeer, C., Nilsson, H. et al. (1998). Mechanisms of Ca^{2+} sensitization of force production by noradrenaline in rat mesenteric small arteries. *J. Physiol. (Lond.)*, **510**, 577–90.

Calder, J.A., Schachter, M. & Sever, P.S. (1993). Ion channel involvement in the acute vascular effects of thiazide diuretics and related compounds. *J. Pharmacol. Exp. Ther.*, **265**, 1175–80.

Catterall, W.A. (1998). Structure and function of neuronal Ca^{2+} channels and their role in neurotransmitter release. *Cell Calcium*, **24**, 307–23.

Collier, M.L., Ji, G., Wang, Y. & Kotlikoff, M.I. (2000). Calcium-induced calcium release in smooth muscle. Loose coupling between the action potential and calcium release. *J. Gen. Physiol.*, **115**, 653–62.

Coussin, F., Macrez, N., Morel, J.L. & Mironneau, J. (2000). Requirement of ryanodine receptor subtypes 1 and 2 for $Ca^{(2+)}$-induced $Ca^{(2+)}$ release in vascular myocytes. *J. Biol. Chem.*, **275**, 9596–603.

Dohlman, H.G. & Thorner, J. (1997). RGS proteins and signaling by heterotrimeric G proteins. *J. Biol. Chem.*, **272**, 3871–4.

Doyle, D.A., Morais Cabral, J., Pfuetzner, R.A. et al. (1998). The structure of the potassium channel: molecular basis of K$^+$ conduction and selectivity. *Science*, **280**, 69–77.

Dumas, J.P., Bardou, M., Goirand, F. & Dumas, M. (1999). Hypoxic pulmonary vasoconstriction. *Gen. Pharmacol.*, **33**, 289–97.

Feron, O., Octave, J.N., Christen, M.O. & Godfraind, T. (1994). Quantification of two splicing events in the L-type calcium channel alpha-1 subunit of intestinal smooth muscle and other tissue. *Eur. J. Biochem.*, **222**, 195–202.

Francis, S.H. & Corbin, J.D. (1994). Structure and function of cyclic nucleotide-dependent protein kinases. *Annu. Rev. Physiol.*, **56**, 237–72.

Ganitkevich, V.Y. & Isenberg, G. (1995). Efficacy of peak Ca^{2+} currents (ICa) as trigger of sarcoplasmic reticulum Ca^{2+} release in myocytes from the guinea-pig coronary artery. *J. Physiol. (Lond.)*, **484**, 287–306.

Garcha, R.S. & Hughes, A.D. (1997). Action of ryanodine on neurogenic responses in rat isolated mesenteric small arteries. *Br. J. Pharmacol.*, **122**, 142–8.

Griffith, T.M., Edwards, D.H., Davies, R.L.I., Harrison, T.J. & Evans K.T. (1987). EDRF coordinates the behaviour of vascular resistance vessels. *Nature*, **329**, 442–5.

Gustafsson, F. & Holstein-Rathlou, N. (1999). Conducted vasomotor responses in arterioles: characteristics, mechanisms and physiological significance. *Acta Physiol. Scand.*, **167**, 11–21.

Hai, C.M. & Murphy, R.A. (1988). Regulation of shortening velocity by cross-bridge phosphorylation in smooth muscle. *Am. J. Physiol.*, **255**, C86–94.

Hall, A. (1999). Signal transduction pathways regulated by the Rho family of small GTPases. *Br. J. Cancer*, **80**(suppl. 1), 25–7.

Han, J., Luby-Phelps, K., Das, B. et al. (1998). Role of substrates and products of PI 3-kinase in regulating activation of Rac-related guanosine triphosphatases by Vav. *Science*, **279**, 558–60.

Hancock, J.T. (1997). Superoxide, hydrogen peroxide and nitric oxide as signalling molecules: their production and role in disease. *Br. J. Biomed. Sci.*, **54**, 38–46.

Harder, D.R. (1984). Pressure-dependent membrane depolarization in cat middle cerebral artery. *Circ. Res.*, **55**, 197–202.

Hartshorne, D.J. (1998). Myosin phosphatase: subunits and interactions. *Acta Physiol. Scand.*, **164**, 483–93.

Hawes, B.E., Luttrell, L.M., van-Biesen, T. & Lefkowitz, R.J. (1996). Phosphatidylinositol 3-kinase is an early intermediate in the G beta gamma-mediated mitogen-activated protein kinase signaling pathway. *J. Biol. Chem.*, **271**, 12133–6.

Hermsmeyer, K. (1982). Electrogenic ion pumps and other determinants of membrane potential in vascular smooth muscle. *Physiologist*, **25**, 454–65.

Hildebrandt, J.D. (1997). Role of subunit diversity in signaling by heterotrimeric G proteins. *Biochem. Pharmacol.*, **54**, 325–39.

Hockerman, G.H., Peterson, B.Z., Johnson, B.D. & Catterall, W.A. (1997). Molecular determinants of drug binding and action on L-type calcium channels. *Annu. Rev. Pharmacol. Toxicol.*, **37**, 361–96.

Hofmann, F., Ammendola, A. & Schlossmann, J. (2000). Rising behing NO: cGMP-dependent protein kinases. *J. Cell Sci.*, **113**, 1671–6.

Holman, M.E., Neild, T.O. & Lang, R.J. (1990). On the passive properties of smooth muscle. In

Frontiers in Smooth Muscle Research, ed. Sperelakis, N. & Wood, J.D., pp. 379–98. New York: Alan R. Liss.

Horowitz, A., Menice, C.B., Laporte, R. & Morgan, K.G. (1996). Mechanisms of smooth muscle contraction. *Physiol. Rev.*, **76**, 967–1003.

Hughes, A.D. (1995). Calcium channels in vascular smooth muscle cells. *J. Vasc. Res.*, **32**, 353–70.

Hughes, A.D. & Bolton, T.B. (1995). Action of angiotensin II, 5-hydroxytryptamine and adenosine triphosphate on ionic currents in single ear artery cells of the rabbit. *Br. J. Pharmacol.*, **116**, 2148–54.

Hughes, A.D. & Schachter, M. (1994). Hypertension and blood vessels. *Br. Med. Bull.*, **50**, 356–70.

Hughes, A.D. & Wijetunge, S. (1998). Role of tyrosine phosphorylation in excitation–contraction coupling in vascular smooth muscle. *Acta Physiol. Scand.*, **164**, 457–69.

Hughes, A.D., Clunn, G.F., Refson, J. & Demoliou, M.C. (1996). Platelet-derived growth factor (PDGF): actions and mechanisms in vascular smooth muscle. *Gen. Pharmacol.*, **27**, 1079–89.

Ignarro, L.J., Cirino, G., Casini, A. & Napoli, C. (1999). Nitric oxide as a signaling molecule in the vascular system: an overview. *J. Cardiovasc. Pharmacol.*, **34**, 879–86.

Jaggar, J.H., Wellman, G.C., Heppner, T.J. et al. (1998a). Ca^{2+} channels, ryanodine receptors and $Ca^{(2+)}$-activated K^+ channels: a functional unit for regulating arterial tone. *Acta Physiol. Scand.*, **164**, 577–87.

Jaggar, J.H., Stevenson, A.S. & Nelson, M.T. (1998b). Voltage dependence of Ca^{2+} sparks in intact cerebral arteries. *Am. J. Physiol.*, **274**, C1755–61.

Jentsch, T.J., Friedrich, T., Schriever, A. & Yamada, H. (1999). The CLC chloride channel family. *Pflugers Arch.*, **437**, 783–95.

Kadambi, V.J. & Kranias, E.G. (1997). Phospholamban: a protein coming of age. *Biochem. Biophys. Res. Common.*, **239**, 1–5.

Kamishima, T. & McCarron, J.G. (1996). Depolarization-evoked increases in cytosolic concentration in isolated smooth muscle cells of rat portal vein. *J. Physiol. (Lond.)*, **492**, 61–74.

Kamishima, T. & McCarron, J.G. (1997). Regulation of the cytosolic Ca^{2+} concentration by Ca^{2+} stores in single smooth muscle cells from rat cerebral arteries. *J. Physiol. (Lond.)*, **501**, 497–508.

Kamishima, T. & McCarron, J.G. (1998). Ca^{2+} removal mechanisms in rat cerebral resistance size arteries. *Biophys. J.*, **75**, 1767–73.

Karaki, H., Ozaki, H., Hori, M. et al. (1997). Calcium movements, distribution, and functions in smooth muscle. *Pharmacol. Rev.*, **49**, 157–230.

Kawahara, Y., Kawata, M., Sunako, M. et al. (1991). Small GTP-binding proteins in bovine aortic smooth muscle. *Jpn Circ. J.*, **55**, 1036–43.

Khalil, R.A., Menice, C.B., Wang, C.-L.A. & Morgan, K.G. (1995). Phosphotyrosine-dependent targeting of mitogen-activated protein kinase in differentiated contractile vascular cells. *Circ. Res.*, **6**, 1101–18.

Kimura, K., Ito, M., Amano, M. et al. (1996). Regulation of myosin phosphatase by Rho and Rho-associated kinase (rho-kinase). *Science*, **273**, 245–8.

Klockner, U. (1993). Intracellular calcium ions activate a low-conductance chloride channel in smooth-muscle cells isolated from human mesenteric artery. *Pflugers Arch.*, **424**, 231–7.

Kozasa, T., Jiang, X., Hart, M.J. et al. (1998). p115 RhoGEF, a GTPase activating protein for Galpha12 and Galpha13. *Science*, **280**, 2109–11.

Lamb, F.S., Clayton, G.H., Liu, B.X. et al. (1999). Expression of CLCN voltage-gated chloride channel genes in human blood vessels. *J. Mol. Cell Cardiol.*, **31**, 657–66.

Large, W.A. & Wang, Q. (1996). Characteristics and physiological role of the $Ca^{(2+)}$-activated Cl^- conductance in smooth muscle. *Am. J. Physiol.*, **271**, C435–54.

Lee, M.W. & Severson, D.L. (1994). Signal transduction in vascular smooth muscle: diacyl-glycerol second messengers and PKC action. *Am. J. Physiol.*, **267**, C659–78.

Lefkowitz, R.J. (1998). G protein-coupled receptors. III. New roles for receptor kinases and beta-arrestins in receptor signaling and desensitization. *J. Biol. Chem.*, **273**, 18677–80.

Loirand, G., Pacaud, P., Baron, A., Mironneau, C. & Mironneau, J. (1991). Calcium-activated cation channel in rat portal vein myocytes. *Z. Kardiol.*, **80**(suppl. 7), 59–63.

Lymn, J.S. & Hughes, A.D. (2000). Phospholipase C isoforms, cytoskeletal organization, and vascular smooth muscle differentiation. *N.I.P.S.*, **15**, 41–5.

Marrero, M.B., Paxton, W.G., Duff, J.L., Berk, B.C. & Bernstein, K.E. (1994). Angiotensin II stimulates tyrosine phosphorylation of phospholipase C-gamma 1 in vascular smooth muscle cells. *J. Biol. Chem.*, **269**, 10935–9.

Marston, S., Burton, D., Copeland, O. et al. (1998). Structural interactions between actin, tropomyosin, caldesmon and calcium binding protein and the regulation of smooth muscle thin filaments. *Acta Physiol. Scand.*, **164**, 401–14.

McCulloch, K.M., Osipenko, O.N. & Gurney, A.M. (1999). Oxygen-sensing potassium currents in pulmonary artery. *Gen. Pharmacol.*, **32**, 403–11.

Mogford, J.E., Davis, G.E. & Meininger, G.A. (1997). RGDN peptide interaction with en-dothelial alpha5beta1 integrin causes sustained endothelin-dependent vasoconstriction of rat skeletal muscle arterioles. *J. Clin. Invest.*, **100**, 1647–53.

Moore, E.D., Etter, E.F., Philipson, K.D. et al. (1993). Coupling of the Na^+/Ca^{2+} exchanger, Na^+/K^+ pump and sarcoplasmic reticulum in smooth muscle. *Nature*, **365**, 657–60.

Morgan, K.G. & Leinweber, B.D. (1998). PKC-dependent signalling mechanisms in differenti-ated smooth muscle. *Acta Physiol. Scand.*, **164**, 495–505.

Morris, A.J. & Malbon, C.C. (1999). Physiological regulation of G protein-linked signaling. *Physiol. Rev.*, **79**, 1373–430.

Mulvany, M.J., Aalkjaer, C. & Jensen, P.E. (1991). Sodium–calcium exchange in vascular smooth muscle. *Ann. N.Y. Acad. Sci.*, **639**, 498–504.

Nakamura, M., Ichikawa, K., Ito, M. et al. (1999). Effects of the phosphorylation of myosin phosphatase by cyclic GMP-dependent protein kinase. *Cell Signal*, **11**, 671–6.

Nilsson, H. (1998). Interactions between membrane potential and intracellular calcium concen-tration in vascular smooth muscle. *Acta Physiol. Scand.*, **164**, 559–66.

Nixon, G.F., Mignery, G.A. & Somlyo, A.V. (1994). Immunogold localization of inositol 1,4,5-trisphosphate receptors and characterization of ultrastructural features of the sarco-plasmic reticulum in phasic and tonic smooth muscle. *J. Muscle Res. Cell Motil.*, **15**, 682–700.

Ohanian, V., Ohanian, J., Shaw, L. et al. (1996). Identification of protein kinase C isoforms in rat mesenteric small arteries and their possible role in agonist-induced contraction. *Circ. Res.*, **78**, 806–12.

Ohanian, J. Liu, G., Ohanian, V. & Heagerty, A.M. (1998). Lipid second messengers derived from glycerolipids and sphingolipids, and their role in smooth muscle function. *Acta Physiol. Scand.*, **164**, 533–48.

Pfitzer, G. & Arner, A. (1998). Involvement of small GTPase in the regulation of smooth muscle contraction. *Acta Physiol. Scand.*, **164**, 449–56.

Raeymaekers, L. & Wuytack, F. (1993). Ca^{2+} pumps in smooth muscle cells. *J. Muscle Res. Cell Motil.*, **14**, 141–57.

Rembold, C.M. & Murphy, R.A. (1993). Models of the mechanism for crossbridge attachment in smooth muscle. *J. Muscle Res. Cell Motil.*, **14**, 325–34.

Ross, R. (1999). Atherosclerosis – an inflammatory disease. *N. Engl. J. Med.*, **340**, 115–26.

Senba, S., Eto, M. & Yazawa, M. (1999). Identification of trimeric myosin phosphatase (PP1M) as a target for a novel PKC-potentiated protein phosphatase-1 inhibitory protein (CPI17) in porcine aorta smooth muscle. *J. Biochem. (Tokyo)*, **125**, 354–62.

Shimamoto, H., Shimamoto, Y., Kwan, C.Y. & Daniel, E.E. (1992). Participation of protein kinase C in endothelin-1-induced contraction in rat aorta: studies with a new tool, calphostin C. *Br. J. Pharmacol.*, **107**, 282–7.

Small, J.V. (1995). Structure–function relationships in smooth muscle: the missing links. *Bioessays*, **17**, 785–92.

Small, J.V. & Gimona, M. (1998). The cytoskeleton of the vertebrate smooth muscle cell. *Acta Physiol. Scand.*, **164**, 341–8.

Somlyo, A.P. & Somlyo, A.V. (2000). Signal transduction by G-proteins, rho-kinase and protein phosphatase to smooth muscle and non-muscle myosin II. *J. Physiol. (Lond.)*, **522**, 177–85.

Somlyo, A.V., Matthew, J.D., Wu, X, Khromov, A.S. & Somlyo, A.P. (1998). Regulation of the cross-bridge cycle: the effects of MgADP, LC17 isoforms and telokin. *Acta Physiol. Scand.*, **164**, 381–8.

Standen, N.B. & Quayle, J.M. (1998). K^+ channel modulation in arterial smooth muscle. *Acta Physiol. Scand.*, **164**, 549–57.

Stull, J.T., Lin, P.J., Krueger, J.K., Trewhella, J. & Zhi, G. (1998). Myosin light chain kinase: functional domains and structural motifs. *Acta Physiol. Scand.*, **164**, 471–82.

Surks, H.K., Mochizuki, N., Kasai, Y. et al. (1999). Regulation of myosin phosphatase by a specific interaction with cGMP-dependent protein kinase Ialpha. *Science*, **286**, 1583–7.

Tomita, T. (1990). Spread of excitation in smooth muscle. In *Frontiers in Smooth Muscle Research*, ed. Sperelakis, N. & Wood, J.D., pp. 361–73. New York: Alan R. Liss.

Tribe, R.M., Borin, M.L. & Blaustein, M.P. (1994). Functionally and spatially distance Ca^{2+} stores are revealed in cultured vascular smooth muscle cells. *Proc. Natl Acad. Sci. U.S.A.*, **94**, 5908–12.

Uehata, M., Ishizaki, T., Satoh, H. et al. (1997). Calcium sensitization of smooth muscle mediated by a Rho-associated protein kinase in hypertension [see comments]. *Nature*, **389**, 990–4.

van Breemen, C., Chen, Q. & Laher, I. (1995). Superficial buffer barrier function of smooth muscle sarcoplasmic reticulum. *Trends Pharmacol. Sci.*, **16**, 98–104.

Walker, L.A., Gailly, P., Jensen, P.E., Somlyo, A.V. & Somlyo, A.P. (1998). The unimportance of being (protein kinase C) epsilon. *FASEB J.*, **12**, 813–21.

Wang, Q., Hogg, R.C. & Large, W.A. (1993). A monovalent ion-selective cation activated by noradrenaline in smooth muscle cells of rabbit ear artery. *Pflugers Arch.*, **423**, 28–33.

Watts, S.W. (1996). Serotonin activates the mitogen-activated protein kinase pathway in vascular smooth muscle: use of the mitogen-activated protein kinase inhibitor PD098059. *J. Pharmacol. Exp. Ther.*, **279**, 1541–50.

Welling, A., Ludwig, A., Zimmer, S. et al. (1997). Alternatively spliced IS6 segments of the alpha 1C gene determine the tissue-specific dihydropyridine sensitivity of cardiac and vascular smooth muscle L-type Ca^{2+} channels. *Circ. Res.*, **81**, 526–32.

Wilkinson, S.E. & Hallam, T.J. (1994). Protein kinase C: is its pivotal role in cellular activation over-stated? *Trends Pharmacol. Sci.*, **15**, 53–7.

Winder, S.J., Allen, B.G., Clement-Chomienne, O. & Walsh, M.P. (1998). Regulation of smooth muscle actin–myosin interaction and force by calponin. *Acta Physiol. Scand.*, **164**, 415–26.

Wu, X., Somlyo, A.V. & Somlyo, A.P. (1996). Cyclic GMP-dependent stimulation reverses G-protein-coupled inhibition of smooth muscle myosin light chain phosphate. *Biochem. Biophys. Res. Commun.*, **220**, 658–63.

Wu, X., Mogford, J.E., Platts, S.H. et al. (1998a). Modulation of calcium current in arteriolar smooth muscle by alphav beta3 and alpha5 beta1 integrin ligands. *J. Cell Biol.*, **143**, 241–52.

Wu, X, Haystead, T.A., Nakamoto, R.K., Somlyo, A.V. & Somlyo, A.P. (1998b). Acceleration of myosin light chain dephosphorylation and relaxation of smooth muscle by telokin. Synergism with cyclic nucleotide-activated kinase. *J. Biol. Chem.*, **273**, 11362–9.

Yamaguchi, H. & Jensen, P.E. (1993). Spike generating smooth muscle cells in mesenteric artery of rats. *Pflugers Arch.*, **425**, 187–9.

Yamazaki, J., Duan, D., Janiak, R. et al. (1998). Functional and molecular expression of volume-regulated chloride channels in canine vascular smooth muscle cells. *J. Physiol. (Lond.)*, **507**, 729–36.

Yip, K.P. & Marsh, D.J. (1997). An Arg-Gly-Asp peptide stimulates constriction in rat afferent arteriole. *Am. J. Physiol.*, **273**, F768–76.

Vascular compliance

Brenda A. Kelly[1] and Philip Chowienczyk[2]

[1]Maternal and Fetal Research Unit/Centre for Cardiovascular and Vascular Biology, King's College, London
[2]Department of Clinical Pharmacology, St Thomas' Hospital, London

Introduction

Compliance of a vessel is the amount by which it will increase in volume for a given increase in distending pressure and is determined by the elastic properties of the vessel wall. A compliant vessel will accommodate a large volume of blood at low pressure and show little rise in pressure when a large volume of blood is ejected into it. It has long been appreciated that vascular compliance has an important influence on circulatory haemodynamics. The compliance of the large veins enables them to accommodate blood returning to the heart and thus influences preload on the heart and hence cardiac output. Similarly, the compliance of the aorta and large arteries enables them to accommodate blood ejected from the left ventricle. This reduces afterload, preventing an excessive rise in systolic blood pressure, and increases flow to the peripheral and coronary circulation when the aorta contracts as distending pressure falls during diastole. In this context the aorta has been referred to as the 'second heart'. It has recently been appreciated that reduced compliance of the aorta may represent one of or, in certain groups, the most important predictor of cardiovascular mortality. This has renewed interest in the determinants and consequences of large artery compliance. In this chapter we focus on large artery compliance, reviewing its measurement, influence on haemodynamics, biomechanical determinants, alterations in physiological and pathophysiological conditions, importance as a cardiovascular risk factor and interventions which may modify large artery compliance.

Definitions and terminology

The terms arterial 'compliance' and 'distensibility' tend to be used interchangeably but have distinct definitions. Compliance (C) of a segment of a vessel is the increase in volume (ΔV) of the segment per unit increase in distending pressure (ΔP) across the segment:

$$C = \Delta V / \Delta P$$

Whereas distensibility (D) is the proportionate increase in volume per unit increase in distending pressure:

$$D = [\Delta V / V] / \Delta P$$

Distensibility is more closely related to the intrinsic elasticity of the vessel wall, whereas compliance depends, in addition, upon vessel diameter. As vessel diameter increases, compliance increases. Thus, a larger artery may exhibit greater compliance than a smaller artery even if the intrinsic elasticity of the large artery wall is lower than that of the small artery. In recent years the term 'arterial stiffness' has been coined. Stiffness does not have a strict definition but loosely is the inverse of distensibility. 'Stiffness' has the appeal of being an intuitive term encapsulating the idea that a reduction in compliance is associated with a rigid vessel, which will dilate very little even when subject to a large distending pressure.

Influence of large artery compliance on systemic haemodynamics

Blood pressure and organ perfusion are often regarded as being determined by cardiac output and total peripheral vascular resistance. This is true in as much as cardiac output and total peripheral resistance determine mean arterial blood pressure. However, large artery compliance has an important influence on dynamic changes in blood pressure and flow during the cardiac cycle, such changes being dependent on the interaction between the left ventricle and the large arteries (Nichols and O'Rourke, 1998). A poorly compliant or stiff aorta will result in an excessive rise in systolic blood pressure and precipitous fall in blood pressure during early diastole. Conversely, a compliant aorta acts as a cushion or windkessel, reducing the rise in systolic blood pressure. Reanalysis of the results of large blood pressure-lowering trials has drawn attention to the importance of systolic blood pressure and pulse pressure as being predictive of cardiovascular mortality and this underlines the potential importance of large artery compliance (Franklin et al., 1999; Millar et al., 1999). The windkessel effect has importance not only in reducing systolic blood pressure but also in increasing diastolic blood pressure. This, in turn, may have important implications for coronary artery blood flow which occurs mainly during diastole.

These windkessel effects can be explained simply by the ability of the aorta to stretch and accommodate an increased blood volume during systole. However, large artery compliance also influences systemic haemodynamics through its effects on the transmission of pressure throughout the vascular tree. Pressure is not transmitted instantaneously but at a rate dependent on the pulse wave velocity (PWV: Bramwell and Hill, 1922). Thus, the pressure pulse at the femoral artery arrives momentarily after that at the carotid artery due to the finite speed of transmission of pressure along the aorta. The difference in conduit artery length from the heart to these two peripheral sites divided by the difference in time of arrival of the pressure pulse at these two sites is the PWV. PWV is determined by the distensibility of the aorta. A more compliant or distensible aorta is associated with a lower PWV.

In addition to providing a useful means for measuring aortic distensibility (see below), PWV determines the timing of reflected pressure waves. The pressure wave caused by ventricular contraction propagates away from the heart along the arterial tree, reaching large and medium-sized arteries in peripheral parts of the vascular tree at a later time during systole. In addition this pressure wave is reflected at various points along the vascular tree, causing pressure wave reflections which travel in the opposite direction towards the heart. Some degree of pressure wave reflection occurs at all points along the vascular tree but the majority occurs from small arteries in the lower body. To a first approximation one can consider a single site of pressure wave reflection in the lower body, from which a backward-going pressure wave returns towards the heart. This pressure wave will travel with the same PWV as the forward-going wave and the timing of its arrival at the aortic root relative to the forward-going wave will depend upon PWV. The total pressure in the vasculature at any point in time is the sum of the pressure contributions from both the forward- and backward-going waves. In the case of a compliant aorta the reflected wave arrives at the aortic root in diastole and adds little to systolic pressure but tends to increase early diastolic pressure. The former effect keeps pulse pressure to a minimum and the latter may be important with regard to coronary perfusion. A poorly compliant or stiff aorta will result in a higher PWV and the arrival of a greater proportion of reflected waves during systole. This will cause an augmentation of systolic blood pressure, often generating a peak systolic blood pressure exceeding that which would be generated by forward propagation of blood pressure alone (Nichols and O'Rourke, 1998).

Measurement of arterial compliance

The most direct approach to determining arterial compliance would seem, at first sight, to measure the change in volume of an arterial segment occurring during the cardiac cycle and to relate this to corresponding pressure changes. High-resolution duplex ultrasound provides the ability to measure changes in diameter and hence in cross-sectional area and volume. Sophisticated systems exist which allow tracking of the vessel wall and give accurate measurements of diameter changes during the cardiac cycle. Arterial pressure can be measured invasively or noninvasively to relate diameter and hence volume changes to those of pressure and hence determine compliance. This method allows for the nonlinearity of the pressure–diameter relationship and also provides for determinations at isobaric pressure (Stefanadis et al., 1995). Disadvantages with this method are that only a small segment of the artery (that which can be imaged) can be measured and, depending on the artery of interest, it is not always possible to determine blood pressure in the artery directly. This may introduce an error since blood pressure differs between central and peripheral arteries as a result of pressure wave reflection. This method can, however, be used to good effect in the carotid artery which is easily accessible for imaging and in which carotid artery tonometry can provide a noninvasive registration of blood pressure through the cardiac cycle (Giannattasio et al., 1996).

An alternative method for determining arterial compliance/distensibility is to measure PWV. PWV is the velocity with which the pressure pulse propagates along an artery and is inversely related to the square root of arterial distensibility (Bramwell and Hill, 1922). PWV can be determined by measuring the time delay (ΔT) between the foot of velocity or pressure waveforms measured at two accessible sites in the arterial tree, such as the carotid and femoral arteries. Carotid to femoral PWV (PWV_{cf}) is given by:

$$PWV_{cf} = L_{cf}/\Delta T$$

where L_{cf} is the difference in length from the aortic root to the carotid artery and the length from the aortic root to the femoral artery and is estimated from surface markings. This method provides an integrated measure of distensibility over the arterial conduit of interest (usually the aortofemoral). Although it requires some user experience it is less demanding than approaches which use direct imaging and does not depend upon simultaneous blood pressure measurement (although this influences PWV). The method is of particular interest because PWV_{cf} has been shown to be a predictor of mortality in certain groups (Blacher et al., 1999). In animal studies transducers placed along the aorta can be used to measure PWV.

In addition to these relatively direct methods for determining PWV there are several indices of arterial stiffness which can be determined by contour analysis of the peripheral arterial pulse. The peripheral pulse can be recorded noninvasively by applying a tonometer to the radial artery. This is an instrument in which deflection of a piezoelectric transducer is used to record radial artery pressure. A peripheral pulse may also be obtained by measuring the transmission of infrared light through the finger pulp. This yields a volume pulse which is closely related to the peripheral pressure pulse. The contour of the pressure and volume pulse is determined by the ejection characteristics of the left ventricle and by the bio-mechanical properties of the systemic circulation. Reflection of pressure waves from peripheral parts of the circulation influences the contour of both the systolic and diastolic components of the pulse waveform.

The timing of the reflected wave depends mainly upon large artery PWV. A high PWV is associated with a greater proportion of wave reflection arriving in systole augmenting systolic blood pressure. Measurement of an aortic augmentation index (AIx) derived from pulse contour analysis has therefore been advocated to determine arterial stiffness (O'Rourke and Mancia, 1999). However, although AIx is influenced by PWV and hence by large artery compliance, it is important to note that there are other important determinants of AIx, namely the site and amount of pressure wave reflection (Nichols and O'Rourke, 1998). The latter may vary widely according to arterial tone. Another type of pulse wave analysis involves the assumption that the diastolic decay of the arterial pressure pulse is due to a 'systemic' (mainly large) artery compliance and estimating this from measurements taken from the diastolic portion of the pressure wave or by fitting the wave to a mathematical Windkessel model (Cohn et al., 1995). This method requires an estimation of cardiac output and neglects the possible influence of wave reflection on the pressure wave. Whether the latter is a quantitatively important confounding factor, however, remains to be determined.

Biomechanical determinants of compliance: arterial wall structure

Arterial compliance is determined by arterial diameter and the intrinsic elasticity of the artery wall. This in turn is determined by individual components of the vessel wall. The vessel wall cannot be considered simply as a collection of cells and extracellular matrix (ECM). Rather, it is a dynamic organ composed of en-dothelial, medial smooth muscle and fibroblast cells invested in ECM and is subject to remodelling in response to haemodynamic conditions and pathological states. Remodelling can be viewed as an active process of structural alteration dependent on a continual interaction between locally generated growth factors, vasoactive substances and haemodynamic stimuli. The endothelium is particularly suited to play a central part in vessel adaptation, being strategically located to serve in a sensory capacity, assessing haemodynamic and humoral signals as well as eliciting responses that may eventually affect the structure and mechanical properties of the vessel. It is capable of releasing locally active mediators such as nitric oxide (NO) and endothelin, which have immediate vasoactive properties and longer-term trophic effects on the medial smooth muscle cells. Vascular smooth muscle cells (VSMCs) not only actively control wall tension but also synthesize the major structural components of the vessel wall. The ECM accounts for up to 60%

of the intimal volume and is composed of the scaffolding elements of collagen (types I, III, IV and V) and elastin embedded in glycoproteins such as fibronectin and proteoglycans such as heparin sulphate. This matrix also acts as a repository for several potent growth factors. Certain matrix proteins bind growth factors such as basic fibroblast growth factor, transforming growth factor-β_1 (TGF-β_1) and thrombin (Taipale and Keski-oja, 1997). Alteration in matrix spatial arrangement and composition may additionally modulate the growth of the vascular cells via release of stored growth factor. Thus, the matrix, contrary to previous expectation, cannot be considered simply as an inert supportive tissue for surrounding cells but a dynamic structure central to the control of vascular reorganization.

In muscular arteries compliance is inextricably linked to vascular smooth muscle (VSM) tone. Usually a decrease in tone is associated with an increase in compliance. This is not always the case, however, since a large decrease in VSM tone may transfer stress to more rigid elements in the vessel wall so that when the VSM is fully relaxed, compliance may decrease. In large elastic arteries such as the aorta, compliance is dependent less on VSM tone but rather on the intrinsic elasticity of the ECM. This in turn will depend on the characteristics and relative proportions of elastin, collagen and other components of the ECM. Although the amount of collagen or collagen subtypes/elastin may be important, changes in the connective tissue of the vessel wall may prove to be more subtle, involving reorganization of existing collagen and elastin matrices. This could be achieved through altered matrix–matrix interactions involving proteoglycans such as decorin or through changes in the attachment properties of proteins such as integrins or fibronectins in cell–matrix interactions. Central to controlled reorganization of ECM at any level is the activity of a unique family of enzymes, the matrix metalloproteinases (MMPs). MMPs, beyond their previously described functions as extracellular degrading enzymes, may also exert effects on cellular growth and proliferation (Dollery et al., 1995). This may occur indirectly through evoking release of ECM-associated growth factors such as fibroblast growth factor (FGF) and TGF-β (Taipole and Keski-oja, 1997) during matrix turnover or directly via degradation of growth factors or of growth factor-binding proteins such as insulin-like growth factor-binding protein (IGFBP-3: Fowlkes et al., 1994).

Alterations in large artery compliance in physiological conditions

Ageing, pregnancy and the menopause

The major physiological conditions associated with changes in large artery compliance are ageing and pregnancy. Many investigators have reported an inverse association between large artery distensibility and age (Avolio et al., 1983, 1985;

Safar, 1990). This association with age is much less marked in muscular arteries, suggesting that it may relate to structural changes in the elastin, which comprises a major element of the vascular wall of large arteries. Indeed, electron microscopy studies show that elastin fibres are subject to degenerative changes akin to the stress fracturing seen in many mechanical elements subject to repeated stress (Nichols and O'Rourke, 1998). Such degenerative changes are unlikely to be reversible and are most unlikely to account for alterations in large arterial compliance associated with pregnancy and perimenopausal changes. Alterations in pregnancy are particularly marked and may thus offer a unique insight into physiological determinants of arterial compliance.

It has long been appreciated that normal pregnancy is associated with profound haemodynamic changes beginning early in the first trimester. These include an increase in intravascular volume and cardiac output and decrease in peripheral vascular resistance (which may precede the other changes). The fall in peripheral resistance is sufficiently large to result in a fall in mean blood pressure despite the increase in cardiac output. An active state of peripheral vasodilation of resistance arteries, whether through decreased constriction or enhanced dilation, provides the most obvious explanation for the fall in peripheral resistance. Such a decrease in tone of resistance arteries would, as discussed above, be likely to lead to an increase in arterial compliance and this has indeed been observed in animal gestations (Hart et al., 1986; Slangen et al., 1997). More recently, an increase in large artery compliance has been observed in uncomplicated human pregnancies (Poppas et al., 1997; Edouard et al., 1998) and may contribute to the adaptation to an increased cardiac output, preventing an excessive rise in systolic blood pressure. In preeclampsia, a syndrome unique to pregnancy (defined clinically by an elevation in blood pressure and the presence of proteinuria), there appears to be a failure or reversal of maternal vascular adaptation with potential deleterious consequences for both mother and fetus. A preliminary study has reported reduced arterial compliance in such hypertensive pregnancies (Hibbard et al., 1998). The relatively short-term changes in large artery compliance associated with pregnancy suggest that oestrogen may modulate the structure of large arteries. This hypothesis is further supported by the observation that large artery compliance is higher in post-menopausal women taking hormone replacement therapy (HRT) and decreases following withdrawal of HRT (Rajkumar et al., 1997).

Vascular structural change in pregnancy

Dramatic remodelling of wall structure has been described in the uteroplacental circulation, with a more complaint vascular bed facilitating perfusion of the placental intervillous space with maternal blood. Alterations in endothelial function and VSM tone in these arteries undoubtedly contribute to an increase in compliance. However, the incidence or degree of restructuring in larger arteries has been less frequently addressed. This is perhaps surprising given the magnitude and duration of change in cardiovascular function observed in normal pregnancy and the observation that structural reorganization of the vasculature is generally manifest whenever functional changes persist for more than a few days. What information exists is limited and largely confined to animal studies. In an extensive histological investigation of different vascular beds in the pregnant rat, Awal et al. (1995) described an increase in wall thickness and in lumen diameter in muscular arteries. In contrast, these dimensions appeared unchanged in the elastic aorta. In a further study, using electron microscopy, the aortic intimal cross-sectional area of the pregnant guinea pig was shown to decrease (Jovanovic and Jovanovic, 1997) and, in the absence of changes in intrinsic elasticity of the vessel wall, this would be expected to result in *decreased* compliance. However, in addition to the inevitable artefacts that may occur in tissue fixation and processing, vessels studied in this way are not subjected to transmural (physiological) pressure. In normal pregnant women aortic diameter over a range of aortic pressures was reported to increase in an early study by Hart et al. (1986). The changes appear more marked in multiparous women compared to primiparae, which is consistent with the findings of a later study (Easterling et al., 1991). Clapp and Capeless (1997) additionally show that systemic vascular resistance, while gradually returning *towards* baseline, differed significantly from prepregnancy values for up to a year postpartum. The persistence of vascular remodelling beyond delivery, when one would have expected that endocrine-associated functional changes would have regressed, and the observation of larger and more compliant aortas in multiparous pregnant women suggest that intrinsic modification in the arterial wall may occur as a result of pregnancy in humans.

Dramatic remodelling of the ECM has been described in the reproductive system in pregnancy. In contrast, little information is available on vascular matrix turnover in pregnancy. A reduction in wall collagen to elastin ratio specific to certain resistance vascular beds has been described (Griendling et al., 1985; Mackey et al., 1992). In an early study, increased collagen synthesis was observed in aortas of pregnant rats maintained in organ culture; and interestingly, this was exaggerated in hypertensive pregnant animals (Foidart et al., 1978). This study would appear to contradict the hypothesis that a reduction in arterial collagen accompanies an increase in aortic compliance in normal pregnancy. However, in addition to the limitations of organ culture, it is not possible from this study to conclude what proportion of the newly synthesized collagen would be deposited in the vessel wall and therefore functionally relevant. Nor is it possible to estimate which subtypes of collagen are synthesized. Another possibility is that pregnancy-induced changes in the connective tissue of the vessel wall may involve reorganization of existing collagen and elastin matrices through the action of MMPs. A role for these enzymes in the adaptation of nonvascular ECM to pregnancy is well established in several tissues including the cervix, uterus and fetal membranes. Compared to the number of investigations ascribing a role for MMPs in structural remodelling of spiral arteries, and the numerous studies advocating a role for MMPs in pathological cardiovascular remodelling (Dollery et al., 1999), the potential role of MMPs in the adaptation of maternal vasculature to normal pregnancy has been remarkably neglected. Preliminary data from our laboratory show increased expression of MMP-3 in aortas from late-gestation pregnant rats compared to those from virgin rats. There was no significant difference in the expression of MMP-2 between the groups studied. These data advocates a role for proteoglycan turnover in the vascular matrix, suggesting that a mechanism of reorganization might be through altered matrix–matrix interaction.

Influence of oestrogen

Many of the haemodynamic changes observed in normal pregnancy can be induced in animal models by chronic exposure of the nonpregnant animal to oestrogen (Hart et al., 1985; Magness et al., 1993). Human endothelial and VSMCs contain functional oestrogen receptors. The mechanisms by which changes in arterial compliance are accomplished are unclear but, importantly, their elucidation might well provide further insight into the cardioprotective effects of oestrogens in premenopausal women and in those postmenopausal women on oestrogen replacement therapy. Oestrogen treatment of ovariectomized rats affects the rate of collagen and elastin accumulation in the aortic wall in favour of a reduction in the collagen to elastin ratio (Fischer, 1972). In addition, aortic smooth muscle cells cultured in the presence of estradiol produce an altered ratio of type I: type III collagen. It is interesting that neither the $\alpha_1(I)$ nor the $\alpha_2(I)$ collagen genes contain an oestrogen-response element. More recent work by Neugarten et al. (1999) has shown that oestrogen suppression of type I collagen synthesis can occur via an upregulation of the MAP kinase cascade. Oestrogenic effects on vascular collagen turnover might well be mediated through a NO-dependent pathway as this steroid is also known to stimulate NO synthesis, through both genomic and nongenomic pathways (Chen et al., 1999). The evidence supporting enhanced NO synthesis in pregnancy is growing and herein may lie a link between a stimulus for vasodilatation and for remodelling in pregnancy. NO has been shown specifically to increase type III collagen synthesis in cultured VSMCs (Westerhausen-Larson et al., 1997) and, in the renal vessels of transgenic mice, inhibition of NOS induces type I collagen gene expression (Chatziantoniou et al., 1998). Interestingly, this stimulation of collagen I gene activation was abolished when animals were treated with bosentan, an endothelin receptor antagonist. This substantiates another recent report suggesting interactions occur between endothelin receptors (particularly ET-B) and NO in the renal vasculature in pregnancy (Conrad et al., 1999).

Alterations in arterial compliance in vascular disease

Hypertension

The mechanical/structural relationship in arteries has been studied extensively with respect to the development and treatment of hypertension. Small resistance-sized arteries have received most attention, in view of the elevated total peripheral resistance that characterizes essential hypertension. Sustained hypertension has been extensively reported to induce an increased arterial wall thickness and media-to-lumen ratio (Folkow, 1982; Mulvany and Aalkjaer, 1990). The data on small arteries and arterioles (Laurent, 1995) have been confirmed by clinical studies performed on isolated subcutaneous arterioles (Aalkjaer et al., 1987). The observed morphological changes have been distinguished either as 'remodelling' ('eutrophic') or 'hypertrophy' depending on the decrease or increase in external diameter respectively. This reconfiguration of the media has also been associated with an increased amount of collagen relative to elastin (Brayden et al., 1983). The data on how these changes in vessel geometry are related to altered arterial stiffness, however, are conflicting. In experimental hypertensive models in the rat, similar changes in wall structure have been associated with a reduction, no change or an increase in the stiffness of the vessel wall (Lew and Angus, 1992; Intengan et al., 1999a,b). In resistance arteries isolated from untreated essential hypertensive patients, the media-to-lumen ratio and media width were greater in hypertensive vessels reducing wall stress. While analysis of the media showed a greater collagen-to-elastin ratio in these arteries, the stiffness of wall components (derived from incremental elastic modulus versus stress) was significantly *lower* in hypertensive vessels compared to vessels isolated from control normotensive volunteers (Intengan et al., 1999b). One interpretation of this is that the wall adapts to maintain a physiologically relevant buffering capacity despite stiffer wall components and that this may be attained through more subtle spatial reorganization of other matrix elements and their interactions.

In large arteries most studies demonstrate an increase in stiffness (Nichols and O'Rourke, 1998; Safar et al., 1998). The pressure dependence of arterial compliance complicates the evaluation of mechanical properties of large arteries in hypertension, with difficulty in establishing whether a change in arterial compliance is a consequence of increased blood pressure or reflects intrinsic alterations in the arterial wall. This issue of 'cause or consequence' has been addressed in two recent studies. van Gorp et al. (2000) showed that decreases in distensibility and compliance precede the development of hypertension in spontaneously hypertensive rats (SHRs), in which hypertension develops gradually over weeks. While media hypertrophy was evident at this stage the authors report no significant difference in total collagen content. It is not possible from this study to know whether media hypertrophy in SHR developed after birth or was already present in fetal life. Further, with this limited information, it would be premature to discount the hypothesis that ECM changes contribute to alterations in compliance. For instance, while *total* collagen content may be unaltered, there may be changes in collagen subtypes. An alteration in the proportion of the 'stiffer' type 1 compared to the more extensible type III might contribute to altered passive mechanical properties. Abnormalities of extracellular degradation of collagen type I have been reported in essential hypertension (Laviades et al., 1998). Modification of vascular matrix may occur by other means, such as through altered cell–matrix or matrix–matrix attachment sites and interactions without change in total amounts of the major matrix proteins. Interestingly, an increase in $\alpha_v\beta_3$ and $\alpha_5\beta_1$ integrins has been reported in vessels from SHRs in established hypertension (Intengan et al., 1999a,b).

The relationship between arterial compliance and hypertension has been examined prospectively in a cohort of nearly 7000 normotensive men and women by Liao et al. (1999). Arterial elasticity was measured using high-resolution ultrasound of the left common carotid artery simultaneously controlling for blood pressure and arterial diameter. The data suggest that impaired elasticity of larger arteries is an antecedent factor in the natural history of blood pressure elevation at the population level.

Of the many neurohormonal factors which might be responsible for structural changes in hypertension leading to increased arterial stiffness, increased local angiotensin production possibly within the vascular wall itself seems a likely mechanism. Angiotensin II promotes collagen production from aortic smooth muscle cells in culture (Kato et al., 1991) and an association has been reported between increased arterial stiffness and the presence of angiotensin II type 1 receptor gene (Benetos et al., 1995). Several reports have indicated that angiotensin converting enzyme (ACE) blockade has specific effects on the arterial connective tissue, producing substantial modifications in fibronectin expression and collagen content (Albaladejo et al., 1994; Himeno et al., 1994). The latter changes were shown to be more related to ACE inhibition than to blood pressure reduction.

Other conditions associated with altered large artery stiffness

Decreased arterial distensibility (measured mainly by aortic PWV) has been reported in association with other risk factors for cardiovascular disease, in particular hypercholesterolaemia and diabetes. Lehmann et al. (1998) have shown aortic PWV to be related to the number of cardiovascular risk factors. However, many of these subjects had established atherosclerosis (and many more may have had silent disease) and it is unclear whether the observed association of aortic PWV with risk factors reflects the effects of atherosclerosis or the risk factors per se. It is noteworthy that in young subjects with familial hypercholesterolaemia, the same investigators observed a decreased aortic PWV (Lehmann et al., 1992). This suggests that the development of atherosclerosis may be the main factor influencing aortic stiffness in hypercholesterolaemia but interventional studies will be required to help resolve this issue.

Increased aortic stiffness as a cardiovascular risk factor

As discussed above, increased aortic stiffness (assessed by PWV) has been shown to be predictive of cardiovascular events in patients with renal failure and of cardiovascular risk in hypertensive subjects. Furthermore, the observation that arterial pulse pressure is a better predictor of cardiovascular mortality than systolic or diastolic blood pressure (Franklin et al., 1999) suggests that arterial stiffness is likely to be highly predictive of mortality in hypertensive subjects. Aortic stiffness may act as a marker for established atherosclerosis or other factors associated with cardiac events or it may be that the risk associated with increased aortic stiffness results from adverse haemodynamic effects. These include increased left ventricular load and an altered pressure and flow pattern within the aorta and hence coronary arteries. This may result in altered shear forces, with increased pulsatility leading to atherosclerosis within the aorta, carotid and coronary arteries.

Interventions to modify large artery stiffness

There have been surprisingly few studies of interventions to modify large artery stiffness. Withdrawal of HRT leads to an increase in large artery stiffness (Rajkumar et al., 1997), suggesting that HRT may be an effective treatment to improve large artery distensibility in postmenopausal women. Exercise is associated with greater aortic distensibility and may be an intervention which can reverse increases in arterial stiffness (Cameron and Dart, 1994; Kingwell et al., 1997). Antihypertensive drugs may affect large artery stiffness over and above effects due to blood pressure reduction and, in view of the accelerated age-related increases in aortic stiffness seen in hypertensive subjects, may prove to be effective in preventing a decline in arterial distensibility. Of the various antihypertensive agents, ACE inhibitors appear most promising, for the reasons discussed above.

Other interventions to reduce cardiovascular risk factors, such as smoking cessation and lipid-lowering therapy, may reduce arterial stiffness. In view of the possible regulation of vessel wall structure by NO, interventions which improve endothelial function and especially basal release of NO may reduce arterial stiffness. This is an area of intense research and there are many possible interventions being pursued, including L-arginine (the substrate for NO synthase) and antioxidant therapy.

Conclusion

Large artery stiffness is dependent on the characteristics of arterial smooth muscle and the ECM. Both may be influenced by chemical mediators, including endothelium-derived NO. The major physiological determinants of large artery stiffness are ageing and pregnancy. Hypertension, and possibly other atherogenic conditions and/or atherosclerosis itself, are associated with increased stiffness. Aortic and large artery stiffness has an important influence on haemodynamics, influencing the load on the left ventricle, the dynamic component of arterial flow and the distribution of shear stress within the arterial tree and coronary arteries. Increased aortic stiffness is a risk factor for cardiac events. Whether this results from adverse haemodynamic consequences or as a result of increased stiffness being a marker for atherosclerosis or both remains to be determined.

REFERENCES

Aalkjaer, C., Heagerty, A.M., Petersen, K.K., Swales, J.D. & Mulvany, M.J. (1987). Evidence for increased media thickness, increased neuronal amine uptake, and depressed excitation – contraction coupling in isolated resistance vessels from essential hypertensives. *Circ. Res.*, **61**, 181–6.

Albaladejo, P., Bouaziz, H., Duriez, M. et al. (1994). Angiotensin converting enzyme inhibition prevents the increase in aortic collagen in rats. *Hypertension*, **23**, 74–82.

Avolio, A.P., Chen, S.G., Wang, R.P. et al. (1983). Effects of aging on changing arterial compliance and left ventricular load in a northern Chinese urban community. *Circulation*, **68**, 50–8.

Avolio, A.P., Deng, F.Q., Li, W.Q. et al. (1985). Effects of aging on arterial distensibility in populations with high and low prevalence of hypertension: comparison between urban and rural communities in China. *Circulation*, **71**, 202–10.

Awal, M.A., Matsumoto, M. & Nishinakagawa, H. (1995). Morphometrical changes of the arterial walls of main arteries from heart to the abdomino-inguinal mammary glands of rat from virgin through pregnancy, lactation and post-weaning. *J. Vet. Med. Sci.*, **57**, 251–6.

Benetos, A., Topouchian, J., Ricard, S. et al. (1995). Influence of angiotensin II type 1 receptor polymorphism on aortic stiffness in never-treated hypertensive patients. *Hypertension*, **26**, 44–7.

Blacher, J., Guerin, A.P., Pannier, B., Marchais, S.J. & Safar, M.E. (1999). Impact of aortic stiffness on survival in end-stage renal disease. *Circulation*, **99**, 2434–9.

Bramwell, J.C. & Hill, A.V. (1922). Velocity of transmission of the pulse and elasticity of arteries. *Lancet*, **1**, 891–2.

Brayden, J.E., Halpern, W. & Brann, L.R. (1983). Biochemical and mechanical properties of resistance arteries from normotensive and hypertensive rats. *Hypertension*, **5**, 17–25.

Cameron, J.D. & Dart, A.M. (1994). Exercise training increases total systemic arterial compliance in humans. *Am. J. Physiol.*, **266**, H693–H701.

Chatziantoniou, C., Boffa, J.J., Ardaillou, R. & Dussaule, J.C. (1998). Nitric oxide inhibition induces early activation of type I collagen gene in renal resistance vessels and glomeruli in transgenic mice. *J. Clin. Invest.*, **101**, 2780–9.

Chen, Z., Yuhanna, I.S., Galcheva-Gargova, Z. et al. (1999) Estrogen receptor α mediates the nongenomic activation of endothelial nitric oxide synthase by estrogen. *J. Clin. Invest.*, **103**, 401–6.

Clapp, J.F. III & Capeless, E. (1997). Cardiovascular function before, during, and after the first and subsequent pregnancies. *Am. J. Cardiol.*, **80**, 1469–73.

Cohn, J.N., Finklestein, S., Mcveigh, G. et al. (1995). Noninvasive pulse-wave analysis for the early detection of vascular disease. *Hypertension*, **26**, 503–8.

Conrad, K.P., Gandley, R.E., Ogawa, T., Nakanishi, S. & Danielson, L.A. (1999). Endothelin mediates renal vasodilation and hyperfiltration during pregnancy in chronically instrumented conscious rats. *Am. J. Physiol.*, **276**, F767–F776.

Dollery, C.M., McEwan, J.R. & Henney, A.M. (1995). Matrix metalloproteinases and cardiovascular disease. *Circ. Res.*, **77**, 863–8.

Dollery, C.M., Humphries, S.E., McClelland, A., Latchman, D.S. & McEwan, J.R. (1999). Expression of tissue inhibitor of matrix metalloproteinases 1 by use of an adenoviral vector inhibits smooth muscle cell migration and reduces neointimal hyperplasia in the rat model of vascular balloon injury. *Circulation*, **99**, 3199–205.

Easterling, T.R., Benedetti, T.J., Schmucker, B.C., Carlson, K. & Millard, S.P. (1991). Maternal hemodynamics and aortic diameter in normal and hypertensive pregnancies. *Obstet. Gynecol.*, **78**, 1073–7.

Edouard, D.A., Pannier, B.M., London, G.M., Cuche, J.L. & Safar, M.E. (1998). Venous and arterial behavior during normal pregnancy. *Am. J. Physiol.*, **274**, H1605–12.

Fischer, G.M. (1972). In vivo effects of estradiol on collagen and elastin dynamics in rat aorta. *Endocrinology*, **91**, 1227–31.

Foidart, J.M., Rorive, G. & Nusgens, B. (1978). Aortic collagen biosynthesis during renal hypertension, pregnancy and hypertension during pregnancy in the rat. *Biomedicine*, **28**, 215–19.

Folkow, B. (1982). Physiological aspects of primary hypertension. *Physiol Rev.*, **62**, 347–504.

Fowlkes, J.L., Enghild, J.J., Suzuki, K. & Nagase, H. (1994). Matrix metalloproteinases degrade insulin-like growth factor-binding protein-3 in dermal fibroblast cultures. *J. Biol. Chem.*, **269**, 25742–6.

Franklin, S.S., Khan, S.A., Wong, N.D., Larson, M.G. & Levy, D. (1999). Is pulse pressure useful in predicting risk for coronary heart disease? The Framingham heart study. *Circulation*, **100**, 354–60.

Giannattasio, C., Failla, M., Mangoni, A.A. et al. (1996). Evaluation of arterial compliance in humans. *Clin. Exp. Hypertens.*, **18**, 347–62.

Griendling, K.K., Fuller, E.O. & Cox, R.H. (1985). Pregnancy-induced changes in sheep uterine and carotid arteries. *Am. J. Physiol.*, **248**, H658–65.

Hart, M.V., Hosenpud, J.D., Hohimer, A.R. & Morton, M.J. (1985). Hemodynamics during pregnancy and sex steroid administration in guinea pigs. *Am. J. Physiol.*, **249**, R179–85.

Hart, M.V., Morton, M.J., Hosenpud, J.D. & Metcalfe, J. (1986). Aortic function during normal pregnancy. *Am. J. Obstet. Gynecol.*, **154**, 887–91.

Hibbard, J.U., Korcarz, C., Giardet, N.G. et al. (1998). Arterial circulation in pregnancy complicated by hypertension. Abstract 11th World Congress of the International Society for the Study of Hypertension in Pregnancy, Japan, 1998. OS13–4, p. 131.

Himeno, H., Crawford, D.C., Hosoi, M., Chobanian, A.V. & Brecher, P. (1994). Angiotensin II alters aortic fibronectin independently of hypertension. *Hypertension*, **23**, 823–6.

Intengan, H.D., Thibault, G., Li, J.S. & Schiffrin, E.L. (1999a). Resistance artery mechanics, structure, and extracellular components in spontaneously hypertensive rats: effects of angiotensin receptor antagonism and converting enzyme inhibition. *Circulation*, **100**, 2267–75.

Intengan, H.D., Deng, L.Y., Li, J.S. & Schiffrin, E.L. (1999b). Mechanics and composition of human subcutaneous resistance arteries in essential hypertension. *Hypertension*, **33**, 569–74.

Jovanovic, S. & Jovanovic, A. (1997). Remodelling of guinea-pig aorta during pregnancy: selective alteration of endothelial cells. *Hum. Reprod.*, **12**, 2297–302.

Kato, H., Suzuki, H., Tajima, S. et al. (1991). Angiotensin II stimulates collagen synthesis in cultured vascular smooth muscle cells. *J. Hypertens.*, **9**, 17–22.

Kingwell, B.A., Arnold, P.J., Jennings, G.L. & Dart, A.M. (1997). Spontaneous running increases aortic compliance in Wistar-Kyoto rats. *Cardiovasc. Res.*, **35**, 132–7.

Laurent, S. (1995). Arterial wall hypertrophy and stiffness in essential hypertensive patients. *Hypertension*, **26**, 355–62.

Laviades, C., Varo, N., Fernandez, J. et al. (1998). Abnormalities of the extracellular degradation of collagen type I in essential hypertension. *Circulation*, **98**, 535–40.

Lehmann, E.D., Watts, G.F., Fatemi-Langroudi, B. & Gosling, R.G. (1992). Aortic compliance in young patients with heterozygous familial hypercholesterolaemia. *Clin. Sci. (Colch.)*, **83**, 717–21.

Lehmann, E.D., Hopkins, K.D., Rawesh, A. et al. (1998). Relation between number of cardiovascular risk factors/events and noninvasive Doppler ultrasound assessments of aortic compliance. *Hypertension*, **32**, 565–9.

Lew, M.J. & Angus, J.A. (1992). Wall thickness to lumen diameter ratios of arteries from SHR and WKY: comparison of pressurised and wire-mounted preparations. *J. Vasc. Res.*, **29**, 435–42.

Liao D., Arnett, D.K., Tyroler, H.A. et al. (1999). Arterial stiffness and the development of hypertension. The ARIC study. *Hypertension*, **34**, 201–6.

Mackey, K., Meyer, M.C., Stirewalt, W.M., Starcher, B.C. & McLaughlin, M.K. (1992). Composition and mechanics of mesenteric arteries from pregnant rats. *Am. J. Physiol.*, **263**, R8.

Magness, R.R., Parker, C.R. & Rosenfeld, C.R. (1993). Systemic and uterine responses to chronic infusion of estradiol-17 beta. *Am. J. Physiol.*, **265**, E690–8.

Millar, J.A., Lever, A.F. & Burke, V. (1999). Pulse pressure as a risk factor for cardiovascular events in the MRC Mild Hypertension Trial. *J. Hypertens.*, **17**, 1065–72.

Mulvany, M.J. & Aalkjaer, C. (1990). Structure and function of small arteries. *Physiol. Rev.*, **70**, 921–61.

Neugarten, J., Medve, I., Lei, J. & Silbiger, S.R. (1999). Estradiol suppresses mesangial cell type I collagen synthesis via activation of the MAP kinase cascade. *Am. J. Physiol.*, **277**, F875–81.

Nichols, W.W. & O'Rourke, M.F. (1998). *McDonald's Blood Flow in Arteries. Theoretical, Experimental and Clinical Principles.* London: Arnold, 1998.

O'Rourke, M.F. & Mancia, G. (1999). Arterial stiffness. *J. Hypertens.*, **17**, 1–4.

Poppas, A., Shroff, S.G., Korcarz, C.E. et al. (1997). Serial assessment of the cardiovascular system in normal pregnancy. *Circulation*, **95**, 2407–15.

Rajkumar, C., Kingwell, B.A., Cameron, J.D. et al. (1997). Hormonal therapy increases arterial compliance in postmenopausal women. *J. Am. Coll. Cardiol.*, **30**, 350–6.

Safar, M. (1990). Ageing and its effects on the cardiovascular system. *Drugs*, **39** (suppl. 1), 1–8.

Safar, M.E., London, G.M., Asmar, R. & Frohlich, E.D. (1998). Recent advances on large arteries in hypertension. *Hypertension*, **32**, 156–61.

Slangen, B.F.M., Ingen Schenau, D.S., van Gorp, A.D.W., De Mey, J.G.R. & Peeters, L.L.H. (1997). Aortic distensibility and compliance in conscious pregnant rats. *Am. J. Physiol.*, **272**, H1260–5.

Stefanadis, C., Stratos, C., Vlachopoulos, C. et al. (1995). Pressure–diameter relation of the human aorta. A new method of determination by the application of a special ultrasonic dimension catheter. *Circulation*, **92**, 2210–19.

Taipale, J. & Keski-oja, J. (1997). Growth factors in the extracellular matrix. *FASEB J*, **11**, 51–9.

van Gorp, A.D.W., van Ingen Schenau, D.S., Hoeks, A.P.G. et al. (2000). In spontaneously hypertensive rats alterations in aortic wall properties precede the development of hypertension. *Am. J. Physiol.*, **278**, H1241–7.

Westerhausen-Larson, A., Collura, L.C., Rizzo, C.F., Ojimba, J. & McLaughlin, M.K. (1997). Nitric oxide increases type III collagen secretion in vascular smooth muscle cells. *J. Soc. Gynecol. Invest.*, **4**, 532.

3

Flow-mediated responses in the circulation

Lucilla Poston

Department of Obstetrics and Gynaecology, Guy's, King's and St Thomas' School of Medicine, King's College London, London

Introduction

Haemodynamic forces are now well established as important modulators of vascular tone and vascular wall remodelling, and are increasingly implicated in atherogenesis. Blood vessels are under the influence of two primary haemodynamic forces: firstly, the circumferential force, the wall tension, which originates from the blood pressure and, secondly, the frictional force or shear stress which results from blood flow along the vessel wall. Although the circumferential force has important influences on vascular tone, it is the intention of this short review to concentrate upon flow-associated events in the vasculature. The shear stress experienced by the endothelium is a function of the 'axial' pressure gradient (Figure 3.1) which occurs as blood flows through the vessel (Malek and Izumo, 1994) and, physiologically, is of the order of 0–50 dyn/cm^2 (Figure 3.2).

Until recently, little was known of the mechanisms whereby the physical force of flow could be transduced into a wide range of associated intracellular biochemical events. It is now recognized that the endothelial cell, uniquely situated at the interface between the blood and the vascular wall, is effectively a biological mechanotransducer which senses shear forces and converts these physical stimuli to intracellular biochemical signals.

Flow and vascular tone

Amongst the myriad of events now known to be triggered by shear stress, the first to be investigated in any depth was the observation that flow through isolated arteries, more particularly the conduit vessels, leads to relaxation and dilatation. Flow was first recognized to be important in the control of vascular tone in 1933 (Schretzenmayr, 1933), when it was observed that the femoral artery in the dog hind limb dilates in response to a hyperaemic stimulus. Experimentally, the effects of shear stress have most frequently been investigated by determining the response

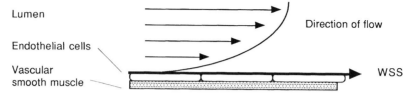

Figure 3.1   Wall shear stress. Wall shear stress (WSS) is the force per unit area acting in the direction of blood flow (Q) at the endothelial surface dependent on the blood's viscosity, μ. In laminar flow, the magnitude of the shear stress is proportional to the third power of the internal radius of the vessel (r): $\text{WSS} = \dfrac{4 \times \mu \times Q}{\pi \times r^3}$.

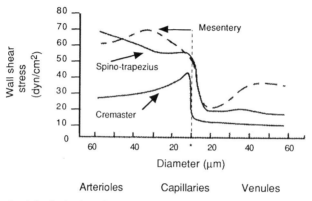

Figure 3.2   Physiological values for wall shear stress. Representative arteriovenous distributions of wall shear stress from measurements of red cell velocity in the microcirculation of mesentery, spinotrapezius muscle and cremaster muscle from studies in cat, rat and rabbit. Reproduced from Lipowsky (1995) with permission.

to flow in vitro in isolated conduit arteries (Rubanyi et al., 1986; Cooke et al., 1991) or in isolated vascular beds (Smiesko et al., 1989; Griffith and Edwards, 1990; Matrougui et al., 1997). Whilst there are many reports of flow-mediated dilatation in isolated resistance-sized arteries (Koller et al., 1994; Cockell and Poston, 1996, 1997; Izzard and Heagerty, 1999; Huang et al., 2000), numerous laboratories have failed to find substantial dilatation in small arteries. Flow-mediated dilatation in small vessels seems to be sensitive to experimental conditions and to be vascular bed-dependent. In our laboratory we have routinely observed substantial dilatation in small arteries from pregnant women (Learmont and Poston, 1996; Cockell and Poston, 1997) and animals (Cockell and Poston, 1996), but have shown absent or only very modest dilatation in small arteries from nonpregnant women (Cockell and Poston, 1997) and animals (Tribe et al., 1998). Flow-mediated dilatation in larger arteries in vivo can be observed using an entirely noninvasive method which has become popular in recent years for investigations of endothelial function in humans. This technique employs high-resolution Doppler ultrasound of the brachial arteries (Meredith et al., 1996) to evaluate flow-mediated dilatation evoked by a downstream hyperaemic stimulus.

The endothelium dependence of flow-induced dilatation has been proven in isolated conduit arteries from experimental animals (Pohl et al., 1986; Rubanyi et al., 1986) and in resistance-sized arterioles (Koller and Kaley, 1991; Koller et al., 1993). There is evidence for some variability amongst species and/or vascular beds as flow-induced relaxation may persist after endothelium removal in some circulations, e.g. rabbit ear resistance artery (Bevan et al., 1988). The brachial artery response to hyperaemia has also been shown to be, at least in part, dependent on the endothelium as the relaxation is blunted by infusion of the nitric oxide synthase inhibitor L-nitroarginine methyl ester (L-NAME: Meredith et al., 1996).

Shear evokes relaxation through nitric oxide and prostacyclin release

Relaxation to flow is widely considered to result from release of nitric oxide (NO) and, to a lesser extent, prostacyclin (PGI_2), although NO independence has occasionally been reported (Izzard and Heagerty, 1999). Involvement of PGI_2 has been implicated by the demonstration of flow-induced synthesis of 6-ketoprostaglandin $F_{1\alpha}$, a stable metabolite of PGI_2 (Rubanyi et al., 1986; Hecker et al., 1993), or by showing blunted responses in the presence of indometacin (Sun et al., 1999). The contribution of NO is usually evaluated by determining responses to flow in the presence and absence of specific inhibitors of NO synthase (NOS: Cooke et al., 1990; Koller et al., 1994; Cockell and Poston, 1997; Kublickiene et al., 1997; Huang et al., 1998). Others have implicated NO by showing that the effluent emerging from perfused arteries stimulates soluble guanylyl cyclase (Hecker et al., 1993), the enzyme activated by NO to form cyclic guanosine 3,5-monophosphate (cGMP), which relaxes the vascular smooth muscle. In addition to activation of vascular smooth muscle, NO acts in an autocrine fashion to stimulate guanylyl cyclase in endothelial cells and measurement of endothelial cell cGMP provides an alternative endpoint for the estimation of NO synthesis. Thus, endothelial cGMP has been shown to be increased in a graded fashion with laminar flow in cultured endothelial cells (Ohno et al., 1993). Laminar and pulsatile flow have also been found to increase the expression of nitric oxide synthase III (NOS-III) mRNA in endothelial cells (Noris et al., 1995; Ranjan et al., 1995), but turbulent flow had no effect when NOS-III was assessed by a biochemical assay (Noris et al., 1995).

'Cross-talk' between PGI_2 and NO has also been suggested, since inhibition or the absence of one of the two vasodilators seems to be compensated by increased synthesis of the other. This was first demonstrated in the NOS-III knockout mouse, in which flow-mediated dilatation in gracilis muscle arterioles was shown to be maintained by a compensatory increase in PGI_2 (Sun et al., 1999). Similarly, inhibition of NOS in cultured human umbilical venous endothelial cells leads to upregulation of flow-mediated PGI_2 synthesis (Osanai et al., 2000).

Another vasodilator, the endothelium-derived hyperpolarizing factor (EDHF), undoubtedly plays a major role in endothelium-dependent relaxation despite lack of agreement regarding its chemical identity. Cyclical stress induced by rhythmic vessel distension has been shown to evoke EDHF-mediated relaxation (Busse and Fleming, 1998) but few studies have attempted to define a role for EDHF in flow-mediated relaxation, probably because most investigations show complete inhibition of dilatation after NOS and prostaglandin inhibition. However, EDHF has been implicated in relaxation to flow in the rat mesenteric circulation (Takamura et al., 1999).

Vasodilatation to flow in vascular disease

The recognition of the important role of flow in the maintenance of vascular dilatation and hence in the control of peripheral resistance has led to the proposal that impaired dilatation to flow in patients with known endothelial cell dysfunction may contribute to the pathogenesis of the disease. Studies of isolated arteries from patients have been few, although in our laboratory we have shown flow-induced dilatation to be reduced in small arteries from pregnant women with preeclampsia (Cockell and Poston, 1997). In animal models of disease, poor dilatation to flow has also been reported in isolated arterioles from hypertensive rats (Koller and Huang, 1994; Matrougui et al., 1997; Izzard and Heagerty, 1999) and in the coronary circulation of the atherosclerotic pig (Kuo et al., 1992). The abnormality of flow-mediated relaxation in the male spontaneously hypertensive rat has recently been shown to be reversed by 17β-estradiol (Huang et al., 2000).

The estimation of flow-induced responses in vivo in humans has been extensively investigated using high-resolution Doppler ultrasound imaging of the brachial artery. The flow stimulus is induced by provoking reactive hyperaemia in the hand or forearm with the use of an inflated cuff, and measuring changes in the artery diameter. The stimulus is therefore distal to the site of measurement and the ensuing dilatation of the brachial artery cannot be attributed to locally produced metabolites. Accuracy in the measurement of diameter is essential as the flow-induced dilatation is small (in the order of 8–10% of artery diameter). It must be considered, however, that the brachial artery is not a common site of atherosclerotic plaque formation and, being a conduit artery, plays little role in the control of peripheral resistance. Failure of the brachial artery to dilate to flow may therefore have little pathophysiological consequence; the wider implications rest on the assumption that the brachial artery is a reliable model of 'global' endothelial function. The method is undoubtedly the most reliable technique currently available for noninvasive assessment of flow-mediated dilatation and also offers the possibility of evaluating endothelial function in response to dietary and pharmacological interventions. Abnormal responses have been identified in a wide variety of subjects, including children and adults at risk of atherosclerosis (Celermajer et al., 1992), children with low birth weight (Leeson et al., 1997), patients with noninsulin-dependent diabetes (Goodfellow et al., 1996), cigarette smokers and passive smokers (Celermajer et al., 1996), patients with hyper-homocysteinaemia (Woo et al., 1997), patients with coronary heart disease (Stein et al., 1999), postmenopausal women (Bush et al., 1998) and in subjects undergo-ing haemodialysis (Miyazaki et al., 2000). Interventions reported to increase flow-mediated dilatation include folate supplements in patients with hyper-homocysteinaemia (Woo et al., 1999), red wine in subjects eating a high-fat diet (Cuevas et al., 2000), dietary supplementation with $\omega 3$ fatty acids in hypercholes-terolaemic subjects (Goodfellow et al., 2000), grape juice in patients with coronary artery disease (Stein et al., 1999), vitamin E (acutely) in smokers (Neunteufl et al., 2000), vitamin E-coated haemodialysers in patients with renal failure (Miyakazi et al., 2000) and oestrogen replacement in postmenopausal women (Bush et al., 1998; Koh et al., 1999).

The endothelial cell as a mechanotransducer

The cytoskeleton as a mechanotransducer

The complexity of the mechanotransduction pathways by which the frictional force is detected in endothelial cells is gradually being unravelled. The frictional force is obviously experienced initially at the luminal surface of the cell, but it is questionable whether this is the principal site of flow detection. Evidence now points to an important role for transduction of the frictional force through the cytoskeleton to focal adhesion sites on the basal side of the cell, implying that cell–matrix interactions may be pivotal in the detection process (Figure 3.3). The dramatic realignment of filamentous actin (F-actin) stress fibres (Figure 3.4) which occurs 12–15 h after the onset of increased shear implicates cytoskeletal proteins as the principal force transmission structure of endothelial cells. In the presence of low shear, the intermediate filament, F-actin, is predominantly located in the periphery of the cell, particularly at cell–cell junctions where it is thought to play a role in cell permeability. In the presence of higher shear long, thicker strands of F-actin are observed centrally in association with elongation of the cell in the direction of flow (Davies, 1995; Noria et al., 1999). Most studies investigating realignment of the cytoskeleton in response to flow have been limited by the need to fix the cells for immunohistochemical procedures after exposure to flow (Galbraith et al., 1998; Noria et al., 1999) and have generally only shown

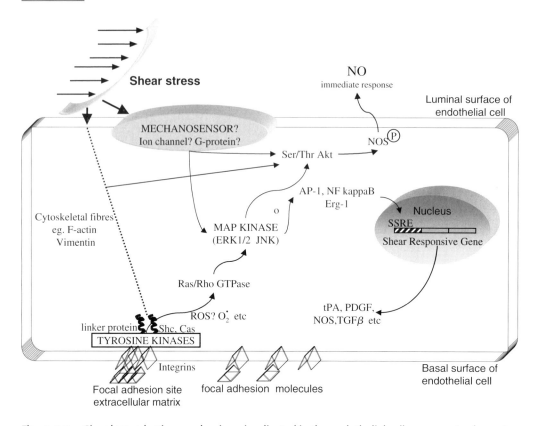

Figure 3.3   Signal transduction mechanisms implicated in the endothelial cell response to shear stress. Mechanisms for the mechanotransduction pathways in the endothelial cell. The cytoskeleton plays an important role in the transmission of the force stimulus. MAP-kinase, mitogen-activated protein kinase; Erg-1, early response-1; NFκB, Nuclear factor κB; Ser/thr Akt, serine/threonine protein kinase Akt; NOS-III, nitric oxide synthase III; PDGF, platelet derived growth factor; SSRE, shear stress response element; TGFβ, transforming growth factor β; ROS, reactive oxygen species; Shc, Cas adaptor proteins.

alterations in the cytoskeleton after prolonged exposure to shear. Recently the use of green fluorescent proteins (GFPs) has enabled the direct visualization of spatiotemporal dynamics in living cells. Helmke et al. (2000) have used a GFP-vimentin fusion protein to evaluate changes in position of this intermediate filament in response to shear stress. Their study revealed a very rapid regional displacement of vimentin filaments in response to flow, which indicates that the cytoskeleton may mediate acute as well as prolonged responses to flow. It was of interest that the cell nucleus (no flow and flow) was surrounded by a clear ring of vimentin filaments which might possibly link with the nuclear laminar, and the authors speculated that transmisssion of flow responses to the nucleus might occur via these thin filaments.

Cell morphology   F-actin

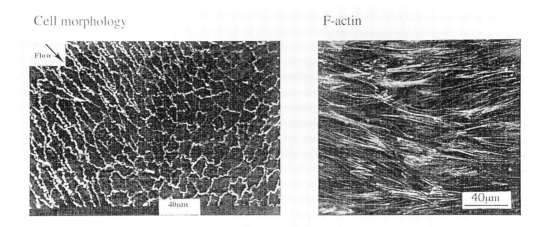

Figure 3.4   Left. Outlines of endothelial cells in primate thoracic aorta adjacent to an intercostal branch artery. A region of predicted flow separation is shown in which the shapes of the cells change abruptly from elongated to polygonal. The polygonal morphology is believed to be caused by flow separation and vortices that subject the endothelial surface to shear stress in several different directions during the cardiac cycle. The adjacent cells are subjected to markedly different shear stress profiles. The gradients of shear stress are steepest on cells located at the edge of the flow separation region. Scanning electron micrograph after silver staining. From Davies, 1995 with permission. Right. F actin stress fibre distribution in confluent endothelial cells. Flow from left to right of section. From Davies et al., 1993, with permission.

The role of focal adhesion sites is implied by their remodelling, which occurs in response to flow. This has been observed in elegant experiments in which focal adhesion sites have been 'visualized' using tandem scanning confocal image analysis in cultured endothelial cells (Davies et al., 1994). Focal adhesion sites are rich in β-integrins. The integrin family are transmembrane proteins that span the plasma membrane and bind to extracellular adhesion proteins, connecting to the cytoskeleton via linker proteins on the inside of the cell (Figure 3.3). The importance of the integrins in mechanotransduction was strengthened by the observation that a synthetic integrin 'inhibiting' peptide prevented flow-mediated dilatation of coronary arterioles, as did a β-integrin antibody (Muller et al., 1997). The method by which flow, integrins and cellular responses are interrelated has yet to be fully elucidated, although certain elements of the pathway have been identified (Davies, 1995), particularly the tyrosine kinases (Corson et al., 1996; Muller et al., 1997). Tyrosine kinases (and therefore tyrosine phosphorylation) play an important role in many signal transduction pathways, leading to a myriad of responses, in turn mediated through a complex network of signalling molecules. Many of these signalling molecules are expressed in response to shear in cultured endothelial cells. Those implicated include the Rho and Ras family of guanosine triphos-phatase (GTPase) and the mitogen-activated protein (MAP) kinase family (Tseng et al., 1995) particularly the stress-activated protein kinase, c-Jun NH(2)-terminal kinase (JNK) (Go et al 1999) and the extracellular signal-regulated kinases (ERKs) (Takahashi and Berk, 1996). Flow-mediated activation of integrins has been shown to be associated with phosphorylation of focal adhesion kinase (FAK, a 125 kDa tyrosine kinase). One proposal suggests that activation of this tyrosine kinase leads to recruitment and activation of other protein kinases which in turn phosphorylate the focal adhesion molecule protein, paxillin. Paxillin changes its alignment in response to flow, suggesting a probable role in mechanotransduction (Davies, 1995). More details are now emerging of the intricacies of the signalling network. A recent report (Chen et al., 1999) has suggested an important role for the adaptor protein Shc in the mediation of the tyrosine kinase responses. Shc has recently been recognized to be an intrinsic component in the coupling of tyrosine kinases to the Ras/MAP kinase pathway. Shear was found to induce the association of Shc with $\alpha_v\beta_3$ integrin in endothelial cells and introduction of a plasmid containing a Shc mutant led to failure of shear-mediated expression of ERKs. The same group (Li et al., 1999) have implicated the Rho, a small GTPase in the cytoskeletal reorganization, by showing that mutants of Rho prevent the flow-induced alignment of cellular stress fibres. Another group has suggested involve-ment of the Ras-related small GTP-binding protein, Rac1 (Yeh et al., 1999). Additionally, Okuda et al. (1999) have proposed that Cas, an adaptor protein associated with focal adhesion sites and important in actin filament assembly, is rapidly phosphorylated by flow through a tyrosine kinase and is likely to play an important role in downstream signalling.

In common with several other cell-signalling pathways, activation of some shear-mediated events in endothelial cells is dependent upon local synthesis of reactive oxygen species (ROS). Thus, NO and nitric superoxide, which together form peroxynitrite, are required for activation of JNK in cultured endothelial cells in response to flow, and the addition of peroxynitrite stimulates JNK (Go et al., 1999). Therefore – and remarkably so, because it is more frequently associated with ROS-induced cell dysfunction – peroxynitrite may act as a flow-signalling molecule. Yeh et al. (1999) have similarly suggested a dependence on ROS of the Rac1-mediated phosphorylation of MAP kinase in response to flow.

The shear-mediated activation of the MAP kinase, ERK, is dependent upon the presence of cholesterol in the plasma membrane. Caveolae are microdomains in the plasma membrane-rich in cholesterol, caveolin and signalling molecules. Park et al. (2000), investigating the possibility that the caveoli might be influential in mechanotransduction-cultured endothelial cells, found that antibodies which bind to the scaffolding and oligomerization domains of the caveolin molecule (and therefore the site likely to be influential in the interaction of caveoli with signalling molecules) led to reversal of flow-mediated ERK activation.

G proteins as mechanosensors

The cell membrane-associated G proteins have also been implicated as mechanosensors in the response to flow, but whether G protein activation is secondary to deformation of the cytoskeleton or to activation of hitherto unidentified luminal membrane receptors is unknown. Recently it has been proposed that G protein activation could be achieved through shear-mediated alteration in membrane fluidity (Haidekker et al., 2000). Originally, a role for G proteins was inferred because it was found that intracellular messengers associated with G protein-dependent pathways were also generated in response to flow. These included inositol triphosphate (IP_3), diacylglycerol (DAG), protein kinase C (PKC) and a rise in cell calcium. Involvement of the G_i subtype of G proteins was suggested by the observation in some, but not all, experiments of the pertussis toxin sensitivity of NO release (Ohno et al., 1993) and PGI_2 release (Berthiaume and Frangos 1992). Later studies showed directly that increases in expression of the G protein subunits $G_{\alpha q/\alpha 11}$ and $G_{\alpha i3/\alpha o}$ occur in response to flow (Gudi et al., 1996). MAP kinase activation in response to flow may also be mediated through PKC (Ishida et al., 1996). Therefore, if the G proteins are important mechanosensors, distinct from the cytoskeletal system of detection, then at least one of the signalling pathways (the MAP kinases) may be common to both detector mechanisms.

Ion channels as mechanosensors

Shear stress evokes an immediate increase in current through endothelial cell potassium channels (Nakache and Gaub, 1988; Cooke et al., 1991), one of the fastest recorded responses to shear stress. The immediacy of the response has led some to suggest that K channels may be effective mechanosensors. The exact trigger is unknown but could result from direct displacement of the luminal channel protein by shear stress or as a secondary response to stimulation of another mechanoreceptor, e.g. a G protein. Opening of potassium channels leads to hyperpolarization, but this is short-lived, probably because of the simultaneous yet unrelated opening of chloride channels, recently reported by Barakat et al. (1999). Chloride channel opening leads to depolarization and therefore counteracts the K channel-associated hyperpolarization. Sodium channels have also been implicated in shear-mediated responses. Traub et al. (1999) have suggested a tonic inhibition of flow-mediated MAP kinase (ERK) stimulation by sodium channels, since shear-mediated ERK1/2 stimulation was enhanced by addition of the sodium channel inhibitor, tetrodotoxin.

Hyperpolarization in endothelial cells leads to an increase in cell calcium and the transient rise in cell calcium reported in response to shear (Schwarz et al., 1992; Shen et al., 1992; Corson et al., 1996) is considered to result from the hyperpolarization associated with increased K channel opening. A rise in endothelial cell calcium is a potent stimulus to activation of NOS-III (Luckhoff and Busse, 1990) and was originally considered to be the reason for increased NO release. However, it is now widely appreciated that the maintained flow-induced NO-mediated relaxation in endothelial cells is largely calcium-independent (Ayajiki et al., 1996). This calcium independence of NOS synthesis was a novel and intriguing observation when first reported. Calcium-independent NO release is now known to be associated with phosphorylation of NOS (Corson et al., 1996), recently proposed to involve the serine/threonine protein kinase Akt, which phosphorylates the NOS molecule at the ser 1177 residue (Dimmeler et al., 1999). Since experimentally induced serine phosphorylation of NOS confers calcium independence on the activity of the enzyme (Dimmeler et al., 1999; Fisslthaler et al., 2000), this would seem to be the likely mechanism underlying the rapid effect of flow on NO synthesis. Additionally, heat shock protein 90 (hsp90) is thought to play a facilitatory or coordinating role in this acute NO response as hsp90 rapidly associates with NOS-III when shear is applied to cultured endothelial cells (Garcia-Cardena et al., 1998).

Shear stress-sensitive gene expression

As outlined above, the mechanotransduction pathways in response to shear are rapidly being elucidated, and it is apparent that a complex network of cell-signalling pathways contributes to a wide range of functional responses. As detailed above, the immediate 'nongenomic' stimulation of NO is the classic acute response, and other vasoactive agonists such as adenosine triphosphate (ATP) and substance P are also rapidly released in response to flow. Sustained flow, however, leads to a host of responses resulting from altered gene expression. The first gene implicated was the tissue plasminogen activator (tPA) gene, as tPA mRNA expression was found to be upregulated when cultured endothelial cells were exposed to laminar shear stress (Diamond et al., 1990).

The mechanism of upregulation of tPA mRNA and many other 'shear-responsive' genes is now broadly understood. Shear stress, through activation of the mechanosensitive tyrosine kinase and MAP kinase pathways, leads to activation of a number of transcription factors which include the early growth response genes early growth response-1 (Egr-1), AP-1 (composed of c-*jun*/c-*jun* and c-*jun*/c-*fos* dimers) and nuclear factor κB (NF-κB) (Chien et al., 1998). These are responsible for the subsequent upregulation of many endothelial cell genes, probably achieved in the majority by binding to a shear stress response element (SSRE) on the promoter region of the susceptible gene (e.g. Khachigian et al., 1995). The SSRE was first identified in the platelet-derived growth factor B (PDGF-B) gene and was found to be a 6 base pair stretch with the sequence GAGACC (Resnick and Gimbrone, 1995). This sequence is now known to be common to many other endothelial shear-sensitive genes, including NOS-III, tPA, transforming growth factor β_1 (TGF-β1), c-fos and intercellular cell adhesion molecule (ICAM-1). However, this SSRE does not explain all flow-mediated de novo protein synthesis. Some genes have an apparently functionless GAGACC sequence, e.g. monocyte chemotactic protein-1 (MCP-1), and others are responsive to shear in the absence of this sequence, e.g. PDGF-A (Resnick and Gimbrone, 1995). This and other genes possess different SSREs, e.g. the MCP-1 gene has a shear stress element with the sequence TGACTCC which is critical for shear responses, and which is a divergent TRE (phorbol ester tissue 12-O-tetradecanoylphorbol 13 acetate-responsive element), the site which binds AP-1 (Chien et al., 1998). Other recognized shear-responsive sites are the Sp1 site on the promoter region of the tissue factor (TF) gene and the Erg-1 site on the PDGF-A gene (Chien et al., 1998).

NOS-III is one of the many genes now recognized to be upregulated by shear (Uematsu et al., 1995), and NO itself may act as an intermediate second messenger in other flow-sensitive pathways. For example, NO has been implicated as a potential inhibitor of growth through negative modulation of Egr-1, a promoter of the expression of the growth factor PDGF-A (Chiu et al., 1999). Indeed, shear modulates the expression of a number of growth factors, including both PDGF-A, PDGF-B and TGF-β_1). Shear also affects expression of angiotensin-converting enzyme (ACE) (Gosgnach et al., 2000), possibly relevant to growth and remodelling through angiotensin II. Expression of some molecules shows a biphasic response to shear stress, with higher expression at low flow rates (e.g. ET-1) and others show the greater responses at very high rates of shear (30 dyn/cm^2), e.g. the heat shock protein HSP60 (Hochleitner et al., 2000), implicated as an autoantigen involved in atherogenesis. An increasing literature shows that very different responses are observed in response to steady shear when compared with turbulent or abrupt onset of shear, and many of the original observations on gene expression have been revisited with the knowledge that temporal gradients may have profound effects on endothelial cell gene expression. These will be discussed in relation to the origins of atherosclerosis (see below). None the less, it is reasonable to summarize that, at steady flow, with physiological rates of shear, the expression of endothelial genes favours an antithrombotic, antiproliferative and anti-antherogenic phenotype (for reviews, see Davies, 1995; Resnick and Gimbrone, 1995; Chien et al., 1998; Traub and Berk, 1998).

Vascular permeability and hydraulic conductivity in response to shear

Increments in shear stress are now recognized to have important effects on the ion permeability of the vasculature. Increasing shear in perfused microvessels from the mesenteric circulation of the frog leads to an increase in potassium permeability, independent of NO and prostanoids, and inversely related to cellular cyclic adenosine monophosphate (cAMP: Kajimura and Michel, 1999). Disturbances of barrier function to larger molecules and to fluid have also been reported in response to shear. Cultured endothelial cells exposed to disturbed flow or to high flow rates demonstrate increased permeability to dextran (molecular weight 70 000: Phelps and DePaola, 2000) and an NO-dependent increase in hydraulic conductivity (Lp) of bovine aortic endothelial cells in response to shear has been reported (Chang et al., 2000). The proteins which contribute to cell–cell connections and so to integrity of the endothelial barrier have also been studied. Noria et al. (1999) have shown dramatic effects of shear stress on a group of proteins which mediate cell–cell adhesion. Several of the proteins (e.g. vascular endothelial-cadherin) which form the adherens junction were evenly distributed around the cell in static conditions but were shown to be disassembled by shear stress. The resultant adherens 'plaques' were seen to colocalize with the ends of the F-actin fibres. Others (DePaola et al., 1999) have investigated the effect of shear on regulation of the gap junction protein connexin 43 (Cx43). Cells exposed to laminar flow demonstrated a transient increase in Cx43 expression, whereas in cells exposed to disturbed flow Cx43 expression was persistently elevated. The altered Cx43 expression was reflected in sustained inhibition of cell–cell communication as assessed by dye transfer. These and many more observations highlight the differences emerging in responses to laminar and disturbed flow. As detailed below, these may have implications in the origins of atherosclerosis.

Flow, vascular remodelling and atherosclerosis

Arteries develop structural reorganization in response to flow. The most obvious example is the alignment and elongation of the endothelial cells in the direction of flow (Flaherty et al., 1972). The rearrangement may not only be involved in mechanosignal transduction, as discussed above, but the associated adhesion to components of the extracellular matrix would also confer stability on the cell (Davies, 1995).

If increased flow is maintained for any length of time, arteries become permanently dilated. This is a result of structural modification associated with an increase in lumen diameter and a greater medial cross-sectional area (Zarins et al., 1987). Flow-induced structural changes occur in several physiological and pathophysiological situations (for review, see Langille, 1995). Shear stress may play an important role in the remodelling which occurs in the uterine vascular bed during the menstrual cycle and in many different vascular beds during pregnancy, although the relative contribution of haemodynamic and hormonal influences is not known. Elegant experiments in chick embryos (Rychter, 1962) have shown the importance of flow in the normal development of the aortic arch. Furthermore, the abrupt changes in blood flow which occur in some vascular beds at the time of birth may have profound influences on vessel development. This is suggested by the strong correlation with blood flow and vessel growth observed in the weeks following birth (Langille et al., 1991).

The relationship between shear stress, vascular restructuring and/or growth has led to speculation of an association between shear and the formation of atherosclerotic lesions. The distribution of shear in the aorta, carotid and femoral arteries is, however, complex. The shear at any given point is influenced by many factors, such as the vessel size, wall elasticity, curvature, local geometry and branching. Separations of the flow 'streamlines' at branches, bifurcations and points of curvature lead to regions of disturbed flow, complicated by the imposition of the cardiac cycle. Rapidly changing gradients of shear will occur and the turbulent flow is, on average, associated with lower levels of shear stress. These spatially defined flow patterns are postulated to give rise to the focal origins of atherosclerosis by creating focused groups of endothelial cells in which differential protein expression leads to a proatherosclerotic phenotype.

Endothelial cell heterogeneity through the vascular tree was first recognized by Wright (1972), who recognized that there were more mitotic areas of endothelial cells at points of curvature and near branches. There is also good evidence for an association between low levels of shear stress and focal areas of disease. Intimal thickening in human arteries is greater in areas of low shear (Friedman et al., 1986) and, in a pig model of atherosclerosis (Gerrity et al., 1985), focal areas of disease have been associated with nonaligned endothelial cells (indicative of low shear). Substantial reductions in flow rates have also been shown to stimulate remodelling of the carotid artery of immature rabbits (Cho et al., 1997) and to promote hypertrophy in carotid arteries of hypertensive but not normotensive rats (Ueno et al., 2000). Studies in cultured cells have now shown clearly that turbulent flow (with an average low shear rate) stimulates increases in cell cycle entry (Davies et al., 1986; Tardy et al., 1997) and that steady flow suppresses G_0–G_1 phase transition (Levesque et al., 1990; Akimoto et al., 2000). The mechanisms by which steady flow suppresses growth are now under scrutiny. Akimoto et al. have recently proposed that flow induces the synthesis of the cyclin-dependent kinase (cdk) inhibitor, p21[Sdil/Cip1/Waf1]. The role of cdks in G_1–S transition in other cell types is well established. These kinases promote G_1–S transition through phosphorylation of retinoblastoma protein (pRb). Whether this cdk inhibitor is directly upregulated by shear or increases in response to another shear stress sensory pathway remains to be determined, although it is highly relevant that NO increases expression of p21$^{Sdil/Cip1/Waf1}$, causing inhibition of S-phase transition (Ishida et al., 1997). An important role for NO is also emphasized in the well recognized property of this radical as an inhibitor of smooth muscle proliferation and migration and by the recent implication of reduced NOS activity in low-flow hypertrophy (Ueno et al., 2000). Others have shown increased rates of apoptosis at low flow rates (Cho et al., 1997; Tardy et al., 1997; Ueno et al., 2000) and have proposed that this process may contribute to vascular remodelling.

Many laboratories have now turned their attention to different patterns of flow (Davies et al., 1997). Various methods have been employed to apply different forms of shear stress to endothelial cells by generating laminar flow, laminar pulsatile flow and turbulent flow. Pulsatile flow seems to have similar effects to those of laminar flow. Responses of endothelial genes to laminar flow is generally a function of the magnitude of the shear stimulus. Turbulent flow induces endothelin-1, PDGF-B, basic fibroblast growth factor and thrombomodulin (for review, see Chien et al., 1998). Nagel et al. (1999) have recently reported that the transcription factors NF-κB, Erg-1, c-*jun* and c-*fos* respond differentially to laminar and disturbed shear patterns; expression is always greater with disturbed shear. Similarly, Bao et al. (1999) have shown that MCP-1 and PDGF-A expression is greatly increased in cells exposed to 'step flow' and 'impulse' flow, i.e. to cells exposed to rapid changes in gradient, but that laminar flow depressed expression of these potentially atherogenic factors. Additionally, laminar flow induces a sustained increase in antiatherogenic factors through induction of NOS, cyclooxygenase-2 and Mn superoxide dismutase (Chien et al., 1998).

The failure of therapeutic angioplasty procedures is frequently due to subsequent intimal proliferation and changes in shear stress may play a role. In a rat model of carotid artery angioplasty, in which vascular damage was induced by balloon catheter injury, increasing the blood flow (and therefore the shear stress) was found to reduce early neointimal proliferation (Kohler and Jaiwien, 1992). Another practical application of shear responses was recently reported by a group from Johns Hopkins University which showed that polyurethane vascular grafts seeded with endothelial cells, and exposed to high shear rates before implantation in rats, showed a considerable reduction of neonintimal thickness when compared with grafts not exposed to shear (Dardik et al., 1999). In light of the likely role of PDGFs in flow-mediated neointimal proliferation, another group has investigated whether inhibition of PDGF receptors might reduce neointimal thickening in polytetafluoroethylene grafts implanted in baboons (Davies et al., 2000). Antibodies to both α and β PDGF receptors were given intravenously and it was found that inhibition of the PDGF β receptor, but not the α receptor, was effective in reducing neointimal formation in grafts subjected to high shear rates. These and other practical approaches are exciting developments which may lead to important advances in clinical management.

Conclusion

Despite the recognition more than 60 years ago that flow was an important modulator of vascular tone, it has only been in the last decade that the extent and physiological importance of flow-mediated responses have been appreciated. The flow-mediated release of potent vasodilators in response to shear stress suggests that flow tonically reduces the blood pressure. Furthermore, we are now beginning to appreciate the complexity of the underlying pathways involved in the transduction of the flow signal to cellular responses. The role played by spatial and temporal gradients of flow in endothelial cell gene expression is likely to offer considerable insight into mechanisms of atherosclerosis. In the clinical setting, it is becoming increasingly apparent that abnormal responses to flow or abnormal flow patterns within arteries may contribute to cardiovascular dysfunction. A more detailed understanding of the physical and biochemical events underlying flow-mediated responses is likely to have an important role to play in the prevention and treatment of cardiovascular disease.

REFERENCES

Akimoto, S., Mitsumata, M., Sasaguri, T. & Yoshida, Y. (2000). Laminar shear stress inhibits cell proliferation by inducing cyclin-dependent kinase inhibitor p21 (Sdi1/Cip1/Waf1). *Circ. Res.*, **86**, 185–90.

Ayajiki, K., Kindermann, M., Hecker, M., Fleming, I. & Busse, R. (1996). Intracellular pH and tyrosine phosphorylation but not calcium determine shear stress-induced nitric oxide production in native endothelial cells. *Circ. Res.*, **78**, 750–8.

Bao, X., Luc, C. & Frangos, J.A. (1999). Temporal gradient in shear but not steady shear stress induces PDGF-A and MCP-1 expression in endothelial cells. *Arterioscl., Thromb. Vasc. Biol.*, **19**, 996–1003.

Barakat, A.I., Leaver, E.E., Pappone, P.A. & Davies, P.F. (1999). A flow activated chloride-selective membrane current in vascular endothelial cells. *Circ. Res.*, **85**, 820–8.

Berthiaume, F. & Frangos, J.A. (1992). Flow-induced prostacyclin production is mediated by a pertussis toxin-sensitive G protein. *FEBS Lett.*, **308**, 277–9.

Bevan, J.A., Joyce, E,H. & Wellman, G.C. (1988). Flow-dependent dilation in a resistance artery still occurs after endothelium removal. *Circ. Res.*, **63**, 980–5.

Bush, D.E., Jones, C.E., Bass, K.M. et al. (1998) Estrogen replacement reverses endothelial dysfunction in post-menopausal women. *Am. J. Med.*, **104**, 552–8.

Busse, R. & Fleming, I. (1998). Pulsatile stretch and shear stress: physical stimuli determining the production of endothelium-derived relaxing factors. *J. Vasc. Res.*, **35**, 73–84.

Celermajer, D.S., Sorenson, K.E., Gooch, V.M. et al. (1992). Non-invasive detection of endothelial dysfunction in children and adults at risk of atherosclerosis. *Lancet*, **340**, 1111–15.

Celermajer, D.S., Adams, M.R., Clarkson, P. et al. (1996). Passive smoking and impaired endothelium-dependent arterial dilatation in healthy young adults. *N. Engl. J. Med.*, **334**, 150–4.

Chang, Y.S., Yaccino, J.A., Lakshimarayanan, S., Frangos, J.A. & Tarbell, J.M. (2000). Shear-induced increase in hydraulic conductivity in endothelial cells is mediated by a nitric oxide dependent mechanism. *Arterioscl. Thromb. Vasc. Biol.*, **20**, 35–42.

Chen, K.D., Li, Y.S., Kim, M. et al. (1999). Mechanotransduction in response to shear stress. Roles of receptor tyrosine kinases, integrins, and Shc. *J. Biol. Chem.*, **274**, 18393–400.

Chien, S., Song, L. & Shyy, J.Y-J. (1998). Effects of mechanical forces on signal transduction and gene expression in endothelial cells. *Hypertension*, **31**, 162–9.

Chiu, J.J., Wung, B.S., Hsieh, H.J., Low, L.W. & Wang, D.L. (1999). Nitric oxide regulates shear stress-induced early growth response-1. Expression via the extracellular signal-regulated kinase pathway in endothelial cells. *Circ. Res.*, **85**, 238–46.

Cho, A., Mitchell, L., Koopmans, D. & Langille, B.L. (1997). Effects of changes in blood flow rate on cell death and cell proliferation in carotid arteries of immature rabbits. *Circ. Res.*, **81**, 328–37.

Cockell, A.P. & Poston, L. (1996). Isolated mesenteric arteries from pregnant rats show enhanced flow-mediated relaxation but normal myogenic tone. *J. Physiol.*, **495**, 545–51.

Cockell, A.P. & Poston, L. (1997). Flow mediated vasodilatation is enhanced in normal pregnancy but reduced in pre-eclampsia. *Hypertension*, **30**, 247–51.

Cooke, J.P., Stamler, J., Andon, N.A. et al. (1990). Flow stimulates endothelial cells to release a nitrovasodilator that is potentiated by reduced thiol. *Am. J. Physiol.*, **259**, H804–12.

Cooke, J.P., Rossitch, E., Andon, N.A., Loscalzo, J. & Dzau V.J. (1991). Flow activates an endothelial potassium channel to release an endogenous nitrovasodilator. *J. Clin. Invest.*, **88**, 1663–71.

Corson, M.A., James, N.L., Latta, S.E. et al. (1996). Phosphorylation of endothelial nitric oxide synthase in response to fluid shear stress. *Circ. Res.*, **79**, 984–91.

Cuevas, A.M., Guasch, V. & Castillo, O. (2000). A high-fat diet induces and red wine counteracts endothelial dysfunction in human volunteers. *Lipids*, **35**, 143–8.

Dardik, A., Liu, A. & Ballermann, B.J. (1999). Chronic in vitro shear stress stimulates endothelial cell retention on prosthetic grafts and reduces subsequent in vivo neointimal thickness. *J. Vasc. Surg.*, **29**, 157–67.

Davies, P.F. (1995). Flow-mediated endothelial mechanotransduction. *Physiol. Rev.*, **75**, 519–60.

Davies, P.F., Remuzzi, A., Dewey, C.F. & Gordon, M.A. (1986). Turbulent shear stress induces vascular endothelial cell turnover in vitro. *Proc. Nat. Acad. Sci. USA*, **83**, 2114–18.

Davies, P.F, Robotewskyj, A. & Griem, M.L. (1993). Endothelial cell adhesion in real time. Measurements in vitro by tandem scanning confocal image and analysis. *J. Clin. Invest.*, **91**, 2649–52.

Davies, P.F, Robotewskyj, A. & Griem, M.L. (1994). Quantitative studies of endothelial cell adhesion: directional remodelling of focal adhesion sites in response to flow forces. *J. Clin. Invest.*, **93**, 2031–8.

Davies, P.F., Barbee, K.A., Volin, M.V. et al. (1997). Spatial relationships in early signalling events of flow-mediated endothelial mechanotransduction. *Annu. Rev. Physiol.*, **59**, 527–49.

Davies, M.G., Owens, E.L. Mason, D.P. et al. (2000). Effect of platelet-derived growth factor receptor-alpha and-beta blockade on flow-induced neointimal formation in endothelialized baboon vascular grafts. *Circ. Res.*, **86**, 779–86.

DePaola, N., Davies, P.F., Pritchard, W.F., Florez, L. & Polacek, D.C. (1999). Spatial and temporal regulation of gap junction connexin43 in vascular endothelial cells exposed to controlled disturbed flows in vitro. *Proc. Nat. Acad. Sci. USA*, **96**, 3154–9.

Diamond, S.L., Sharefkin, J.B, Dieffenbach, C. et al. (1990). Tissue plasminogen activator messenger RNA levels increase in cultured human endothelial cells exposed to laminar shear stress. *J. Cell Physiol.*, **143**, 364–71.

Dimmeler, S., Fleming, I., Fisslthaler, B. et al. (1999). Activation of nitric oxide synthase in endothelial cells by Akt-dependent phosphorylation. *Nature*, **399**, 601–5.

Fisslthaler, B., Dimmeler, S., Hermann, C., Busse, R. & Fleming, I. (2000). Phosphorylation and activation of endothelial nitric oxide synthase by fluid shear stress. *Acta Physiol. Scand.*, **168**, 81–8.

Flaherty, J.J., Pierce, J.E, Ferrans, V.J. et al. (1972). Endothelial nuclear patterns in the canine arterial tree with particular reference to hemodynamic events. *Circ. Res.*, **30**, 23–33.

Friedman, M.H., Peters, O.J., Bargeron, C.B., Hutchins, G.M. & Mark, F.F. (1986). Shear-dependent thickening of the human arterial intima. *Atherosclerosis*, **60**, 161–71.

Galbraith, C.G., Skalak, R. & Chien, S. (1998) Shear stress induces spatial reorganization of the endothelial cell cytoskeleton. *Cell Motil. Cytoskeleton*, **40**, 317–30.

Garcia-Cardena, G., Fan, R., Shah, V. et al. (1998). Dynamic activation of endothelial nitric oxide synthase by HSP90. *Nature*, **392**, 821–4.

Gerrity, R.V., Goss, J.A. & Soby, L. (1985). Control of monocyte recruitment by chemotactic factors in lesion prone areas of swine aorta. *Atherosclerosis*, **5**, 55–66.

Go, Y.M., Patel, R.P., Maland, M.C. et al. (1999). Evidence for peroxynitrite as a signaling molecule in flow-dependent activation of c-Jun NH(2)-terminal kinase. *Am. J. Physiol.*, **277**, H1647–53.

Goodfellow, J., Ramsey, M.W., Luddington, L.A. et al. (1996). Endothelium and inelastic arteries: an early marker of vascular dysfunction in non-insulin dependent diabetes. *Br. Med. J.*, **312**, 744–5.

Goodfellow, J., Bellamy, M.F., Ramsey, M.W., Jones, C.J. & Lewis, M.J. (2000). Dietary supplementation with marine omega-3 fatty acids improve systemic large artery endothelial function in subjects with hypercholesterolaemia. *J. Am. Coll. Cardiol.*, **35**, 265–70.

Gosgnach, W., Challah, M., Coulet, F., Michel, J.B. & Battle, T. (2000). Shear stress induces angiotensin converting enzyme expression in cultured smooth muscle cells; possible involvement of bFGF. *Cardiovasc. Res.*, **45**, 486–92.

Griffith, T.M. & Edwards, D.H. (1990). Myogenic autoregulation of flow may be inversely related to endothelium-derived relaxing factor activity. *Am. J. Physiol.*, **258**, H1171–80.

Gudi, S.R.P., Clark., C.B. & Frangos, J.A. (1996). Fluid flow rapidly activates G proteins in human endothelial cells: involvement of G proteins in mechanotransduction. *Circ. Res.*, **79**, 834–9.

Haidekker, M.A., L'Heureux, N. & Frangos, J.A. (2000). Fluid shear stress increases membrane fluidity in endothelial cells: a study with DCVJ fluorescence. *Am. J. Physiol.*, **278**, H1401–6.

Hecker, M., Mülsch, A., Bassenge, E. & Busse, R. (1993). Vasoconstriction and increased flow: two principal mechanisms of shear stress-dependent endothelial autocoid release. *Am. J. Physiol.*, **265**, H828–33.

Helmke, B.P., Goldman, R.D. & Davies, P.E. (2000). Rapid displacement of vimentin intermediate filaments in living endothelial cells exposed to flow. *Circ. Res.*, **86**, 745–52.

Hochleitner, B.W., Hochleitner E.O., Obrist P. et al. (2000). Fluid shear stress induces heat shock protein 60 expression in endothelial cells in vitro and in vivo. *Arterioscl. Thromb. Vasc. Biol.*, **20**, 617–23.

Huang, A., Sun, D., Koller, A. & Kaley, G. (1998). Gender differences in flow-induced dilation and regulation of shear stress: role of estrogen and nitric oxide. *Am. J. Physiol.*, **275**, R1571–7.

Huang, A., Sun, D., Koller, A. & Kaley, G. (2000). 17beta estradiol restores endothelial nitric oxide release to shear stress in arterioles of male hypertensive rats. *Circulation*, **101**, 94–100.

Ishida, T., Peterson, T.E, Kovach, N.L. & Berk, B.C. (1996). MAP kinase activation by flow in endothelial cells. *Circ. Res.*, **79**, 310–16.

Ishida, A., Sasaguri, T., Kosaka, C., Nojima, H. & Ogata, J. (1997). Induction of the cyclin-dependent kinase inhibitor p21 [Sdi1/Cip1/Waf1] by nitric oxide-generating vasodilator in vascular smooth muscle cells. *J. Biol. Chem.*, **272**, 10050–7.

Izzard, A.S. & Heagerty, A.M. (1999). Impaired flow-dependent dilatation in distal mesenteric arteries from the spontaneously hypertensive rat. *J. Physiol.*, **518**, 239–45.

Kajimura, M. & Michel, C.C. (1999). Inhibition of effects of flow on potassium permeability in single perfused frog mesenteric capillaries. *J. Physiol.*, **516**, 201–7.

Khachigian, L.M., Resnick, N., Gimbrone, M.A. & Collins, T. (1995). Nuclear factor -κB interacts functionally with the PDGF-B chain shear-stress-response-element in vascular endothelial cells exposed to shear stress. *J. Clin. Invest.*, **96**, 1169–75.

Koh, K.K., Cardillo, C., Bui, M.N. et al. (1999). Vascular effects of estrogen and cholesterol-lowering therapies in hypercholesterolaemic postmenopausal women. *Circulation*, **99**, 354–60.

Kohler, T.R. & Jaiwien, A. (1992). Flow affects development of intimal hyperplasia after arterial injury in rats. *Arterioscl. Thromb.*, **12**, 963–71.

Koller, A. & Huang, A. (1994). Impaired nitric oxide-mediated flow-induced dilation in arterioles of spontaneously hypertensive rats. *Circ. Res.*, **74**, 416–21.

Koller, A. & Kaley, G. (1991). Endothelial regulation of wall shear stress and blood flow in skeletal muscle microcirculation. *Am. J. Physiol.*, **260**, H862–8.

Koller, A., Sun, D. & Kaley, G. (1993). Role of shear stress and endothelial prostaglandins in flow- and viscosity-induced dilatation of arterioles in vitro. *Circ. Res.*, **72**, 1276–84.

Koller, A., Sun, D., Huang, A. & Kaley, G. (1994). Corelease of nitric oxide and prostaglandins mediates flow-dependent dilation of rat gracilis muscle arterioles. *Am. J. Physiol.*, **267**, H326–32.

Kublickiene, K.R., Cockell, A.P. & Poston, L. (1997) Role of nitric oxide in the regulation of vascular tone in pressurized and perfused resistance myometrial arteries from term pregnant women. *Am. J. Obstet. Gynecol.*, **177**, 1263–9.

Kuo, L., Davis, M.J., Cannon, M.S. & Chilian, W.M. (1992). Pathophysiological consequences of atherosclerosis extend into the coronary microcirculation. Restoration of endothelium-dependent responses by L-arginine. *Circ. Res.*, **70**, 465–76.

Langille, B.L. (1995). Blood flow-induced remodelling of the artery wall. In *Flow-dependent Regulation of Vascular Function*, ed. Bevan, J. Kaley, G. & Rubanyi, G., pp. 277–99. New York: Oxford University Press.

Langille, B.L., Brownlee, R.D. & Adamson, S.L. (1991). Perinatal aortic growth in lambs: relation to blood flow changes at birth. *Am. J. Physiol.*, **259**, H1247–53.

Learmont, J.G. & Poston, L. (1996). Nitric oxide is involved in flow-induced dilation of isolated human small fetoplacental arteries. *Am. J. Obstet. Gynecol.*, **174**, 583–8.

Leeson, C.P., Whincup, P.H., Cook, D.G. et al. (1997) Flow-mediated dilatation in 9–11-year-old children: the influence of intrauterine and childhood factors. *Circulation*, **96**, 2233–8.

Levesque, M.J., Nerem, R.M. & Sprague, E.A. (1990). Vascular endothelial cell proliferation in culture and the influences of flow. *Biomaterials*, **11**, 702–7.

Li, S., Chen, B.P., Azuma, N. et al. (1999). Distinct roles for the small GTPases CDs42 and Rho in endothelial cells. *J. Clin. Invest.*, **103**, 1141–50.

Lipowsky, H.L. (1995). Shear stress in the circulation. In *Flow-dependent Regulation of Vascular Function*, ed. Bevan, J., Kaley, G. & Rubanyi, G.M. New York: Oxford University Press.

Luckhoff, A. & Busse, R. (1990). Calcium influx into endothelial cells and formation of endothelium-derived relaxing factor is controlled by the membrane potential. *Pflugers Arch.*, **416**, 305–11.

Malek, A.M. & Izumo, S. (1994). Molecular aspects of signal transduction of shear stress in the endothelial cell. *J. Hypertens.*, **12**, 989–99.

Matrougui, K., Maclouf, J., Levy, B.I. & Henrion, D. (1997). Impaired nitric oxide- and prostaglandin-mediated responses to flow in resistance arteries of hypertensive rats. *Hypertension*, **30**, 942–7.

Meredith, I.T., Currie, K.E., Anderson, T.J. et al. (1996). Post-ischaemic vasodilation in human forearm is dependent on endothelium-derived nitric oxide. *Am. J. Physiol.*, **270**, H1435–40.

Miyazaki, H., Matsuoka, H., Itabe, H. et al. (2000). Hemodialysis impairs endothelial function via oxidative stress: effects of vitamin E-coated dialyzer. *Circulation*, **101**, 1002–6.

Muller, J.M., Chilian, W.M. & Davies, M.J. (1997). Integrin signaling transduces shear stress dependent vasodilatation of coronary arterioles. *Circ. Res.*, **80**, 320–6.

Nagel, T., Resnick, N., Dewey, C.F. & Gimbrone, M.A. (1999). Vascular endothelial cells respond to spatial gradients in fluid by enhanced activation of transcription factors. *Arteriosl. Thromb. Vasc. Biol.*, **19**, 1825–34.

Nakache, M. & Gaub, H.E. (1988). Hydrodynamic hyperpolarisation of endothelial cells. *Proc. Nat. Acad. Sci. USA*, **85**, 1841–1843.

Neunteufl, T., Preiglinger, U., Heher, S. et al. (2000). Effects of vitamin E on chronic and acute endothelial dysfunction in smokers. *J. Am. Coll. Cardiol.*, **35**, 277–83.

Noria, S., Cowan, D.C., Gotlieb, A.I. & Langille, B.L. (1999). Transient and steady state shear stress on endothelial cell adherens junctions. *Circ. Res.*, **85**, 504–14.

Noris, M., Morigi, M., Dondelli, R. et al. (1995). Nitric oxide synthesis by cultured endothelial cells is modulated by flow conditions. *Circ. Res.*, **76**, 536–43.

Ohno, M., Gibbons, G.H, Dzau, V.J. & Cooke, J.P. (1993). Shear stress elevates endothelial cGMP. Role of a potassium channel and G protein coupling. *Circulation*, **88**, 193–7.

Okuda, M., Takahashi, M., Suero, J. et al. (1999). Shear stress stimulation of p130 (cas) tyrosine phosphorylation requires calcium-dependent c-Src activation. *J. Biol. Chem.*, **274**, 26803–9.

Osanai, T., Fujite, N., Fujiwara, N. et al. (2000). Cross talk of shear-induced production of prostacyclin and nitric oxide in endothelial cells. *Am. J. Physiol.*, **278**, H233–8.

Park, H., Go, Y.M., Darji, R. et al. (2000). Caveolin-1 regulates shear stress-dependent activation of extracellular signal-regulated kinase. *Am. J. Physiol.*, **278**, H1285–93.

Phelps, J.E. & DePaola, N. (2000). Spatial variations in endothelial barrier function in disturbed flows in vitro. *Am. J. Physiol.*, **278**, H469–76.

Pohl, U., Holtz, J., Busse R. & Bassenge, E. (1986). Crucial role of endothelium in the vasodilator response to increased flow in vivo. *Hypertension*, **8**, 37–44.

Ranjan, V., Xiao, Z. & Diamond, S.L. (1995). Constitutive NOS expression in cultured endothelial cells is elevated by fluid shear stress. *Am. J. Physiol.*, **269**, H550–5.

Resnick, N. & Gimbrone, J.R. (1995). Hemodynamic forces are complex regulators of endothelial gene expression. *FASEB J*, **9**, 874–82.

Rubanyi, G.M., Romero, J.C. & Vanhoutte, P.M. (1986). Flow-induced release of endothelium-derived relaxing factor. *Am. J. Physiol.*, **250**, H1145–9.

Rychter, Z. (1962). Experimental morphology of the aortic arches and heart loop in chick embryos. *Adv. Morphol.*, **2**, 333.

Schretzenmayr, A. (1933). Uber kreislaufregulatorische vorgange an den großen arterien bei der muskelarbeit. *Pflugers Arch. Ges. Physiol.*, **232**, 743–8.

Schwarz, G., Callewaert, G., Droogmans, G. & Nilius, B. (1992). Shear stress-induced calcium transients in endothelial cells from human umbilical cord veins. *J. Physiol.*, **458**, 527–38.

Shen, J., Luscinskas, F.W., Connolly, A., Dewey, C.F. & Gimbrone, M.A. (1992). Fluid shear stress modulates cytosolic free calcium in vascular endothelial cells. *Am. J. Physiol.*, **262**, C384–90.

Smiesko, V., Lang, D.J. & Johnson, P.C. (1989). Dilator response of rat mesenteric arcading arterioles to increased blood flow velocity. *Am. J. Physiol.*, **257**, H1958–65.

Stein, J.H., Keevil, J.G., Wiebe, D.A., Aaeschilmann, S. & Folts, J.D. (1999). Purple grape juice improves endothelial function and reduces the susceptibility to LDL cholesterol to oxidation in patients with coronary artery disease. *Circulation*, **100**, 1050–5.

Sun, D., Huang, A., Smith, C.J. et al. (1999). Enhanced release of prostaglandins contributes to flow-induced arteriolar dilation in eNOS knockout mice. *Circ. Res.*, **85**, 288–93.

Takahashi, M. & Berk, B.C. (1996). Mitogen-activated protein-kinase (ERK1/2) activation by shear stress and adhesion in endothelial cells: essential role for a herbimycin-sensitive kinase. *J. Clin. Invest.*, **96**, 2623–31.

Takamura, Y., Shimokawa, H., Zhao, H. et al. (1999). Important role of endothelium derived hyperpolarizing factor in shear-stress induced endothelium-dependent relaxations in rat mesenteric artery. *J. Cardiovasc. Pharmacol.*, **34**, 381–7.

Tardy, Y., Resnick, N., Nagel, T., Gimbrone, M.A. & Dewey, C.F. (1997). Shear stress gradients remodel endothelial monolayers in vitro via a cell proliferation–migration–loss cycle. *Arterioscl. Thromb. Vasc. Biol.*, **17**, 3102–6.

Traub, O. & Berk, B.C. (1998). Laminar shear stress mechanisms by which endothelial cells transduce an atheroprotective force. *Arterioscl. Thromb. Vasc. Biol.*, **18**, 677–85.

Traub, O., Ishida., T., Ishida, M., Tupper, J.C. & Berk, B.C. (1999). Shear-stress-mediated extracellular signal-regulated kinase activation is regulated by sodium in endothelial cells. *J. Biol. Chem.*, **274**, 20144–50.

Tribe, R.M., Thomas, C.R. & Poston, L. (1998). Flow-induced dilatation in isolated resistance arteries from control and streptozotocin-diabetic rats. *Diabetologia*, **41**, 34–9.

Tseng, H., Peterson, T.E. & Berk, B.C. (1995). Fluid shear stress stimulates mitogen-activated protein kinase in endothelial cells. *Circ. Res.*, **77**, 869–78.

Uematsu, M., Ohara, Y., Navas, J.P. et al. (1995). Regulation of endothelial cell nitric oxide synthase mRNA expression by shear stress. *Am. J. Physiol.*, **269**, C1371–8.

Ueno, H., Kanellakis, P., Agrotis, A. & Bobik, A. (2000). Blood flow regulates the development of vascular hypertrophy, smooth muscle cell proliferation, and endothelial cell nitric oxide synthase in hypertension. *Hypertension*, **36**, 89–96.

Woo, K.S., Chook, P., Lolin, Y.I. et al. (1997). Hyperhomocyst(e)inaemia is a risk factor for arterial endothelial dysfunction in humans. *Circulation*, **96**, 2542–4.

Woo, K.S., Chook, P., Lolin, Y.I. et al. (1999). Folic acid improves arterial endothelial function in adults with hyperhomocystinaemia. *J. Am. Coll. Cardiol.*, **43**, 2002–6.

Wright, H.P. (1972). Mitosis patterns in aortic endothelium. *Atherosclerosis*, **15**, 93–100.

Yeh, L.H., Park, Y.J., Ahmed, I.S. et al. (1999). Shear-induced tyrosine phosphorylation in endothelial cells requires Rac1-dependent production of ROS. *Am. J. Physiol.*, **276**, C838–47.

Zarins, C.K., Zatina, M.A. Giddens, D.P., Ku, D.N. & Glagov, S. (1987). Shear stress regulation of artery lumen diameter in experimental atherogenesis. *J. Vasc. Surg.*, **5**, 413–20.

4

Neurohumoral regulation of vascular tone

Kirsty M. McCulloch[1] and John C. McGrath[2]

[1]Department of Pharmacology, Quintiles Ltd, Edinburgh
[2]Institute of Biomedical and Life Sciences, University of Glasgow, Glasgow

Introduction

The primary factors which govern blood flow to organs and tissues are perfusion pressure and the overall calibre of the small-resistance arteries and arterioles, which together constitute the major resistance to blood flow. The total active tension of the vascular smooth muscle in a segment of blood vessel wall, i.e. vascular tone, is influenced in vivo by numerous factors which fall into two broad categories: firstly, local or intrinsic control, which includes physical forces, myogenic responses, tissue metabolites and autocoids; and secondly, extrinsic neurohumoral regulation, which involves the action of autonomic nerves and circulating endocrine secretions.

Historically, the investigation of neurohumoral regulation of vascular tone has essentially centred, since the start of the twentieth century, on the action of catecholamines and acetylcholine (ACh) released from perivascular nerves, and catecholamine release from the adrenal medulla into the blood stream (Bevan et al., 1980; Burnstock, 1980), although it took well into the century before it was appreciated that these were the issues involved. With hindsight, this can be attributed to the early identification of adrenaline (epinephrine) in the adrenal gland and to the early availability of blocking drugs which turned out to be antagonists of adrenergic and cholinergic receptors, and to the rather later ability to identify ACh and noradrenaline (NA: norepinephrine). The approach was largely pharmacological. As in other areas of the autonomic nervous system, from the start it was clear that there were many examples where the blockers were ineffective and, therefore, it was difficult to explain neurotransmission solely by adrenergic or cholinergic hypotheses. The recent history of the study of neuro-humoral vascular modulation has involved the gradual accrual of information on the roles of further neurotransmitters and endogenous modulators as methods have emerged for their identification and localization and as antagonists of their

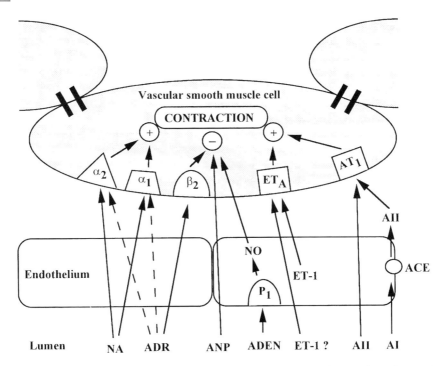

Figure 4.1   Schematic representation demonstrating some of the important humoral regulators of
vascular tone. Agents may act directly upon receptors present on the vascular smooth
muscle, or through interaction with receptors present on the vascular endothelium to
cause the release of a secondary factor. NA, noradrenaline; ADR, adrenaline; ADEN,
adenosine; ANP, atrial natriuretic peptide; AII, angiotensin II; AI, angiotensin I; ACE,
angiotensin-converting enzyme; ET-1, endothelin-1 (? role of circulating ET-1 in control of
vascular tone still controversial); NO, nitric oxide; P_1, P_1-purinoceptor; α_1, α_2 and β_2, α_1- β_2-
and β_2-adrenoceptors; ET_A, endothelin type A receptor; AT_1, angiotensin type 1 receptor.
Dashed lines indicate actions of adrenaline at high concentrations. For additional
explanation see text.

actions have been developed. This gives rise to a constantly emerging picture of the
importance of nonadrenergic, noncholinergic (NANC) components of the autonomic nervous system, with a number of peptides, purines and amines being
implicated in neurohumoral control of the vasculature.

Hormonal control of the vasculature

Several endocrine secretions have been shown to have acute effects on the vasculature (Figure 4.1). It is a general belief that, in the normal subject, hormones are of
less importance for short-term regulation of vascular tone in comparison to
neural control. Circulating hormones and vasoactive agents modulate vascular

tone via direct action on receptors present on the vascular smooth muscle cells, or via indirect action at the vascular endothelium, which releases secondary vasoconstrictor or vasodilator factors. As a result of such actions on both vascular and endothelial receptors, certain humoral agents may have either vasoconstrictor or vasodilator properties depending on species, preparation studied and the level of preexisting vascular tone. Care is therefore required in interpreting experimental data and in comprehending the past literature, since emphasis alters both with knowledge and with fashion.

The overall control of vascular tone centres on the regulation of intracellular free calcium ion concentration ($[Ca^{2+}]_i$) in the smooth muscle cells. When the concentration of $[Ca^{2+}]_i$ rises in the cell, it triggers the activation of Ca^{2+}-calmodulin-dependent protein kinase, which in turn activates myosin light-chain kinase to phosphorylate myosin light chains. This enables actin and myosin to interact and generate active tension. Vasoconstrictors raise the concentration of $[Ca^{2+}]_i$ in the cytosol by activating or stimulating several pathways. Some of the Ca^{2+} originates from the extracellular space and is transported into the cell through voltage or receptor-operated Ca^{2+} channels on the cell membrane. Another source of Ca^{2+} for contraction is the sarcoplasmic reticulum, which behaves as an intracellular storage site for Ca^{2+}. Therefore, by altering the levels of $[Ca^{2+}]_i$, neurotransmitters and circulating hormones regulate the contractile state and hence vascular tone. As time goes on, the number increases of endogenous substances appreciated to possess such actions.

Localization of vascular receptors

A feature common to both neural and humoral control of the vasculature is the action of many vasoactive agents upon specific receptor proteins present on neuronal, smooth muscle and endothelial cells. Although receptors can be studied biochemically in purified preparations, their cytological localization is an area of weakness, which can lead to erroneous interpretation. The reason for this, which has not yet been overcome, is that the cells of blood vessels are heterogeneous and collecting enough homogeneous tissue, particularly of the more interesting small-resistance vessels, is technically very difficult. For example, if a substance changes the tone of a blood vessel, the first assumption is that it is acting on smooth muscle, but it might be acting indirectly. The most striking example of this is the demonstration by Furchgott in the late 1970s that ACh relaxes vascular smooth muscle by releasing a vasodilator substance from the endothelium. Rubbing off the endothelium abolished the response and attaching a piece of tissue with endothelium restored it (Furchgott and Zawadski, 1980; R. F. Furchgott was awarded the 1998 Nobel Prize for Medicine or Physiology for this research).

Such multiple sites of action continue to bedevil this area of research. For example, there is great current interest in peptides such as vasopressin and endothelin which, with other examples, apparently act on both endothelium and smooth muscle. Going back even further, the ability of α-blockers to increase the nerve-induced release of NA was attributed for 40 years to an effect on smooth muscle α-adrenoceptors, until the concept of prejunctional ($α_2$) receptors was introduced in the 1970s. For many years the arterial media was believed to be composed of a phenotypically homogeneous population of smooth muscle cells. There is now growing evidence to indicate that this is not the case, and that morphologically and immunohistochemically distinct smooth muscle cells exist within the arterial media of various mamalian species (Zanellato et al., 1990; Frid et al., 1993). Frid et al. (1997) identified up to four phenotypically distinct populations of cells in conduit bovine pulmonary artery according to their distribution of contractile and cytoskeletal proteins, detected with *in situ* immunological techniques. Electrophysiological studies have also demonstrated that distinct phenotypes of vascular smooth muscle cells express different types of K^+ channels (Archer et al., 1996; McCulloch et al., 2000), but whether this is also the case for subtypes of vascular receptors is not yet known. The localization and biology of vascular receptors thus remain an area awaiting full exploitation.

This has been facilitated by the development of novel and highly selective agonists and antagonists for vascular receptors, initially for functional studies, but of great value in the past 20 years for the study of isolated receptors and now, potentially, to provide visual evidence for the presence of receptors in blood vessels. First described by Young and Kuhar in 1979, autoradiography has been used for localization of a wide range of receptors using reversibly binding radioligands. Spatial localization is not, however, high enough to be of value in small blood vessels. More recently, fluorescent receptor ligands have been developed, for example, BODIPY fluorescent prazosin which can be utilized for visualization of receptors in live vascular preparations (McGrath et al., 1996). This has much higher spatial resolution than autoradiography, can localize receptors at the subcellular level and since it is a dynamic process can be used in pharmacological competition experiments to measure receptor-binding properties (Mackenzie et al., 2000).

At present, however, assumptions about the site of action of vascular modulators rely almost entirely on interpretation of functional responses.

Catecholamines

The major circulating hormones which play a role in the control of vascular tone are the catecholamines, NA and adrenaline. Central sympathetic activity will not only activate perivascular nerves but stimulates preganglionic sympathetic fibres terminating in the adrenal medulla. This activity promotes exocrine secretions from the adrenal glands. The secretion of adrenaline, and to a lesser extent NA (in humans the adrenal gland contains approximately four times more adrenaline than NA, but this varies widely with species) is initiated by the release of ACh from preganglionic sympathetic nerve fibres. ACh depolarizes the adrenal medullary cells via nicotinic receptors, facilitating Ca^{2+} entry into the cells and triggering the secretory process. The plasma levels of adrenaline and NA are 0.1–0.5 nmol/L and 0.5–3.0 nmol/L respectively at rest, with the higher levels of plasma NA arising from 'spillage' from the tonic activity of sympathetic perivascular nerves, rather than adrenal gland secretion. Experiments using electrical stimulation of the splanchnic nerve have shown that the relative amounts of NA and adrenaline released from the adrenal medulla depend on the pattern of stimulation (Bloom et al., 1987). In normal circumstances the output of the adrenal medulla is relatively small and fluctuates during daily activities. As a rule, release of adrenal catecholamines accompanies any increase in sympathetic activity and occurs particularly during mental stress, exercise and hypoglycaemia. Circulating NA is cleared as it passes through certain vascular beds, predominantly the pulmonary vasculature, and is also filtered in the kidney and excreted in the urine.

Adrenergic receptors have been classified into four main groups: α_1, α_2, β_1 and β_2. In blood vessels the main adrenoceptors are of the α_1 and α_2 subtypes, with the β_2-adrenoceptors found mainly in coronary, cerebral and skeletal vascular smooth muscle. The vascular actions of circulating NA and adrenaline can have similar or differing effects depending on the vascular bed studied. In general these catecholamines mediate vasoconstriction via activation of α_1- and possibly α_2-adrenoceptors. The differing effects of the two major catecholamines are most apparent when studied in vivo. Intravenous administration of NA produces sustained increases in systemic vascular resistance due to the activation of α-adrenoceptors. The administration of adrenaline has a less dramatic effect due to the compound being more efficacious on β_2-adrenoceptors in coronary, skeletal and cerebral vessels. At high concentrations adrenaline also evokes vasoconstriction through activation of α-adrenoceptors. It has recently been shown that β_1-adrenoceptors mediate vasodilatation in large conducting arteries such as the aorta and carotid (Chruscinski et al., 2001). The functional consequences of this are not yet known.

Although both α_1- and α_2-adrenoceptor-mediated pressor responses could be clearly demonstrated in whole animals (Docherty and McGrath, 1980; McGrath et al., 1989), initially there were very few examples of α_2-adrenoceptor-mediated contractions in vitro. It was found that by raising vascular tone in some preparations, responses to α_2-adrenoceptor agonists could be uncovered, showing facilitatory actions between vasoconstrictor agonists (for examples, see MacLean and McGrath, 1990; Dunn et al., 1991).

Attenuation of the effects of catecholamines or strategies to prevent their release from nerves have long been issues for therapeutic intervention to reduce vasocon-striction and hence to lower blood pressure. Nonspecific α-blockers were introduced from the 1950s and the first selective $α_1$-blocker, prazosin, was intro-duced in the 1970s. α-Blockers are currently employed, for their vascular effects, to treat hypertension and heart failure and, for their nonvascular effects, to treat benign prostatic hyperplasia.

Angiotensins

Angiotensin II is a circulating octapeptide with powerful vasoconstrictor proper-ties. Its production is initiated by the enzyme renin, which cleaves the precursor angiotensinogen, which is present in the plasma, to produce the peptide angioten-sin I. The angiotensin I is then modified by angiotensin-converting enzyme (ACE) present on the surface of endothelial cells to form angiotensin II, a process which takes place predominantly in the endothelium of the lungs. Angiotensin II elicits vasoconstriction by direct action of angiotensin II type 1 (AT_1) receptors present on the vascular smooth muscle (Figure 4.1) but will also act in vivo to enhance NA release from the sympathetic nerve fibres (Figure 4.2). Angiotensin I also produces vasoconstriction, being approximately 10–100-fold less potent than angiotensin II, and the action of angiotensin I depends on its cleavage into angiotensin II, which often occurs locally by the ACE present on the systemic vascular en-dothelium (Figure 4.1); in vivo this can involve a rise in plasma levels of angioten-sin II but the importance of local conversion can be demonstrated by the blockade of the vasoconstrictor effects of angiotensin I by ACE inhibitors even in vitro in isolated blood vessels. This is, however, species-dependent. In human resistance arteries there is an alternative enzyme, probably chymase, that converts angio-tensin I to angiotensin II, so ACE inhibitors do not block conversion (Padmanab-han et al., 1999).

Knowledge of the importance of angiotensins in vascular control was greatly accelerated by the development of ACE inhibitors from the late 1970s and of angiotensin receptor antagonists in the late 1980s, resulting in the rapid spread of such agents in treating cardiovascular disease in the 1990s. With the recent developments in molecular cloning, polymorphisms within the renin–angiotensin system genes have been investigated as risk factors for both coronary artery disease and hypertension. Examination of the distribution and the allele frequencies of ACE and AT_1-receptor gene polymorphisms may be linked to an increased incidence of myocardial infarction and essential hypertension (Wang et al., 1997; Alvarez et al., 1998; Fatini et al., 2000).

Vasopressin

Vasopressin is a peptide produced by the magnocellular neurons in the supraoptic and paraventricular nuclei of the hypothalamus and secreted from the posterior

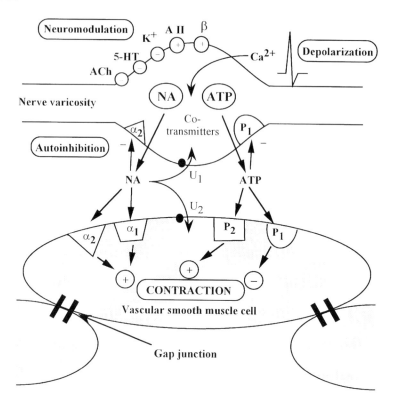

Figure 4.2   Schematic representation of neural regulation of vascular tone by the two main neurotransmitters noradrenaline (NA) and adenosine 5' triphosphate (ATP), which are released from some perivascular nerves as cotransmitters. Main points: (1) NA and ATP released from the varicosity act upon receptors present on the vascular smooth muscle cells initiating the mechanical response. (2) Autoinhibition: released NA and ATP can act prejunctionally to inhibit further transmitter release. (3) Neuromodulation: certain factors can inhibit ($-$) or enhance ($+$) transmitter release from the sympathetic nerve terminals, some examples of which are demonstrated. ACh, acetylcholine; 5-HT, 5-hydroxytryptamine; K^+, potassium ion; AII, angiotensin II; α_1, α_2 and $\beta = \alpha_1$-, α_2- and β-adrenoceptors; P_1 and P_2, P_1- and P_2- purinoceptors; U_1, uptake 1; U_2, uptake 2. For additional explanation see text.

lobe of the pituitary gland. The secretion of vasopressin is regulated partly by hypothalamic cells sensitive to tissue fluid osmolarity and partly by cardiovascular pressure receptors. The major cardiovascular effect of vasopressin is profound vasoconstriction in most tissues, and it remains the most potent known vasoconstrictor of systemic resistance vessels (Figure 4.3). In contrast, cerebral and coronary vessels respond to vasopressin with an endothelium-derived relaxing factor (EDRF)-mediated vasodilatation (Suzuki et al., 1994). This allows vasopressin to help regulate fluid balance without compromising the vital blood flow to the brain and heart. Assessment of vasopressin's importance relative to other agents in

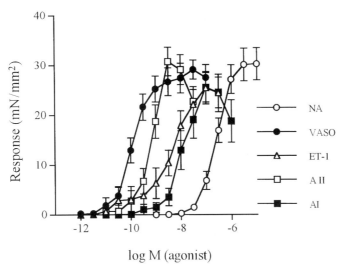

Figure 4.3   Cumulative concentration responses curves to vasoconstrictor agents in rabbit cutaneous arteries (250 μm i.d.) mounted on Mulvany wire myograph indicating the broad range of potencies of vasoactive agents. NA, noradrenaline; VASO, vasopressin; ET-1, endothelin-1; AII, angiotensin II; AI, angiotensin I. Courtesy of J.B. Macmillan, K.M. Smith & J.C. McGrath. Data from Macmillan et al. (1997).

the physiological control of the vasculature has been held up by the lack of potent and selective antagonists. This is an area of current interest.

Endothelin

Since its discovery in the late 1980s the endothelium-derived peptide endothelin-1 (ET-1) has been suggested to play a role in maintenance of systemic vascular tone (Yanagisawa et al., 1988). Endothelins are a family of 21-amino-acid peptides (ET-1, ET-2 and ET-3), which are encoded by three distinct genes (Inoue et al., 1989). The three isoforms are diversely and unevenly distributed, suggesting that endothelin may have multiple functions not just linked to the cardiovascular system. As ET-1 is the only endothelin isoform present in vascular endothelial cells, its involvement in the regulation of vascular tone has been most widely examined. ET-1 is a potent vasoconstrictor of a range of blood vessels from many species, and can also evoke endothelium-dependent relaxation in some vascular preparations (Haynes and Webb, 1993). There are at least two types of vascular receptors at which endothelins act. The ET_A receptor is preferentially activated by ET-1, is expressed predominantly in vascular smooth muscle cells and, when activated, will generally produce vasoconstriction. ET_B receptors, which are nonisopeptide-selective, are expressed on both endothelium and smooth muscle cells and when activated will promote vasodilatation or vasoconstriction depending on the species/preparation and preexisting level of vascular tone.

Haynes and Webb (1994) showed that infusion of the ET_A receptor antagonist BQ-123 into the brachial artery of normal human subjects caused progressive forearm vasodilatation and an increase in blood flow. Although this suggests the presence of endogenous ET-1-induced tone under normal physiological conditions, it is still unclear whether plasma ET-1 levels are sufficiently high to act in an endocrine fashion. Therefore, the actions of ET-1 may be paracrine or autocrine in nature. The possible role of ET-1 in a range of cardiovascular diseases has also been widely examined. Changes in the level of ET-1 and endothelin receptor gene expression may play a significant role in the development of essential hypertension, pulmonary hypertension and heart disease (Stewart et al., 1991; Kiowski et al., 1995; Stevens and Brown, 1995).

Urotensin

Urotensin II (U-II) is a somatostatin-like peptide initially isolated from the spinal cords of fish. The cDNA encoding human U-II has recently been cloned (Coulouarn et al., 1998), and it has subsequently been shown to be an agonist at an orphan human G protein-coupled receptor (analogous to rat GPR14) which is predominantly expressed in vascular tissue (Ames et al., 1999). U-II is a potent vasoconstrictor of isolated vascular tissue (MacLean et al., 2000), produces marked increases in total peripheral resistance in nonhuman primates (Ames et al., 1999) but can also mediate endothelium-dependent vasodilatation in the presence of raised vascular tone (Bottrill et al., 2000; Katano et al., 2000). As human U-II is found within both vascular and cardiac tissue, its involvement in the physiology and pathophysiology of the cardiovascular system is an area of current interest.

Atrial natriuretic peptide

Atrial natriuretic peptide (ANP), an amino acid peptide produced by specialized myocytes in the atria, has been shown to have vasodilator actions in some blood vessel preparations and vascular beds (Januszewicz, 1995). This peptide is secreted in response to increased cardiac filling pressures and mediates vasodilatation via direct action in the vascular smooth muscle, stimulating particulate guanylate cyclase activity and leading to increased cyclic guanosine 3,5-monophosphate (cGMP) levels intracellularly. Study of its roles awaits good antagonists but its levels can now be followed by radioimmunoassay. A rise in its level is an early indication of heart failure and this is likely to lead to increased emphasis on studying its actions.

Purines

Circulating purines may play a role in controlling vascular tone. Purinoceptors have been subdivided into two main classes, P_1 and P_2, both of which may be present in the vasculature (Figures 4.1 and 4.2). In general, adenosine dilates most blood vessels by direct activation of P_1-purinoceptors present on the vascular smooth muscle or through endothelial release of nitric oxide (NO), although in some it may mediate vasoconstriction through indirect release of 5-hydroxytryptamine (5-HT) or angiotensin II. Adenosine triphosphate (ATP) has also been shown to mediate vasodilatation via activation of P_2-purinoceptors present on the vascular endothelium, activation of which releases the vasodilator NO. There is a long-standing literature on the study of the vascular effects of purines. Study of purinoceptors at the molecular level is a topic which is currently of great interest and several subtypes of receptors have been cloned and identified in the vasculature (Kunapuli and Daniel, 1998). However, their functional importance awaits the development of good selective antagonists.

Vascular nerves and neurotransmitters

The localization of vascular nerves can be shown readily by electron microscopy but knowledge of the particular nerve type tends to rely on either a method for conversion of the neurotransmitter into something visible (NA can be converted to a fluorescent analogue), which is limited to a few compounds, or on immunocytochemistry, which depends on the specificity of the antibodies, and again is limited, in practice, to few examples. This limitation has been a major factor in many controversies in this field. For example, the ubiquity of ATP, and the impossibility of demonstrating it satisfactorily by cytochemistry, long delayed its acceptance as a neurotransmitter by the scientific community. Similarly, ACh cannot be localized, except indirectly (and therefore sometimes erroneously) through enzymes which metabolize it. This has led to many controversies as to whether it is a vascular neurotransmitter. On the other hand, the localization in blood vessels, in nerve-like structures, of antibodies to various peptides such as calcitonin gene-related peptide (CGRP) and neuropeptide Y (NPY) was a stimulus to their study as putative transmitters long before any useful pharmacological analysis was possible.

Localization of vascular nerves

It has been observed histologically in a number of blood vessel preparations that the structure and degree of autonomic innervation of the vasculature vary with the size and location of the blood vessel studied. Most large elastic arteries are sparsely innervated, but as the size of the vessel decreases, the innervation density increases, with small arteries and large arterioles being richly innervated. Terminal arterioles are poorly innervated and probably controlled by intrinsic mechanisms, chiefly tissue metabolites. Blood vessels may be innervated by up to three major classes of neurons; most common are the sympathetic vasoconstrictor neurons, with sympathetic or parasympathetic vasodilator neurons and peripheral fibres of small-diameter sensory neurons less commonly observed. The sympathetic out-flow to the heart and the peripheral vessels originates in neurons located in the lateral parts of the ventricular formation. The axons of these neurons form the bulbospinal tract and descend to the preganglionic neurons of the spinal cord. The postganglionic nerve fibres supplying blood vessels are unmyelinated and form a plexus of branching terminal axons (Figure 4.4). In most blood vessels, the nerve plexus is situated in the outer adventitial layer with axons running along the adventitial–medial border (Devine and Simpson, 1967). There are some excep-tions, for example in venous preparations, where axons have been reported to ramify the outer two or three layers of smooth muscle cells in the tunica media. Terminal axons widen at regular intervals into varicosities (1–2 mm diameter) separated by intervaricose regions (0.1–0.3 mm diameter; Burnstock, 1986). Ultrastructural examination using electron microscopy and freeze fractionation shows that the varicosities contain numerous vesicles, some smooth endoplasmic reticulum, mitochondria, neurofilaments and microtubules.

Localization of neurotransmitters

NA can be turned into a fluorescent compound by formaldehyde vapour (for modified technique, see Falck et al., 1982) or glyoxylic acid condensation (Axelsson et al., 1973). This provides a reliable and sensitive fluorescence his-tochemical technique for localizing and visualizing perivascular adrenergic nerves (see also Figure 4.3). Noradrenergic nerves are probably the most important components involved in neural control of vascular tone, and most arteries and arterioles have been shown to be innervated by nerves which contain cate-cholamines. Cholinergic nerves fibres have been identified in some vascular beds (for example, in the brain, tongue, skeletal muscle and external genitalia) using histochemical methods to detect acetylcholinesterase, an enzyme involved in the degradation of ACh, and also by immunohistochemical identification of choline acetyltransferase (Burnstock, 1980).

More recently, immunohistochemical techniques have been utilized to identify not only adrenergic and cholinergic nerves, but also novel vascular neurotransmit-ters, including peptides and purines. Substance P (Furness et al., 1982), vasoactive intestinal polypeptide (VIP: Uddman et al., 1981), NPY (Uddman et al., 1982) and somatostatin (Forssmann et al., 1982) have all been identified in perivascular nerve terminals. A fluorescence histochemical technique using quinacrine has also been used to identify nerves containing purines such as ATP (Burnstock et al., 1979) which, next to NA, is the most-studied neurotransmitter contained in vascular nerves. Recently, nitric oxide synthase (NOS)-containing fibres have also been identified using immunohistochemical techniques in some arteries (e.g.

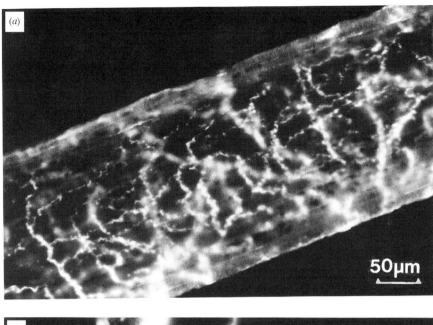

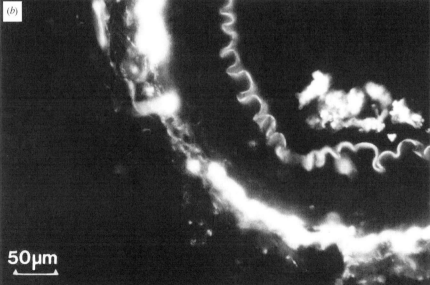

Figure 4.4   (*a*) Segment of rabbit anterior cerebral artery stained using glyoxylic acid condensation technique in which axons containing catecholamines fluoresce when illuminated with ultraviolet light. The nerve fibres can be seen to form a branching varicose network around the vessel. Bar: 50 μm.

(*b*) Cross-section of rabbit cutaneous artery stained using Falck technique, in which adrenergic nerve terminals display fluorescence when illuminated with ultraviolet light. Nerve fibres are restricted to the outer adventitial layer, and do not penetrate the medial smooth muscle layer. The internal elastic lamina is clearly visible due to the autofluorescent nature of elastic tissue. Bar: 50 μm.

cerebral) which, together with functional pharmacological evidence suggests that NO is an inhibitory vascular neurotransmitter in blood vessels (Nozaki et al., 1993; Toda, 2000). 5-HT immunofluorescent nerves have been detected in a number of vessels. However, it appears that 5-HT is not synthesized within the nerve fibre, but is taken up, stored and released, as a false transmitter, from sympathetic nerves (Jackowski et al., 1989). Three types of storage vesicles are found in sympathetic varicosities: many granular and agranular small vesicles and a few dense-cored large vesicles. Both large and small vesicles contain NA and ATP, the relative quantities of which vary in different vessel types (Burnstock, 1990). Neuropeptides and other soluble proteins are found only in large dense-cored vesicles, coexisting with NA and ATP (see section on cotransmission, below).

Fluorescent histochemical and immunohistochemical techniques have also been used to provide semiquantitative analysis of the density of autonomic innervation. This has improved over the years with the development of more sophisticated image analysis techniques, and has been utilized for comparing density of innervation of different vessel sizes and types, and the effects of ageing and disease, all which may affect the degree of innervation, and perhaps the levels, of neurotransmitters (Cowen et al., 1982; Griffith et al., 1982).

Transmitter release and smooth muscle activation

Action potentials are propagated along the nerve fibre to the varicosities via the influx of Na^+ and Ca^{2+} into the neuroplasm. As a consequence of increased intraneuronal $[Ca^{2+}]$, the storage vesicles migrate towards and fuse with the neuronal cell membrane, emptying their contents into the synaptic cleft (Figure 4.5). Once released, the transmitter diffuses across the junctional gap, which can vary between 50 and 2000 nm depending on the size of the vessel. Upon reaching the vascular smooth muscle cells the neurotransmitter interacts with receptors on the postjunctional membrane, leading to changes in the membrane potential and/or intracellular signalling mechanisms. Only vascular smooth muscle cells close to the varicosity are affected directly by the released transmitter. Therefore in richly innervated arterioles most smooth muscle cells are near enough to the nerves to be directly activated, but in larger vessels the innervation is restricted to cells in the medioadventitial border. To affect the deeper noninnervated layers electrical activity must be propagated from cell to cell. This occurs through specialized electrical coupling between neighbouring smooth muscle cells known as nexuses or gap junctions (Bevan et al., 1980). Therefore, although many vascular smooth muscle cells are not directly innervated, they may still be influenced by nerves. This may also be a source of differences between the actions of different neurotransmitters. Those whose signalling includes depolarization of the cell membrane may transfer their effects further through the media than those

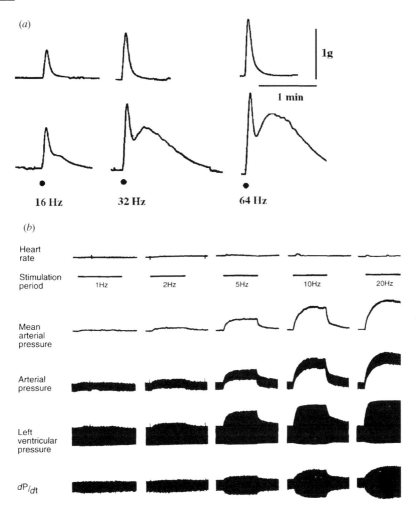

Figure 4.5   (*a*) Representative trace showing frequency-dependent contractions in the rabbit isolated saphenous vein in response to electrical field stimulation. Top panel shows control responses at 16, 32 and 64 Hz stimulation from left to right (stimulation parameters of 0.1 ms pulse width, 1 s train duration, 35 V). Bottom panel shows responses at the same frequencies in the presence of 10 μmol/L cocaine (which blocks U_1 mechanism; see Figure 4.2). Note how the response is prolonged in presence of cocaine. Reproduced from Daly (1993) with permission.

(*b*) Representative trace of heart rate and carotid arterial and left ventricular pressures in a pithed rabbit. The sympathetic outflows in the upper lumbar region were stimulated via the pithing rod. At this level stimulation of the outflow produces direct stimulation of vasoconstrictor nerves without activation of sympathetic nerves to the heart or to the adrenal medulla. Pharmacological analysis showed that this vasoconstrictor response is mediated partly by α_1- and partly by α_2-adrenoceptors. Reproduced from McGrath et al. (1982).

with exclusively 'pharmacomechanical coupling' via nondepolarizing signalling pathways. For example, the effect of NA may stop at the first cell activated, whereas ATP-induced depolarization may propagate further afield. Teleologically this provides a rationale for different neurotransmitters.

Cotransmission

It was initially thought that each neuron synthesized and released only a single neurotransmitter, and this concept became known as Dale's principle. However, there is now substantial evidence both in vitro and in vivo that nerves synthesize, store and release more than one neurotransmitter. An example of such evidence was illustrated by Su (1975), who demonstrated that after priming tissues with tritiated ^{3}H adenosine (a precursor in the synthesis of ATP) and then using tritium efflux as a measure of ATP release, electrical stimulation of the rabbit aorta and portal vein evoked the release of a ^{3}H purine together with NA. The same technique has also been shown to demonstrate cotransmission of ATP and NA in a variety of vascular preparations. The coexistence of NA and the vasoconstrictor peptide NPY in sympathetic nerve terminals also invites the hypothesis that NPY is a vascular neurotransmitter. This has been reinforced by recent evidence that antagonists of NPY can attenuate responses to activation of sympathetic nerves (Hoyo et al., 2000). A parallel hypothesis exists for the vasodilator VIP. To generalize, it appears that ATP and NPY coexist with, and are released with, NA in sympathetic neurons, whereas VIP and ACh are cotransmitters in perivascular nerves (Burnstock, 1990). The physiological significance of this remains to be determined.

Vascular modulation by neurotransmitters

In studying the effects of autonomic nerve activity on the vasculature, probably the most common preparations utilized are isolated blood vessels. These can be set up as perfused or wire-mounted preparations, with the perivascular nerves being selectively stimulated by an electrical field consisting of pulses of short duration – typically 0.1–1 ms, too short to stimulate the smooth muscle cells directly. This elicits a functional response from the blood vessel – a change in perfusion pressure, vessel width or isometric tension, according to the preparation and method of recording (see Figure 4.4a). Direct comparison can be made with the effects of exogenously applied agonists or putative transmitters and pharmacological analysis carried out.

A useful preparation which provides a bridge to the in vivo situation is the pithed animal. Here, the brain and spinal cord are physically destroyed to eliminate all central or reflex activity and the circulation remains functional providing that temperature and respiration are artificially controlled. This allows the study of the effects upon the intact circulation, in the absence of confounding effects of reflexes, of firstly, autonomic nerve stimulation applied to selected spinal outflows via the pithing rod, and secondly, their comparison with exogenously administered neurotransmitters and other substances by appropriate pharmacological analysis. This often enables the demonstration of phenomena which are resistant to study in vitro, perhaps due to the inaccessibility or impracticability of the particular vascular bed or vessels involved or because the in vitro medium lacks some vital characteristic such as the appropriate blood gas conditions, a facilitatory hormone or a necessary enzyme. For example, α_2-adrenoceptor-mediated vasoconstriction is difficult to demonstrate in vitro but was discovered, and is readily studied, in pithed animals. In principle the technique can be applied to any species, and has been used with rats, cats, ferrets and rabbits. The rat is by far the most common, with the rabbit next (see Figure 4.4*b* and McGrath et al., 1982), although some important very early studies at the turn of the twentieth century used pithed cats.

An important general issue in analysing neurotransmission by pharmacological techniques, particularly comparing the effects of antagonists against nerves and putative neurotransmitters, is the nonequilibrium nature of the neurotransmission process. Each junctional release of neurotransmitter causes a rapid rise followed by a slower but still rapid fall in concentration of the transmitter at the region of its target receptors. Although there may be a gradual build-up of transmitter level at high frequencies, the process is essentially one of repetitive rising and falling concentration. This is not appropriate for quantitative comparison with the equilibrium between agonists and antagonists. Indeed, because an antagonist must dissociate from the receptor before an agonist can occupy it, this gives antagonists greater ability to block agonist transmitters from nerves than to block the same agonist at equilibrium when administered exogenously. In practice this means that the identification of receptor subtypes involved in neurotransmission can never be as quantitative as might be expected versus agonists. Consequently, where the relative affinities of antagonists are crucial, controversy is likely.

Vasoconstrictor nerves

To generalize, sympathetic nerve stimulation produces vasoconstriction in most vascular beds. Depolarization of the vasoconstrictor sympathetic nerve terminal releases NA and/or ATP, which acts upon postjunctional adrenoceptors and purinoceptors respectively. Electrophysiological experimentation has shown that in a number of preparations the postjunctional electrical response to sympathetic nerve stimulation involves two distinct phases. The first is a rapid, transient depolarization or excitatory junction potential (e.j.p.) of which several must summate in order to produce depolarization of some 15–20 mV before threshold is reached for voltage-dependent Ca^{2+} channels to be activated, initiating the contractile process (Hirst and Edwards, 1989). These e.j.p.s are rapid in onset, resistant to the action of α-adrenoceptor antagonists, abolished by the blockade of P_2-receptors, and therefore appear to be mediated by the actions of ATP (Vidal et al., 1986). This initial phase is followed by a slow prolonged depolarization, which is mimicked by the effects of exogenous NA and can be abolished by α-adrenoceptor antagonists (Sneddon and Burnstock, 1984). Postsynaptically the α_1-adrenoceptor is the predominant receptor mediating vasoconstriction, but there are also postsynaptic α_2-adrenoceptors which mediate vasoconstriction in some vascular preparations (McGrath et al., 1989).

Although several putative peptide neurotransmitters have been identified in perivascular nerves, their exact role in maintaining vascular tone is not well understood. Release of these peptides may produce persistent vasoconstriction in some vascular preparations (Wharton and Gulbenkian, 1987). The major role of NPY in the vasculature may be that of a pre- or postjunctional modulator of sympathetic transmission (Lundberg et al., 1990).

Measurement of sympathetic nerve firing activity using electrical recordings from the skin of healthy human volunteers showed that sympathetic vasoconstrictor nerves discharge continually at about 1 Hz or less at rest, with the maximum frequency of approximately 8–10 Hz (Bini et al., 1980). Interruption of tonic sympathetic activity in vivo by nerve sectioning or pharmacological blockade results in vasodilatation, as can be demonstrated, for example, in pithed animals in which destruction of spinal sympathetic outflow causes a fall in blood pressure which is partly due to systemic vasodilatation. Therefore the overall degree of vascular tone can be controlled by increasing or decreasing sympathetic nerve firing activity above basal levels to produce vasoconstriction or vasodilatation respectively. The rate of firing of sympathetic neurons can be affected in vivo by a number of factors including rhythm of respiration, temperature and mental activity or stress.

Vasodilator nerves

In a limited number of tissues the arterioles are innervated by vasodilator fibres as well as by the ubiquitous sympathetic vasoconstrictor fibres. Unlike the vasoconstrictor fibres, they are not tonically active. Sympathetic vasodilator nerves are rare but have been suggested to be present in the arterioles of skeletal muscle in carnivores such as the dog and cat. This part of the sympathetic nervous system is activated solely as part of the 'alerting response' to fear and danger and, when activated, elicits a transient vasodilator response mediated via activation of muscarinic receptors by ACh. Evidence for this relies largely on pharmacological analysis using muscarinic antagonists and has long been controversial.

Parasympathetic vasodilator nerves are less widely distributed in comparison to the sympathetic vasoconstrictor fibres. Examples of parasympathetically innervated tissues are blood vessels of the salivary glands and exocrine pancreas, the gastric and colonic mucosa and cerebral and coronary arteries. Most commonly, parasympathetic vasodilatation is mediated via ACh release, hyperpolarizing the vascular smooth muscle; however, cotransmission of ACh and VIP may occur in some tissues, for example, the rabbit lingual artery (Brayden and Large, 1986). Nitric oxide is the parasympathetic postganglionic vasodilator transmitter in several beds, notably penile and cerebral (Toda, 2000).

The ability of antidromic impulses in collateral branches of sensory nerves to cause vasodilatation, forming the flare component of the triple response to mild trauma in the human skin, is well documented. The sensory nerves mediating this response are the nociceptive C fibres which have been shown to contain substance P and CGRP (Gamse et al., 1980).

Modulation of sympathetic neurotransmission

Given a constant activity of the sympathetic neuron, the amount of transmitter released can be either augmented or attenuated by the actions of locally released or circulating factors (Figure 4.2). Angiotensin II is considered to be an important facilitatory modulator of vascular adrenergic transmission. It acts to increase the release of NA from sympathetic nerve terminals. Activation of β-adrenoceptors present on the neuronal membrane can enhance exocytotic release of adrenergic transmitter evoked by nerve impulses. It has been suggested that these effects may play a role in certain forms of hypertension, with increased levels of adrenaline and/or angiotensin II reaching the adrenergic neuronal membrane, facilitating NA release and hence vasoconstriction. Autocoids such as histamine and 5-HT have inhibitory actions on NA release, as does activation by ACh of muscarinic receptors present on the neuronal membrane. Metabolic acidosis, increases in K^+ levels and hyperosmolarity all act to reduce the release of NA from sympathetic nerve terminals (Shepherd and Vanhoutte, 1985).

Released NA is removed from the synaptic cleft by uptake into nerve terminals (uptake$_1$: Borowsky and Hoffman, 1995) and/or uptake into nonneural cells (uptake 2: Gründemann et al., 1998) and will also seep into surrounding capillary networks, clearing the released transmitter from the junctional cleft (Figure 4.2). NA taken up into the nerve terminal cytoplasm may undergo further active uptake into the NA storage vesicles by the vesicular monoamine transporter (VMAT), although most is broken down by enzymes present in the nerve fibres.

The neuronal membrane also 'senses' the concentration of released NA and ATP via prejunctional receptors, which exert a negative-feedback effect on vesicular exocytosis (Figure 4.2). Pharmacological investigation has demonstrated that the receptors responsible for this autoinhibition are the α_2-adrenoceptor and the

P_1-purinoceptor, for NA and ATP respectively. Feedback inhibition of transmitter release can also be initiated by exogenous circulating catecholamines and purines. Postjunctionally the effects of NA and ATP released as transmitters are generally cooperative as both typically act as vasoconstrictors. Their physiological roles may radically differ due to differences in their actions, both temporally (long- and short-acting, respectively) and spatially (due to nonpropagating signalling and propagating action potentials, respectively; see previous section). This also applies to peptide neurotransmitters, which are expected to have long-lived actions. The nature and physiological and pathophysiological roles of purinergic and peptidergic transmission, although potentially of great importance, remain obscure. This could rapidly be clarified if good antagonists became available.

Summary

Vascular tone can be modulated by an ever-growing number of endogenous substances, which can act directly to contract or relax vascular smooth muscle or indirectly by the release of other substances from the endothelium. Nerve terminals, mainly autonomic sympathetic or sensory, release vasoactive substances which modulate smooth muscle tone. Translation of this knowledge of the capability of circulating substances or neurotransmitters to modulate vascular tone into information on the role of particular substances or phenomena in the physiological regulation of vascular tone is dependent on the following: firstly, the availability of appropriate selective antagonist drugs and in vitro preparations responsive to the appropriate stimuli, including nerve stimulation and allowing discrimination between direct (vascular smooth muscle) and indirect (endothelial) effects, and secondly, in vivo preparations amenable to these same manoeuvres. Proof of a role for a given phenomenon in humans requires the further feasibility of testing such antagonists in humans. Paradoxically, this means that the best understood phenomena are those already taken to the level of developing therapeutic blockers rather than blockers which have been developed on the basis of what is physiologically or pathophysiologically most appropriate. This useful symbiosis continues.

REFERENCES

Alvarez, R., Reguero, J.R., Batalla, A. et al. (1998). Angiotensin-converting enzyme and angiotensin II receptor 1 polymorphisms: association with early coronary disease. *Cardiovasc. Res.*, **40**, 375–9.

Ames, R.S., Sarau, H.M., Chambers, J.K. et al. (1999). Human urotensin-II is a potent vasoconstrictor and agonist for the orphan receptor GPR14. *Nature*, **401**, 282–6.

Archer, S.L., Huang, J.M.C., Reeve, H.L. et al. (1996). Differential distribution of electrophysiologically distinct myocytes in conduit and resistance arteries determines their response to nitric oxide and hypoxia. *Circ. Res.*, **78**, 431–42.

Axelsson, S., Bjorklund, A., Falck, B., Lindvall, O. & Svensson, L.A. (1973). Glyoxylic acid condensation: a new fluorescence method for the histological demonstration of biogenic monoamines. *Acta Physiol. Scand.*, **87**, 57–62.

Bevan, J.A., Bevan, R.D. & Duckles, S.P. (1980). Adrenergic regulation of vascular smooth muscle. In *Handbook of Physiology. The Cardiovascular System*, vol. II. Vascular smooth muscle, section 2, ed. Bohr, D.F., Somlyo, A.P. & Sparks, H.V. pp. 515–66. Bethesda, MD: American Physiological Society.

Bini, G., Hagbarth, K.E., Hynninen, P. & Wallin, B.G. (1980). Regional similarities and differences in thermoregulatory vaso- and sudomotor tone. *J. Physiol.*, **306**, 513–26.

Bloom, S.R., Edwards, A.V. & Jones, C.T. (1987). The adrenal contribution to the neuroendocrine responses to splanchnic nerve stimulation in conscious calves. *J. Physiol.*, **397**, 513–26.

Borowsky, B. & Hoffman, B.J. (1995). Neurotransmitter transporters: molecular biology, function and regulation. *Int. Rev. Neurobiol.*, **38**, 139–99.

Bottrill, F.E., Douglas, S.A., Hiley, C.R. & White, R. (2000) Human urotensin-II is an endothelium-dependent vasodilator in rat small arteries. *Br. J. Pharmacol.*, **130**, 1865–70.

Brayden, J.E. & Large, W.A. (1986). Electrophysiological analysis of neurogenic vasodilatation in the isolated lingual artery of the rabbit. *Br. J. Pharmacol.*, **89**, 163–71.

Burnstock, G. (1980). Cholinergic and purinergic regulation of blood vessels. In *Handbook of Physiology. The Cardiovascular System*, vol. II. Vascular smooth muscle, section 2 ed. Bohr, D.F., Somlyo, A.P. & Sparks, H.V., pp. 567–612. Bethesda, MD: American Physiological Society.

Burnstock, G. (1986). Autonomic neuromuscular junctions: current developments and future directions. *J. Anat.*, **146**, 1–30.

Burnstock, G. (1990) Co-transmission. (The fifth Heymans memorial lecture.) *Arch. Int. Pharmacodyn. Ther.*, **304**, 7–33.

Burnstock, G., Crowe, R. & Wong, H.K. (1979). Comparative pharmacological and histological evidence for purinergic inhibitory innervation of the portal vein of the rabbit, but not guinea pig. *Br. J. Pharmacol.*, **65**, 377–88.

Chruscinski, A., Brede, M.E., Meinel, L. et al. (2001). Differential distribution of beta-adrenergic receptor subtypes in blood vessels of knockout mice lacking beta(1)- or beta(2)-adrenergic receptors. *Mol. Pharmacol.*, **60**, 955–62.

Coulouarn, Y., Lihrmann, I., Jegou, S. et al. (1998). Cloning of the cDNA encoding the urotensin II precursor in frog and human reveals intense expression of the urotensin II gene in motoneurons of the spinal cord. *Proc. Natl Acad. Sci.*, **95**, 15803–8.

Cowen, T., Haven, A.J., Wen Qin, C. et al. (1982). Development and ageing of perivascular adrenergic nerves in the rabbit. A quantitative fluorescent histochemical study using image analysis. *J. Auton. Nerv. Syst.*, **5**, 317–36.

Daly, C.J. (1993). The contribution of α_2-adrenoceptors to sympathetic neuroeffector transmission in the rabbit isolated saphenous and plantaris veins. MSc. thesis, University of Glasgow.

Devine, C.E. & Simpson, F.O. (1967). The fine structure of vascular sympathetic neuromuscular contacts in the rat. *Am. J. Anat.*, **121**, 153–74.

Docherty, J.R. & McGrath, J.C. (1980). A comparison of pre- and post-junctional potencies of several α-adrenoceptor agonists in the cardiovascular system and anococcygeus of the rat. Evidence for two types of post-junctional α-adrenoceptor. *Naunyn Schmiedeberg's Arch. Pharmacol.*, **312**, 107–16.

Dunn, W.R., Daly, C.J., McGrath, J.C. & Wilson, V.G. (1991). A comparison of the effects of angiotensin II and Bay K 8644 on responses to noradrenaline mediated via postjunctional α_1- and α_2-adrenoceptors in rabbit isolated blood vessels. *Br. J. Pharmacol.*, **103**, 1475–83.

Falck, B., Björklund, A. & Lindvall, O. (1982). Recent progress in aldehyde fluorescence histochemistry. *Brain Res. Bull.*, **9**, 3–10.

Fatini, C., Abbate, R., Pepe, G. et al. (2000). Searching for a better assessment of the individual coronary risk profile. The role of angiotensin-converting enzyme, angiotensin II type 1 receptor and angiotensinogen gene polymorphisms. *Eur. Heart J.*, **21**, 633–8.

Forssman, W.G., Hock, D. & Metz, J. (1982). Peptidergic innervation of the kidney. *Neurosci. Lett*, **10** (suppl.) S183.

Frid, M.G., Printseva, O.Y., Chiavegato, A. et al. (1993). Myosin heavy-chain isoform composition and distribution in developing and adult human aortic smooth muscle. *J. Vasc. Res.*, **30**, 279–92.

Frid, M.G., Aldashev, A.A., Dempsey, E.C. & Stenmark, K.R. (1997). Smooth muscle cells isolated from discrete compartments of the mature vascular media exhibit unique phenotypes and distinct growth capabilities. *Circ. Res.*, **81**, 940–52.

Furchgott, R.F. & Zawadski, J.V. (1980). The obligatory role of endothelial cells in the relaxation of arterial smooth muscle by acetylcholine. *Nature (Lond.)*, **288**, 373–6.

Furness, J.B., Papka, R.E., Della, N.G., Costa, M. & Eskay, R.L. (1982). Substance P-like immunoreactivity in nerves associated with the vascular system of guinea pigs. *Neuroscience*, **7**, 447–59.

Gamse, R., Holzer, P. & Lembeck, F. (1980). Decrease of substance P in primary afferent neurones and impairment of neurogenic plasma extravasation by capsaicin. *Br. J. Pharmacol.*, **68**, 207–13.

Griffith, S.G., Crowe, R., Lincoln, J., Haven, A.J. & Burnstock, G. (1982). Regional differences in the density of perivascular nerves and varicosities, noradrenaline content and responses to nerve stimulation in the rabbit ear artery. *Blood Vessels*, **19**, 41–52.

Gründemann, D., Schechinger, B., Rappold, G.A. & Schömig, E. (1998). Molecular identification of the corticosterone-sensitive extraneuronal catecholamine transporter. *Nature Neurosci.*, **1**, 349–51.

Haynes, W.G. & Webb, D.J. (1993). The endothelin family of peptides: local hormones with diverse roles in health and disease? *Clin. Sci.*, **84**, 485–500.

Haynes, W.G. & Webb, D.J. (1994). Contribution of endogenous generation of endothelin-1 to basal vascular tone. *Lancet*, **344**, 852–4.

Hirst, G.D.S. & Edwards, R.R. (1989). Sympathetic neuroeffector transmission in arteries and arterioles. *Physiol. Rev.*, **69**, 546–604.

Hoyo, Y., McGrath, J.C. & Vila, E. (2000). Evidence for Y1-receptor-mediated facilitatory, modulatory cotransmission by NPY in the rat anococcygeus muscle. *J. Exp. Pharmacol. Ther.*, **294**, 38–44.

Inoue, A., Yanagisawa, M., Kimura, S. et al. (1989). The human endothelin family: three structurally and pharmacological distinct isopeptides predicted by three separate genes. *Proc. Natl Acad. Sci. USA*, **86**, 2863–7.

Jackowski, A., Crockard, A. & Burnstock, G. (1989). 5-Hydroxytryptamine demonstrated immunohistochemistry in rat cerebrovascular nerves largely represents 5-hydroxytryptamine uptake into sympathetic nerve fibres. *Neuroscience*, **29**, 453–62.

Januszewicz, A. (1995) The natriuretic peptides in hypertension. *Curr. Opin. Cardiol.*, **10**, 495–500.

Katano, Y., Ishihata, A., Aita, T., Ogaki, T. & Horie, T. (2000). Vasodilator effects of urotensin II, one of the most potent vasoconstricting factors, on rat coronary arteries. *Eur. J. Pharmacol.*, **402**, 209–11.

Kiowski, W., Sütsch, G., Hunziker, P. et al. (1995). Evidence for endothelin-1-mediated vasoconstriction in severe chronic heart failure. *Lancet*, **346**, 732–6.

Kunapuli, S.P. & Daniel, J.L. (1998). P_2 receptor subtypes in the cardiovascular system. *Biochem. J.*, **336**, 513–23.

Lundberg, J.M., Franco-Cereceda, A., Hemsen, A., Lacroix, J.S. & Pernow, J. (1990). Pharmacology of noradrenaline and neuropeptide tyrosine (NPY)-mediated sympathetic co-transmission. *Fundam. Clin. Pharmacol.*, **4**, 373–91.

Mackenzie, J.F., Daly, C.J., Pediani, J.D. & McGrath, J.C. (2000). Quantitative imaging in live human cells reveals intracellular α_1-adrenoceptor ligand binding sites. *J. Exp. Pharmacol. Ther.*, **294**, 434–43.

MacLean, M.R. & McGrath, J.C. (1990). Effects of pre-contraction with endothelin-1 on α_2-adrenoceptor and (endothelium-dependent) neuropeptide Y-mediated contractions in the isolated vascular bed of the rat tail. *Br. J. Pharmacol.*, **101**, 205–11.

MacLean, M.R., Alexander, D., Stirrat, A. et al. (2000). Contractile responses to human urotensin-II in rat and human pulmonary arteries: effect of endothelial factors and chronic hypoxia in the rat. *Br. J. Pharmacol.*, **130**, 201–4.

Macmillan, J.B., Smith, K.M. & McGrath, J.C. (1997). Investigation of vasoconstriction responses of rabbit cutaneous resistance arteries. *J. Autonom. Pharmacol.*, **17**, 221.

McCulloch, K.M., Kempsill, F.E.J., Buchanan, K.J. & Gurney, A.M. (2000). Regional distribution of potassium currents in the rabbit pulmonary arterial circulation. *Exp. Physiol.*, **85**, 487–96.

McGrath, J.C., Flavahan, N.A. & McKean, C.E. (1982) α_1 and α_2-adrenoceptor-mediated pressor and chronotropic effects in the rat and rabbit. *J. Cardiovasc. Pharmacol.*, **4**, S101–7.

McGrath, J.C., Brown, C.M. & Wilson, V.G. (1989) Alpha-adrenoceptors : a critical review. *Med. Res. Reviews*, **9**, 407–533.

McGrath, J.C., Arribas, S. & Daly, C.J. (1996) Fluorescent ligands for the study of receptors. *Trends Pharmacol. Sci.*, **207**, 385–427.

Nozaki, K., Moskowitz, M.A., Maynard, K.I. et al. (1993). Possible origins and distribution of immunoreactive nitric oxide synthase-containing nerve fibres in cerebral arteries. *J. Cerebr. Blood Flow Metab.*, **13**, 70–9.

Padmanabhan, N., Jardine, A.G., McGrath, J.C. & Connell, J.M.C. (1999). Angiotensin convert-ing enzyme independent contraction to angiotensin-I in human resistance arteries. *Circula-tion*, **99**, 2914–20.

Shepherd, J.T. & Vanhoutte P.M. (1985). Local modulation of adrenergic neurotransmission in blood vessels. *J. Cardiovasc. Pharmacol.*, **7** (suppl. 3), S167–78.

Sneddon, P. & Burnstock, G. (1984). Inhibition of excitatory junction potentials in guinea-pig vas deferens by $\alpha\beta$-methylene ATP: Further evidence for ATP and noradrenaline as cotran-smitters. *Eur. J. Pharmacol.*, **100**, 85–90.

Stevens, P.A. & Brown, M.J. (1995). Genetic variabilty of the ET-1 and ETA receptor genes in essential hypertension. *J. Cardiovasc. Pharmacol.*, **26**, S9–12.

Stewart, D.J., Levy, R.D., Cernacek, P. & Langleben, D. (1991). Increased plasma endothelin-1 in pulmonary hypertension: marker or mediator of disease? *Ann. Intern. Med.*, **114**, 464–9.

Su, C. (1975) Neurogenic release of purine compounds in blood vessels. *J. Pharmacol. Exp. Ther.*, **195**, 159–66.

Suzuki, Y., Satoh, S., Oyama, H. et al. (1994). Vasopressin mediated vasodilation of cerebral arteries. *J. Auton. Nerv. Syst.*, **49**, S129–32.

Toda, N. (2000). Nitrergic (nitroxidergic) innervation in the blood vessel. In *Nitric Oxide and the Peripheral Nervous System*, ed. Toda, N., Moncada, S., Furchgott, R. & Higgs, E.A. pp. 37–60. London: Portland Press.

Uddman, R., Alumets, J., Edvinsson, L., Hakanson, R. & Sundler F. (1981). VIP nerve fibres around peripheral blood vessels. *Acta Physiol. Scand.*, **112**, 65–70.

Uddman, R., Alumets, J., Edvinsson, L. et al. (1982). Immunohistochemical demonstration of APP (avian pancreatic polypeptide)-immunoreactive nerve fibres around cerebral blood vessels. *Brain Res. Bull.*, **9**, 715–18.

Vidal, M., Hicks, P.E. & Langer, S.Z. (1986). Differential effects of α,β-methylene ATP on responses to nerve stimulation in SHR and WKY tail arteries. *Naunyn-Schmiedebergs's Arch. Pharmacol.*, **332**, 384–90.

Wang, W.Y., Zee, R.Y. & Morris, B.J. (1997). Association of angiotensin II type 1 receptor gene polymorphism with essential hypertension. *Clin. Genet.*, **51**, 31–4.

Wharton, J. & Gulbenkian, S. (1987). Peptides in the mammalian cardiovascular system. *Experientia Basel*, **43**, 821–32.

Yanagisawa, M., Kurihara, H., Kimura, S. et al. (1988). A novel potent vasoconstrictor peptide produced by vascular endothelial cells. *Nature*, **332**, 411–15.

Young, W.S. III & Kuhar, M.J. (1979). A new method for receptor autoradiography: [^{3}H] opioid receptors in rat brain. *Brain Res.*, **179**, 255–70.

Zanellato, A.M., Borrione, A.C., Giuriato, L. et al. (1990). Myosin isoforms and cell heterogene-ity in vascular smooth muscle, I: developing and adult bovine aorta. *Dev. Biol.*, **141**, 431–46.

5

Angiogenesis: basic concepts and the application of gene therapy

John W. Quarmby and Alison W. Halliday

Department of Vascular Surgery, St George's Hospital, London

Introduction

The establishment and maintenance of a vascular supply are necessary for the growth and survival of normal and neoplastic tissues. An important distinction must be made between two types of new vessel formation: vasculogenesis and angiogenesis. The first, vasculogenesis, is the process by which primitive mesenchymal cells differentiate in situ to become the endothelial lining of embryological blood vessels. The second, angiogenesis, describes the endothelial budding and outgrowth into avascular tissue from preexisting capillaries. Vasculogenesis occurs early in embryogenesis and is completed well before independent living is established. Angiogenesis is both a physiological and pathological process that governs the majority of new vessel growth both during embryo development and throughout life.

The term 'angiogenesis' was first used in the 1930s to describe the formation of new blood vessels in the placenta. It has subsequently become clear that angiogenesis is a vital part of all organ growth, both in isolation, as occurs in the uterus during the menstrual cycle, and also as occurs in the normal development of an infant. In pathological states angiogenesis can be beneficial, as in wound healing and inflammation, but also detrimental, as in neoplasia, retinopathies and rheumatoid arthritis, amongst others.

Growth of new capillaries and vessels occurs in conjunction with surrounding mesenchymal tissue and is determined by mechanical, humoral and growth factors. The use of laboratory and clinical methods is rapidly expanding our understanding of the physiology and pathology of angiogenesis. With the application of these scientific principles we are now seeing the development of strategies such as gene therapy which are aimed at either promoting or inhibiting angiogenesis for the therapeutic benefit of patients.

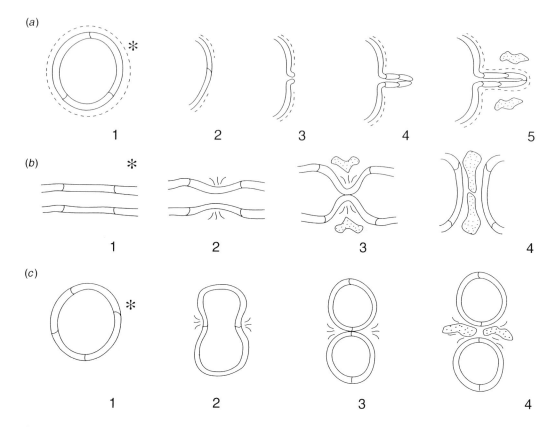

Figure 5.1   (*a*) Classical capillary growth. In response to an angiogenic stimulus (1), basement
membrane disruption (2) occurs, allowing endothelial cell migration (3) followed by
proliferation and tube formation (4) and finally reestablishment of the basement
membrane and migration of pericytes (6). (*b*) Intussusceptive growth. The angiogenic
stimulus (1) induces compression of two opposing endothelial cells towards each other,
accompanied by interstitial cells and filaments (2), which meet (3) and ultimately separate
as two separate daughter capillaries (4). (*c*) Longitudinal growth. As a capillary tube
lengthens, a stimulus (1) induces bulging of the capillary wall into the lumen (2), which
meet (3) and then cause division of the capillary in a longitudinal axis (4).

Basic cellular mechanisms of angiogenesis

For over 70 years observational studies have been used to describe the growth of
new vessels in both health and disease. Classical angiogenesis (Figure 5.1*a*) has
been shown to commence with the migration of endothelial cells into the surrounding extravascular space, followed by proliferation and the formation of
capillary sprouts which eventually connect to neighbouring vessels, thereby establishing flow (Hudlická and Tyler, 1986). This migration is accompanied by a

change in the investing basement membrane of an existing capillary and the accumulation of extravascular fibrin. As a result of matrix proteolysis and chemotaxis endothelial cells are able to migrate, divide and form new capillaries. Nonsprouting or intussusceptive growth (Figure 5.1*b*) is an alternative method of angiogenesis that was first described in lung tissue (Burri and Tarek, 1990) and subsequently in other developing organs. Opposing capillary effacement occurs as a result of mesenchymal proliferation, thus dividing a capillary lumen into two. These two processes have been recently described occurring together in lung, heart and yolk sac (Risau, 1997). A third process (Figure 5.1*c*) has also been described in which longitudinal splitting occurs in existing cardiac capillaries (van Groningen et al., 1991). As growth proceeds, enlarging capillaries are surrounded by both pericytes and contractile smooth muscle units. The process involved is termed 'pruning', as the resulting pattern resembles a tree. These new and more substantial vessels have the histological characteristics of arterioles. There is increasing evidence that embryological endothelial cells are comparatively plastic as far as differentiation is concerned, contrasting with those in mature adults with low turnover rates. Adult endothelium also exhibits age- and organ-specific markers not associated with embryonic endothelium (Risau, 1995). The promoting mechanisms for capillary expansion have been the subject of increasing research in the last 30 years.

Methods of studying angiogenesis

In vitro

Tissue cultures of endothelial cells from multiple sources have been available for years. They have been used to assess motility, migration and cell proliferation in response to mechanical stimuli and to substances with angiogenic potential. Tissue culture systems have the advantage that single factors can be varied and studied both as regards the culture substratum and added angiogenic factors. They are a useful technique for manipulating cellular receptors and signalling mechanisms associated with angiogenesis.

In vitro models of capillary formation have been used to study endothelial cell growth in matrix-containing gels, or tubule formation in two dimensions (Bischoff, 1995). Endothelial cells become quiescent and it has been suggested that this represents the terminal stages of angiogenesis (Kubota et al., 1988). Another model has been developed from rat aortic fragments invading fibrin- or collagen-containing gel, and this model allows tube formation to be studied (Nicosia and Madri, 1987). The disadvantage of tissue cultures is that they oversimplify the complexity of in vivo interactions, and the phenotype of the cultured cell is often very different to that which they are thought to represent. Models of angiogenesis in live animals and humans have been devised to parallel the work with in vitro studies.

In vivo

A long-established and popular choice for the in vivo study of angiogenesis has been the chicken chorioallantoic membrane (CAM) accessed at a week of incubation through a shell window. Substances under scrutiny have then been applied to the surface. Similar models exist for the normally avascular rabbit or rat cornea. Models of observation chambers in rabbit ear, hamster dorsal skin fold and human skin transplanted on to severe combined immunodeficiency (SCID) mice have been used to assess wound healing and regeneration in response to local and systemic applications (Bischoff, 1995; Brooks et al., 1995). The strength of these models lies in coordination of the physiology of complex angiogenic processes.

In situ

The technique of in situ study started over 80 years ago with the observation by Clark (1918) that velocity of blood flow determined the progression and regression in the tadpole tail. Combined with electron microscopy, intravital studies were used by Rhodin and Fujita (1989) to observe the growth of the mesenteric microcirculation in postnatal rats. Intravital models have also been used to study capillary growth in tumours. The main use for this type of study has been to determine the importance of mechanical factors in the initiation of angiogenesis, such as the estimation of wall shear stress and tension.

Larger vessel growth has been studied using techniques that identify structural features of the vasculature such as angiography, vascular casts, histological sectioning with vascular stains and labelling. Increases in maximum vascular conductance (maximal blood flow/blood pressure) have been used to quantify arteriole and conduit artery growth as the capillary bed exerts little resistance to flow. In ischaemic myocardium there is a correlation between the increase in arteriolar density and cross-sectional area and rise in maximum conductance with time (White and Bloor, 1992).

Quantification of angiogenesis

Capillary supply can be estimated from histological sections stained for basement membranes with periodic acid–Schiff/amylase, silver methenamine or with antibodies against laminin, fibronectin and type IV collagen. The enzymatic markers alkaline phosphatase, adenosine triphosphatase (ATPase) and carbonic anhydrase are all variable in their staining and are therefore unreliable.

In human tissue, antibodies to CD34 and von Willebrand factor are reliable methods for staining endothelial cells. They are used clinically along with [^{3}H]-

thymidine, a marker of nuclear division, to assess proliferation and therefore act as a prognostic indicator. The lectin *Ulex europeaus* has been used to stain sugar residues of human endothelial surface glycoproteins.

Quantification of vessel growth, as assessed by change in vessel counts per unit cross-sectional area, is affected by any increase/decrease of the other tissue on the section.

Mediators of angiogenesis and antiangiogenesis

Mechanical

Physical forces, such as exposure to cold, turbulent blood flow, wall shear stress, capillary wall tension, changes in peripheral resistance, capillary pressure, vessel diameter and red cell velocity, have all been implicated in angiogenesis. These forces have been extensively studied in vitro and it is thought that they cause changes in the endothelial cytoskeleton and the extracellular matrix, thus facilitating endothelial cell migration.

Intermediary cytokines (such as prostaglandins and nitric oxide (NO)) are released in vitro by endothelial cells, in response to increased shear stress and may be the effectors. Inhibitors of these cytokines block endothelial growth and migration in vitro.

A single bout of exercise increases the mRNA for vascular endothelial growth factor (VEGF: Breen et al., 1996). In trained subjects this response is attenuated and they have been shown to have developed almost 20% more capillaries in their musculature. Increases in blood flow have some positive influence on capillary supply, as do hypoxia and shear stress. Arterioles can grow by capillary arterialization when some migrate towards capillaries, pericytes form smooth muscle cells or fibroblasts may form capillaries by changing into smooth muscle cells (Figure 5.2). After endurance training an increase in e-nitric oxide synthetase (eNOS) activity leads to a generalized increase in NO production. Dilatation of the affected vessels causes an increase in diameter and circumferential wall stress (Sun et al., 1994; Delp and Laughlin, 1997). In electrically stimulated muscle capillaries proliferate within 2 days and arterioles show growth by 7 days. The whole vascular bed increases within 7–14 days. The capillary increase is due to increased shear stress, NO production and prostaglandin influences, but arteriolar growth is thought to be due to increased wall tension.

Factors

There are increasing numbers of angiogenic factors being described in health and disease (Table 5.1), but there is no doubt that the most important of all are vascular endothelial growth factor (VEGF) and fibroblast growth factor (FGF).

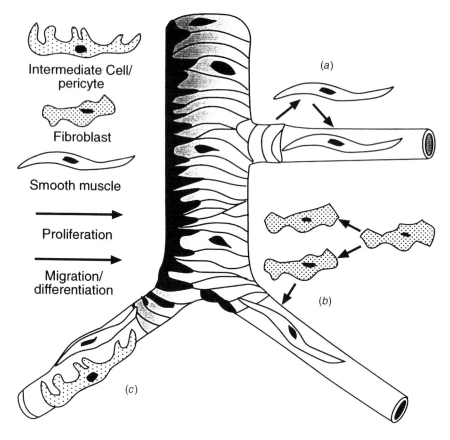

Intermediate Cell/
pericyte

Fibroblast

Smooth muscle

Proliferation

Migration/
differentiation

Figure 5.2   Capillary arterialization. Schematic representation of three possible means of capillary changes into arterioles. (A) 'Arterialization' of capillaries by migrating vascular smooth muscle cells from arterioles towards capillaries. (B) Formation of smooth muscle cells from fibroblasts and (C) from pericytes. Reproduced from Slalak and Price (1996), with permission.

There are now more than 18 different genes involved in mammalian FGFs (Hoshikawa et al., 1998) and the most important of these are FGF1 and FGF2 (also known as α-FGF and β-FGF). These stimulate cell proliferation, modulate differentiated function, delay senescence, inhibit apoptosis and are chemotactic. In vivo they are active in angiogenesis, nerve regeneration, cartilage repair and wound healing, although their inappropriate expression can also result in tumour development (Halaban et al., 1998). The finding that in vitro VEGF and FGF positively regulate many endothelial cellular functions, including proliferation migration, extracellular proteolytic activity and tube formation, has led to the concept that these factors are direct-acting positive regulators with membrane-bound receptors

Table 5.1 Factors promoting or inhibiting angiogenesis based on in vitro studies

Promoters of angiogenesis	Inhibitors of angiogenesis
Angiogenin	Angiostatin
EGF/TGF-α	C-X-C chemokines:
FGFs-1, -2, -5	Platelet factor IV
G-CSF	IP-10, gro-β
HGF	Hyaluronan
Hyaluronan oligosaccharides	IL-12
Hypoxia	Interferons
IL-8	MMP and PA inhibitors
PDGF-BB	16 kDa prolactin fragment
PlGF	Proliferin-related protein
Proliferin	Steroids/metabolites:
Prostaglandins	Glucocorticoids
TGF-β	2-Methoxyestradiol
Tissue factor	Retinoids
TNF-α	Ribonuclease inhibitor
VEGFs	TGF-β
	Thrombospondin
	TNF-α

EGF, endothelial growth factor; TGF-α, transforming growth factor-α; FGFs, fibroblast growth factors; G-CSF, granulocyte colony-stimulating factor; HGF, hepatocyte growth factor; IL-8, interleukin-8; MMP, matrix metalloproteinases; PA, plasminogen activator; PDGF-BB, platelet-derived growth factor BB; PLGF, placental growth factor; TNF-α, tumour necrosis factor-α; VEGFs, vascular endothelial growth factors.

(Dvorak et al., 1995). However, although a role for VEGF in developmental and tumour angiogenesis has been clearly established, much controversy still exists as to whether the FGFs are relevant to the endogenous control of neovascularization in vivo. Experimentally, many factors appear to be active but this does not mean that they are relevant to the endogenous regulation of new vessel formation in the intact organism. In the case of molecules that are active during the phase of endothelial activation, only VEGF meets most criteria for the definition of avasculogenic or angiogenic factor. These other factors may act indirectly on endothelial cells by inducing the production of direct-acting regulators by inflammatory and other nonendothelial cells. In contrast to the direct mitogens (VEGF and FGF), transforming growth factor (TGF-β) and tissue necrosis factor (TNF-α) inhibit endothelial growth in vitro and have therefore been considered as direct-acting negative regulators. In vivo TGF-β and TNF-α are found to be angiogenic by indirectly stimulating the production of direct-acting positive regulators from stromal and chemo-attracted inflammatory cells (Klagsbrun and D'Amore, 1991).

Other cytokines that have been reported to regulate angiogenesis in vivo include hepatocyte growth factor (HGF), EGF/TGF-α, platelet-derived growth factor (PDGF-BB), interleukins (IL-1, IL-6, IL-12), interferons, granulocyte colony-stimulating factor (G-CSF), placental growth factor (PlGF), proliferin and proliferin-related protein. Chemokines that regulate angiogenesis in vivo have to date only been found in the -C-X-C- family and include IL-8, platelet factor IV and gro-β. Angiogenesis can also be regulated by a variety of noncytokine or non-chemokine factors, including the enzymes (angiogenin and platelet-derived endothelial cell growth factor/thymidine phosphorylase (PD-ECGF/TP)), inhibitors of matrix-degrading proteolytic enzymes (tissue inhibitors of meta Hoproteinases: TIMPs) and of plasminogen activators and their inhibitors (PAs and PAIs), extracellular matrix components/coagulation factors or fragments thereof (thrombospondin, angiostatin, hyaluronan and its oligosaccharides), soluble cytokine receptors, prostaglandins, adipocyte lipids and copper ions (Leek et al., 1994).

Among the molecules that are relevant to cell–extracellular matrix interactions are integral membrane proteins, including integrins, which provide a link between the extracellular matrix and the cytoskeleton, and extracellular proteases and their inhibitors, which mediate focal degradation of the extracellular matrix during cellular invasion. One particular integrin, $\alpha_v\beta_3$, has been shown to be particularly important during angiogenesis. It is expressed on vascular endothelial cells preferentially during the proliferative and invasive phases of angiogenesis, once cytokine activation has occurred. $\alpha_v\beta_3$ is a receptor for a number of proteins with an exposed Arg-Gly-Asp subunit, including vitronectin, fibronectin, fibrinogen, laminin, thrombospondin, osteopontin, and von Willebrand factor. The integrin $\alpha_v\beta_3$ is also expressed by smooth muscle cells in postangioplasty restenosis, atherosclerotic plaques and healing arterial wounds (Varner et al., 1996), and is also upregulated in human tumour growth in explants on SCID mice. Antagonists to $\alpha_v\beta_3$ appear to inhibit angiogenesis during development (Brooks et al., 1994), wound healing (Clark et al., 1996), retinal neovascularization (Hammes et al., 1996), and in certain tumour growth causes apoptosis experimentally, thereby inducing regression (Brooks et al., 1995). Many proteases and protease blockers are active during basement membrane degradation, extracellular matrix invasion and capillary loop formation.

Physiological and pathological angiogenesis

The process of angiogenesis must be maintained in a constant state of readiness over long periods of time, in a balance similar to blood coagulation. The microvascular system seems to be quiescent without capillary growth. Endothelial cell turnover in the normal healthy adult is low, apart from angiogenesis associated with the female reproductive organs or in response to tissue injury. The maintenance of endothelial quiescence is thought to be due to the presence of endogenous negative inhibitors suppressing positive regulators. Activation of endothelium is therefore a balance between negative and positive regulators, with angiogenesis occurring when the positive regulators predominate. Angiogenesis has a role in many normal physiological processes such as wound healing, inflammation and reproduction. The concept of the 'angiogenic switch' is applicable in both physiological and pathological angiogenesis.

Table 5.2 lists both the diseases and the areas of specialization that involve angiogenesis as part of the pathological pathway. Wound repair and healing apply to all categories and are therefore not included in the table. It is becoming increasingly apparent that the dominant pathology in many nonneoplastic diseases is as a result of persistent angiogenesis and its consequences. Angiogenesic diseases occur in both men and women and are managed in many branches of medicine and surgery.

Gene therapy and its current application to angiogenesis

Gene therapy can be defined as the transfer of genetic material to prevent or treat a disease. Based on the ever-increasing quantity of published experimental evidence, multiple groups are starting to apply the principles of gene therapy to angiogenesis in the clinical setting.

The first step of this genetic transfer is to isolate the gene that encodes the protein of interest; this is done by extracting mRNA from cultured cells and converting the mRNA into DNA by reverse transcription. This mixture of DNA, called a cDNA library, is therefore screened to identify the cDNA fragments that match the amino acid sequence of the desired protein. The fragment is then inserted into a plasmid expression vector and linked to a sequence, a promoter, that initiates transcription of the gene (Figure 5.3). The technology of genetic engineering has for some time therefore run parallel to angiogenesis research. We are entering an exciting era as the two fields are combined and we are beginning to see the potential of gene therapy being applied to disorders of angiogenesis. Whether transfer is best effected using gene transfer or polypeptide transfer is not yet clear. Nor is it certain which will have the fewest long-term side-effects. With

Table 5.2 Pathological disease processes involving angiogenesis by medical specialty

Medical specialty	Disease process
Cardiology	Myocardial ischaemia/infarction, myocardial hypertrophy
Dermatology	Haemangiomas and other benign vascular proliferations, pyogenic granuloma, squamous cell carcinoma, malignant melanoma, psoriasis
Ear, nose and throat surgery	Leukoplakia, squamous and nasopharyngeal carcinoma
Endocrinology	Diabetes mellitus (proliferative retinopathy and vascular complications)
Gastroenterology	Carcinoma of the oesophagus, stomach, colon, liver and pancreas; peptic ulcer; intestinal ischaemia
Haematology	Leukaemia, lymphoma, multiple myeloma
Infectious diseases	AIDS (Kaposi's sarcoma)
Neurology/neurosurgery	Vascular malformations, cerebral ischaemia/infarction, capillary haemangioblastoma, glial tumours
Obstetrics and gynaecology	Normal reproductive function and infertility; carcinoma of breast, cervix, uterus and ovary
Oncology	Overlaps with virtually all other disciplines
Ophthalmology	Proliferative retinopathy, retinopathy of prematurity, age-related macular degeneration
Paediatrics	Juvenile haemangioma, childhood tumours
Respiratory medicine	Capillary haemangiomas, pulmonary adeno- and small-cell carcinoma
Rheumatology/orthopaedics	Inflammatory arthritis, bone fracture repair and nonunion, Paget's disease, osteosarcoma
Urology	Carcinoma of kidney, prostate and testis
Vascular surgery	Peripheral ischaemia, vascular malformations

AIDS, acquired immunodeficiency syndrome.

the use of gene therapy techniques in early trials, various disease processes are now being treated by promoting or inhibiting angiogenesis. The first application of this new technology involving patients occurred in 1989 when α-interferon was used for the treatment of life-threatening pulmonary haemangiomas in infants (Folkman, 1989; White et al., 1989). The first gene therapy trial attempted in humans was performed in 1990 for sufferers of adenosine deaminase (ADA) deficiency and published 5 years later (Blaese et al., 1995). Listed in Table 5.3 are the clinical fields where angiogenesis technology is currently being investigated.

Following the initial success of the ADA trial, more than 100 clinical gene therapy trials have been initiated, and a proportion of these have been concerned

Table 5.3 Clinical manipulation of angiogenesis currently being explored

Promotion of angiogenesis	Inhibition of angiogenesis
Induction of collateral vessel formation:	Tumour growth and metastases
Myocardial ischaemia	Ocular neovascularization
Peripheral ischaemia	Haemangioma
Cerebral ischaemia	Rheumatoid arthritis
Wound healing and fracture repair	Atherosclerotic plaque neovascularization
Reconstructive surgery including skin flaps	Birth control
Transplantation of islets of Langerhans	

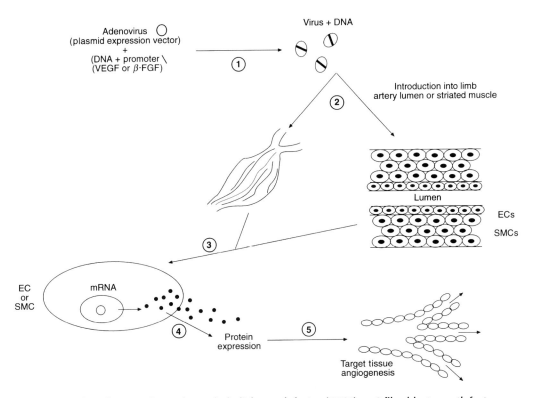

Figure 5.3   Cloned cDNA of vascular endothelial growth factor (VEGF) or β-fibroblast growth factor (β-FGF) combined with a promoter sequence of DNA, are spliced into an adenovirus acting as a vector (1). These are introduced into a limb artery lumen by infusion or on the surface of an angioplasty balloon (2), or into striated limb muscle directly. Distal endothelial cells (EC) or smooth muscle cells (SMC) are transfected by the adenovirus (3), leading to expression of VEGF or β-FGF (4), ultimately inducing angiogenesis (5).

with cardiovascular surgical disease. Gene therapy applications have been explored in restenosis, critical limb ischaemia and graft failure.

Ischaemic heart disease

The first animal models of gene therapy and angiogenesis in ischaemic myocardium used β-FGF. Yanagisawa-Miwa et al. (1992) showed that β-FGF given intraarterially at the time of coronary occlusion and 6 h later reduced the total volume of myocardial infarction. In models of chronic myocardial ischaemia Unger et al. (1994) and Harada et al. (1994) found increased collateral flow and improved myocardial function respectively following the administration of β-FGF. Later, Takeshita et al. (1994) reported using phVEGF$_{165}$ coated on angioplasty balloons which were passed percutaneously into the iliac arteries of rabbits (with previously tied common femoral arteries) and inflated. An improvement in ischaemic blood pressure in the phVEGF$_{165}$-treated group suggested that site-specific arterial gene transfer could be used to achieve physiologically meaningful therapeutic modulation of vascular disorders.

Many patients with ischaemic heart disease are not suitable for conventional bypass procedures or percutaneous revascularization due to the complex nature of the restricting lesions. Therapeutic angiogenesis therefore provides a novel treatment option. Outlined below are the details of one of the first therapeutic trials that followed preliminary trials in rats (Schumacher et al., 1998). β-FGF was genetically engineered from strains of *Escherichia coli* which were isolated and purified. The β-FGF was then injected close to the vessels after completion of coronary artery bypass in 20 patients who had significant disease distal to the anastomoses. Later, angiographic proof of neovascularization was obtained. A capillary network was demonstrated sprouting from the proximal part of the coronary artery and bypassing the stenoses to rejoin the distal parts of the vessel. In the same year direct myocardial injection of phVEGF$_{165}$ was described via a minimally invasive chest wall incision in 5 patients (Losordo et al., 1998). These authors' results suggested improved symptoms as measured by reduced nitrate usage and also improved myocardial perfusion studies and by coronary angiography.

Peripheral vascular disease

Chronic lower-limb ischaemia due to atherosclerosis (Figure 5.4) often ends in amputation. Despite bypass surgery or interventional radiological procedures, the progression of the occlusive arterial exhausts conventional therapy. During the last 10 years many animal models of hind-limb ischaemia have been developed as part of the lead-up to human trials of angiogenic factors. The angiogenic growth

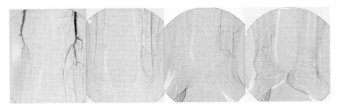

Figure 5.4   Angiogram of severe bilateral lower limb atherosclerosis.

factors first used for this purpose comprised members of the FGF family. In a rabbit model (Baffour et al., 1992), β-FGF was administered in daily intramuscular doses. At the completion of 14 days' treatment, angiography and necropsy measurement of capillary density showed evidence of augmented collateral vessels in the ischaemic limb compared to controls. Using α-FGF in a similar model of rabbit hind-limb ischaemia, Pu et al. (1993) produced improved haemodynamic as well as collateral development in the treated group compared to controls.

In the first published report of arterial gene transfer of naked DNA encoding for VEGF in the presence of limb ischaemia (Isner et al., 1996), a 71-year-old woman had 2000 μg human plasmid phVEGF$_{165}$ administered via a coated angioplasty balloon inflated in the popliteal artery. Subsequent digital subtraction angiography at 4 weeks showed an increase of collateral vessel formation below the knee with symptomatic improvement to match. Three spider angiomas arose in the limb: one was excised 3 weeks after therapy, confirming proliferating endothelium, and the other two were observed to regress. Figure 5.3 is a flow diagram illustrating the basic principles of angiogenesis with an introduced virus acting as the vector. These first attempts at direct intraarterial balloon transfer have been hard to reproduce. In 1997 a small series was reported by the same group using intramuscular injections (Baumgartner et al., 1997). In this series, 9 patients received intramuscular injections of naked plasmid DNA encoding phVEGF$_{165}$ and described improved ankle–brachial index. They reported angiographic evidence of increased collateral vessels in seven limbs, ulcer healing and limb salvage in patients otherwise destined for amputation. In one amputation specimen foci of proliferating endothelial cells were found. Transient lower-limb oedema was seen in over half of the patients: this is consistent with VEGF enhancement of vascular permeability.

The possibility of viruses being used as vectors has been suggested by a report of 10 Finnish patients with impending amputations who had angioplasty balloon transfer of adenovirus-mediated genetic markers a few days prior to amputation (Laitinen et al., 1998). After amputation, transgene expression was detected in smooth muscle cells, endothelial cells, macrophages and in the tunica adventitia of arteries.

Other clinical problems that may benefit from therapeutic angiogenesis in the

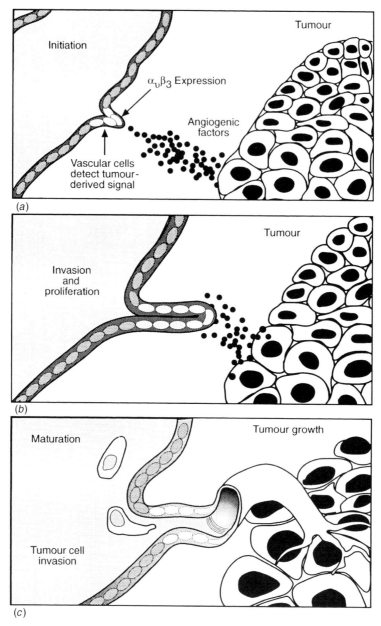

Figure 5.5   Tumour-induced angiogenesis. Angiogenesis can generally be divided into three phases, shown here in tumour-induced angiogenesis. Firstly, angiogenic stimulators, such as β-fibroblast growth factor (β-FGF) and vascular endothelial growth factor (VEGF) are released from the tumour and/or inflammatory cells. These angiogenic signals trigger the invasion/proliferation phase which is characterized by vascular cell proliferation, secretion of proteolytic enzymes and extracellular matrix molecules, as well as altered expression of adhesion molecules. The proteolytic enzymes act to degrade extracellular membrane (ECM) proteins, which, together with new synthesis of ECM molecules, results in

near future include cerebral ischaemia, improved survival of free and pedicle skin flaps and transplantation of islets of Langerhans, as suggested by work on a rat model (Gorden et al., 1997). No clinical trials in humans have yet been reported, but based on the success of animal models, this cannot be far away.

Tumour treatment and the inhibition of angiogenesis

New vessel formation is essential for tumour growth (Figure 5.5). Initiation of vessel growth is controlled by factors released by the tumour (e.g. β-FGF, TGF-α, VEGF) which diffuse towards blood vessels, triggering proliferation and invasion. The endothelial cells secrete components of the extracellular membrane (ECM) and altered adhesion molecules. Proteolytic enzymes degrade the ECM and the environment is gradually remodelled. Endothelial cells invade the remodelled ECM and proliferate, forming a sprout. Adhesive property changes of the vascular cells allow proliferation and invasion. With maturation, endothelial cells change shape and a new basement membrane is formed. The new vessel thus formed provides the tumour with nutrients and allows metastatic cells to invade the body elsewhere.

Both de novo collagen synethesis and proteolysis are involved in tumour angiogenesis. It is possible that elimination of a quiescence signal in the basement membrane or the breakdown of stromal collagen may lead to later changes in the basement membrane, facilitating differentiation. Matrix metalloproteinase-2 (MMP-2) and $\alpha_v\beta_3$ are located on the surface of invasive angiogenic vascular (and melanoma) cells in vivo; and $\alpha_v\beta_3$ agonists and TIMPs can block angiogenesis in vivo. It is possible that MMP-2 and $\alpha_v\beta_3$ functionally cooperate to promote vascular cell invasive behaviour. Invasion of melanoma cells can be inhibited by a natural fragment of MMP-2 (called PEX), and this may be a natural tumour-inhibiting feedback mechanism.

There is good evidence that VEGF and its receptors are crucial in tumour angiogenesis (Dvorak et al., 1995). There are many groups now publishing data describing strategies aimed at inhibiting tumour growth by interfering with cytokine–receptor interactions, including anti-VEGF antibodies, soluble VEGF receptors, antisense VEGF, VEGF-toxin conjugate, and a dominant negative

Caption for Fig. 5.5 (*cont.*)

remodelling of the extracellular microenvironment. The remodelling is crucial since it serves to facilitate vascular cell survival, proliferation and migration, resulting in a vascular invasion of the ECM. The maturation stage involves shape changes of the endothelial cells to achieve the final differentiated luminal structure in contact with a newly synthesized basement membrane. Reproduced from Stromblad and Cheresh (1996) with permission of the authors.

approach using a truncated form of VEGF receptor-2. VEGF therefore seems to have a potential key role in tumour growth suppression, with the important advantage that it seems to have only one target cell, namely, the endothelial cell. Angiostatin has been shown to be a potent angiogenesis inhibitor in vitro. Angiostatin is an internal cleavage product of plasminogen and is now shown to inhibit the growth of a number of tumours in immunoincompetent mice (O'Reilly et al., 1994). The marked increase in tumour cell apoptosis associated with angiostatin became an exponential phase of tumour growth once angiostatin administration was halted and angiogenesis could recommence. This observation suggests that either prolonged and repeated administration of angiostatin may have potential as a therapeutic strategy, or angiostatin could be used in conjunction with other forms of cancer therapy.

Other situations where antiangiogenesis therapy has been successful include juvenile haemangioma, experimental arthritis and proliferative retinopathy, in which interferon-α and thalidomide have been tested (Folkman, 1995). It is uncertain whether the therapeutic effect of interferon-α in childhood haemangioma regression is as a result of a direct antiangiogenic effect on endothelial cells or as an indirect consequence of the reduction of angiogenic factor production by stromal cells (Pepper et al., 1994).

The future of therapeutic angiogenesis and antiangiogenesis

Knowledge of angiogenesis has developed over 30 years, but only in the last few years have therapeutic applications of this technology been explored. Clinical groups have begun to develop treatments aimed at promoting thrombolysis, preventing restenosis after angioplasty and improving the blood supply to ischaemic myocardium and pregangrenous limbs. In oncology, malignant tumours depend on capillary neovascularization and this suggests that new forms of cancer treatment may be devised by inhibiting angiogenesis, perhaps in conjunction with use of conventional cytotoxics.

The therapeutic manipulation of angiogenesis may fall into two forms: firstly, through the use of single or multiple doses of a recombinant protein and, secondly, with the development of gene transfer technology. The factors that may ultimately determine which of these predominates are cost, clinical effectiveness and the avoidance of side-effects. With the reporting of the first trials of angiogenic gene therapy, complications and pitfalls are already coming to light. Recombinant polypeptide use is easier because dose regulation enables the range of efficacy to be balanced against toxicity. If toxicity occurs, it would also be easier to stop or block polypeptide therapy. Against use of polypeptides is the difficulty in producing sufficient quantities of pyrogen-free agents, and the requirement of repeated treatments or a prolonged infusion. In contrast, gene therapy involves the introduction of genetic material into cells aimed at achieving high levels of sustained gene expression without provoking adverse clinical reactions. Restricting the therapeutic effects of gene therapy to the required site (without angiogenic or antiangiogenic effects occurring at ectopic sites) will be an important long-term factor in determining whether or not gene transfer technology is acceptable. Side-effects of antiangiogenesis therapy, including those related to inhibition of physiological angiogenesis, are likely to cause problems, as will the unwanted effects seen with stimulation of angiogenesis.

The best mode of delivery of angiogenic stimuli has not yet been found. There are now trials under way looking at intramuscular as opposed to intravascular depots of angiogenic agents in the treatment of ischaemic heart disease and distal limb ischaemia. With intravascular depots the delivery is dependent on balloon catheter technology. There are three types of balloon currently being used: hydrogel-coated, perforated and double occlusion balloons.

The use of adenoviruses as opposed to retroviruses appears a more efficient vector. There is a lower risk of incorporation into the host genome or reversion to a wild type which is capable of replication. Nonviral vectors that are currently being developed include cationic liposomes and synthetic peptides.

It may be possible to create angiogenesis profiles of patients for conditions with an angiogenesis basis. This could include quantitative histological assessment of tissue in disease processes where blood vessel density secondary to angiogenesis may be an important prognostic indicator, as in breast cancer (Weidner, 1995). Clearly, the blood supply of any metastatic cancer is central to tumour progression and spread, so knowing the angiogenic properties of that metastatic tumour could allow antiangiogenic strategies to be targeted at individual patients. For example, urinary β-FGF may serve as a prognostic indicator for certain solid tumours, and β-FGF urine levels are reduced following surgical resection of the tumour (Nguyen et al., 1994).

There is increasing evidence of a genetic basis to the pathogenesis of certain vascular disorders (Shovlin and Scott, 1996) through disordered angiogenesis. Mutations in endothelial cell receptor tyrosine kinases may underlie developmental vascular malformations and may also play a role in the development of haemangiomas. Possible gene loci for an autosomal-dominant form of venous malformation (Boon et al., 1994) and for Klippel–Trenaunay–Weber syndrome (Whelan et al., 1995) have been identified. What are claimed to be progenitor endothelial cells have been isolated (Asahara et al., 1997) and these may be useful for augmenting collateral vessel growth to ischaemic tissues (therapeutic angiogenesis) and for delivering antiangiogenic agents to sites of pathological angiogenesis.

Gene therapy may also have a role in the related vascular problem of arterial restenosis (along with radiation brachytherapy) after angioplasty. Arterial restenosis involves the migration of activated smooth muscle cells from the arterial media to form a neointima. Using gene therapy, it may be possible to generate a biological attack on the cell-regulatory mechanisms by the introduction of foreign-fragment nuclear material to halt the pathophysiological processes typical of restenosis. This block in theory could be delivered locally as a coating on the angioplasty balloon itself. Graft stenosis secondary to neointimal hyperplasia may be avoidable by the genetic manipulation of cells lining the grafts: this was first investigated in a canine model by Wilson et al. (1989).

Novel gene therapy and pharmacological approaches are continuously being developed both to stimulate and inhibit angiogenesis. This is happening at a rapid pace. It is important that new clinical protocols are backed by sound scientific scrutiny as this new technology may have potentially devastating long-term consequences for young patients being treated in a new field of medicine. As the technology of angiogenesis is relevant to so many disciplines within medicine, it is appropriate that molecular biologists with expertise in gene therapy are closely involved in the management of patients. A close working relationship between clinicians and scientists will help ensure that future clinical applications are developed as quickly and safely as possible.

REFERENCES

Asahara, T., Murohara, T., Sullivan, A. et al. (1997). Isolation of putative endothelial cells for angiogenesis. *Science*, **275**, 964–7.

Baffour, R., Berman, J., Garb, J.L. et al. (1992). Enhanced angiogenesis and growth of collaterals by in vivo administration of recombinant basic fibroblast growth factor in a rabbit model of acute lower limb ischaemia: dose–response effect of basic fibroblast growth factor. *J. Vasc. Surg.*, **16**, 181–91.

Baumgartner, I., Pieczek, A., Manor, O. et al. (1997). Constitutive expression of phVEGF$_{165}$ after intramuscular gene transfer promotes collateral vessel development in patients with critical limb ischaemia. *Circulation*, **97**, 1114–23.

Bischoff, J. (1995). Approaches to studying cell adhesion molecules in angiogenesis. *Trends Cell. Biol.*, **5**, 69–74.

Blaese, R.M., Culver, K.W. & Miller, A.D. (1995). T-lymphocyte directed gene therapy for ADA-SCID: initial trial results after 4 years. *Science*, **270**, 475–80.

Boon, L.M., Mulliken, J.B., Vikkula, M. et al. (1994). Assignment of a locus for dominantly inherited venous malformations to chromosome 9p. *Hum. Mol. Genet.*, **3**, 1583–7.

Breen, E.C., Johnson, E.C., Wagner, H. et al. (1996). Angiogenic growth factor mRNA responses in muscle to a single bout of exercise. *J. Appl. Physiol*, **81**, 355–61.

Brooks, P.C., Clark, R.A.F. & Cheresh, D.A. (1994). Requirement of vascular integrin $\alpha_v\beta_3$ for angiogenesis. *Science*, **264**, 569–71.

Brooks, P.C., Strömblad, S., Klemke, R. et al. (1995). Anti-integrin $\alpha_v\beta_3$ blocks human breast cancer growth and angiogenesis in human skin. *J. Clin. Invest.*, **96**, 1815–22.

Burri, P.H. & Tarek, M.R. (1990). A novel mechanism of capillary growth in the rat pulmonary circulation. *Anat. Record*, **228**, 35–45.

Clark, E.R. (1918). Studies on the growth of blood vessels in the tail of a frog. *Am. J. Anat.*, **23**, 37–88.

Clark, R.A.F., Tonnesen, M.G., Gailit, J. & Cheresh, D.A. (1996). Transient functional expression of $\alpha_v\beta_3$ on vascular cells during wound repair. *Am. J. Pathol.*, **148**, 1407–21.

Delp, M.M. & Laughlin, M.H. (1997). Time course of enhanced endothelium-mediated dilatation in the aorta of trained rats. *Med. Sci. Sports Exerc.*, **29**, 1454–61.

Dvorak, H.F., Brown, L.F., Detmar, M. & Dvorak, A.M. (1995). Vascular permeability factor/vascular endothelial growth factor, microvascular hyper-permeability, and angiogenesis. *Am. J. Pathol.*, **146**, 1029–39.

Folkman, J. (1989). Successful treatment of an angiogenic disease. *N. Engl. J. Med.*, **320**, 1211–12.

Folkman, J. (1995). Clinical applications of research on angiogenesis. *N. Engl. J. Med.*, **333**, 1757–63.

Gorden, D.L., Mandriota, S.J., Montesano, R., Orci, L. & Pepper, M.S. (1997). Vascular endothelial growth factor is increased in devascularised rat islets of Langerhans in vitro. *Transplantation*, **63**, 436–43.

Halaban, R., Kwon, B., Ghosh, S., Delli Bovi, P. & Baird, A. (1998). βFGF as an autocrine growth factor for human melanomas. *Oncogene Res.*, **3**, 177–86.

Hammes, H-P., Brownlee, M., Jonczyk, A., Sutter, A. & Preissner, K.T. (1996). Subcutaneous injection of a cyclic peptide antagonist of vitronectin receptor-type integrins inhibit retinal neovascularisation. *Nature Med.*, **2**, 529–33.

Harada, K., Grossmann, W., Friedman, M. et al. (1994). Basic fibroblast growth factor improves myocardial function in chronically ischaemic porcine hearts. *J. Clin, Invest.*, **94**, 623–30.

Hoshikawa, M., Ohbayashi, N., Yonamine, A. et al. (1998). Structure and expression of a novel fibroblast growth factor, FGF17, preferentially expressed in the embryonic brain. *Biochem. Biophys. Res. Commun.*, **244**, 187–91.

Hudlická, O. & Tyler, K.R. (1986). *Angiogenesis. The Growth of the Vascular System.* London: Academic Press.

Isner, J.M., Pieczek, A., Schainfeld, R. et al. (1996). Clinical evidence of angiogenesis after arterial gene transfer of phVEGF$_{165}$ in patient with ischaemic limb. *Lancet*, **348**, 370–4.

Klagsbrun, M. & D'Amore, P.A. (1991). Regulators of angiogenesis. *Annu. Rev. Physiol.*, **53**, 217–39.

Kubota, Y., Kleinman, H.K., Martin, G.R. & Lawley, T.J. (1988). Role of laminin and basement membrane in the morphological differentiation of human endothelial cells into capillary-like structures. *J. Cell. Biol.*, **107**, 1589–98.

Laitinen, M., Mäkinen, K., Manninen, H. et al. (1998). Adenovirus-mediated gene transfer to lower limb artery of patients with chronic critical leg ischaemia. *Hum. Gene Ther.*, **9**, 1481–6.

Leek, R.D., Harris, A.L. & Lewis, C.E. (1994). Cytokine networks in solid human tumours: regulation of angiogenesis. *J. Leukoc. Biol.*, **56**, 423–35.

Losordo, D.W., Vale, P.R., Symes, J.F. et al. (1998). Gene therapy for myocardial angiogenesis: initial clinical results with direct myocardial injection of phVEGF$_{165}$ as sole therapy for myocardial ischaemia *Circulation*, **98**, 2800–4.

Nguyen, M., Watanabe, H., Budson, A.E. et al. (1994). Elevated levels of the angiogenic peptide, basic fibroblast growth factor, in urine of patients with a wide spectrum of cancers. *J. Natl Cancer Inst.*, **86**, 356–61.

Nicosia, R.F. & Madri, J.A. (1987). The microvascular extracellular matrix. Developmental changes during angiogenesis in the aortic ring-plasma clot model. *Am. J. Pathol.*, **128**, 78–90.

O'Reilly, M.S., Holmgren, L., Shing, Y. et al. (1994). Angiostatin: a novel angiogenesis inhibitor that mediates the suppression of metastases by a Lewis lung carcinoma. *Cell*, **79**, 315–28.

Pepper, M.S., Vassalli, J-D., Wilks, J.W. et al. (1994). Modulation of bovine microvascular endothelial cell proteolytic properties by inhibitors of angiogenesis. *J. Cell. Biochem.*, **55**, 419–34.

Pu, L-Q., Sniderman, A.D., Brassard, R. et al. (1993). Enhanced revascularisation of the ischaemic limb by means of angiogenic therapy. *Circulation*, **88**, 208–15.

Rhodin, J.A.G. & Fujita, H. (1989). Capillary growth in the mesentery of normal young rats. *J. Submicrosc. Cytol. Pathol.*, **21**, 1–34.

Risau, W. (1995). Differentiation of endothelium. *FASEB J.*, **9**, 926–33.

Risau, W. (1997). Mechanisms of angiogenesis. *Nature*, **386**, 671–4.

Schumacher, B., Pecher, P., von Specht, B.U. & Stegmann, T. (1998). Induction of neoangiogenesis in ischaemic myocardium by human growth factor. *Circulation*, **97**, 645–50.

Shovlin, C.L. & Scott, J. (1996). Inherited diseases of the vasculature. *Annu. Rev. Physiol.*, **58**, 483–507.

Slalak, T.C. & Price, R.J. (1996). Mechanical stresses in microvascular remodelling. *Microcirculation*, **3**, 143–165.

Stromblad, S. & Cheresh, D.A. (1996). Cell adhesion and angiogenesis. *Trends Cell. Biol.*, **6**, 462–8.

Sun, D., Huang, A., Koller, A. & Kaley, G. (1994). Short-term daily exercise activity enhances endothelial NO synthesis in skeletal muscle arterioles of rats. *J. Appl. Physiol.*, **76**, 2241–7.

Takeshita, S., Zheng, L. P., Brogi, E. et al. (1994). Therapeutic angiogenesis: a single intra-arterial bolus of vascular endothelial growth factor augments revascularisation in a rabbit ischaemic hindlimb model. *J. Clin. Invest.*, **93**, 662–70.

Unger, E.F., Banai, S., Shou, M. et al. (1994). Basic fibroblast growth factor enhances myocardial collateral flow in a canine model. *Am. J. Physiol.*, **266** (*Heart Circ. Physiol.*, 35) H1588–95.

Van Groningen, J.P., Weninck, A.C. & Testers, L.H. (1991). Myocardial capillaries increase in number by splitting of existing vessels. *Acta Embryol.*, **184**, 65–70.

Varner, J.A., Brooks, P.C. & Cheresh, D.A. (1996). The integrin $\alpha_v\beta_3$: angiogenesis and apoptosis. *Cell Adhes. Commun.*, **264**, 367–74.

Weidner, N. (1995). Intratumour microvessel density as a prognostic factor in cancer. *Am. J. Pathol.*, **147**, 9–19.

Whelan, A.J., Watson, M.S., Porter, F.D. & Steiner, R.D. (1995). Klippel–Trénaunay–Weber syndrome associated with a 5;11 balanced translocation. *Am. J. Med. Genet.*, **59**, 492–4.

White, F.C. & Bloor, C.M. (1992). Coronary vascular remodeling and coronary resistance during chronic ischaemia. *Am. J. Cardiovasc. Pathol.*, **4**, 193–202.

White, C.W., Sonheimer, H.M., Crouch, E.C., Wilson, H. & Fan, L.L. (1989). Treatment of pulmonary haemangiomatosis with recombinant interferon alpha-2a. *N. Engl. J. Med.*, **320**, 1197–200.

Wilson, J.M., Birinyi, L.K., Salomon, R.N. et al. (1989). Implantation of vascular grafts lined with genetically modified endothelial cells. *Science*, **244**, 1344–6.

Yanagisawa-Miwa, A., Uchida, Y., Nakamura, F. et al. (1992). Salvage of infarcted myocardium by angiogenic action of basic fibroblast growth factor. *Science*, **257**, 1401–3.

6

The regulation of vascular smooth muscle cell apoptosis

Nicola J. McCarthy and Martin R. Bennett

Unit of Cardiovascular Medicine, Addenbrooke's Hospital, Cambridge

Introduction

Apoptosis or programmed cell death is a process through which multicellular organisms dispose of cells efficiently. Much has been discovered about the molecular control of apoptosis since its initial description as a series of morphological events (Kerr et al., 1972). The regulation of cell death is critical for the maintenance of tissue homeostasis. Moreover, it is apparent that all cells are programmed to die, and cell death is their default state, which can be suppressed through the expression or presence of intracellular and extracellular survival factors. Although it may seem strange that cells can be lost so easily from tissues, for long-lived multicellular organisms it makes biological sense to have an efficient cellular disposal mechanism, to remove useless or potentially harmful cells.

Apoptosis: defining the mode of cell death

Apoptosis defines a type of cell death distinct from conventional necrotic death, on the basis of characteristic morphological features (Figure 6.1). Specifically, these features are condensation of nuclear chromatin, at first around the inner face of the nuclear membrane, and then clumping of the chromatin. Apoptosis is also associated with loss of cell–cell contact and cell shrinkage and fragmentation, with formation of membrane-bound processes and vesicles containing fragments of nuclear material or organelles. The endproduct, the apoptotic body, may then be phagocytosed by adjacent cells (Figure 6.1). The whole process occurs with minimal disruption of membrane integrity or release of lysosomal enzymes, and consequently little inflammatory reaction. In addition, organelle structure and function appear to be maintained until late into the process.

Necrosis, however, is more commonly used to describe cell death characterized by cell swelling, without chromatin condensation. Moreover, organelle dysfunction occurs early in the process, accompanied by loss of membrane integrity, and

(a)   (b)

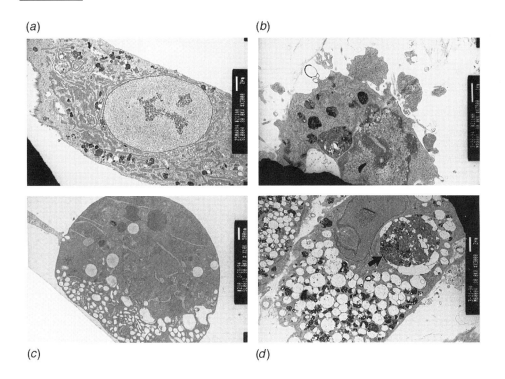

(c)   (d)

Figure 6.1   Electron microscopic appearances of a human vascular smooth muscle cell (VSMC)
             undergoing apoptosis in culture. (*a*) Normal appearance of a human VSMC. (*b*) Intense
             membrane blebbing and vesicle formation in apoptosis, with condensation of the nuclear
             chromatin into clumps. (*c*) An apoptotic body, the endproduct of apoptosis. (*d*) An
             apoptotic body (arrow) ingested by an adjacent human VSMC.

release of lysosomal enzymes with consequent inflammation.

Although the terms are frequently used synonymously, programmed cell death
and apoptosis are not completely interchangeable. They are morphologically and,
in some respects, genetically identical processes, but programmed cell death, in its
truest sense, is cell death occurring at defined times in embryogenesis. This is
clearly 'physiological' cell death that is initiated by a specific genetic programme.
In addition, programmed cell death can be considered to occur in adult organisms
during regression of a variety of hyperplastic tissues, in particular, the hormone-
dependent regression of breast or uterine tissues. Death in this instance is also a
physiological response, but the factor triggering death may be intrinsic or
exogenous, for example removal of a trophic stimulus. Within the vasculature,
true programmed cell death can be said to occur in closure of the ductus
arteriosus, and in many of the changes in vessel calibre and wall thickness which
occur as an adaptation to blood flow in the neonate (see below). In general,

programmed cell death is used to describe cell death observed during embryogenesis in both vertebrates and invertebrates and apoptosis describes death observed in adult tissues.

Cell proliferation and death in the vascular wall

Vascular smooth muscle cells (VSMCs) within the vessel wall are able to proliferate, migrate, synthesize and degrade extracellular matrix upon receiving appropriate stimuli. The normal adult artery shows very low levels of VSMC turnover, and apoptotic and mitotic indices are low in this tissue (Gordon et al., 1990). In diseased tissue additional factors are present both locally, such as inflammatory cytokines, inflammatory cells and the presence of modified cholesterol, and systematically, such as blood pressure and flow. These factors can substantially alter the normal balance of cell proliferation and apoptosis, although the degree to which they are altered is dependent upon the vascular disease under study.

Remodelling

Vessel wall remodelling defines a condition in which alterations in luminal size can occur through processes that do not necessarily require large changes in overall cell number or tissue mass. Thus, redistribution of cells, either towards or away from the lumen, through processes such as selective cell proliferation/apoptosis or matrix synthesis/degradation can significantly alter lumen dimensions. Physiological remodelling by cell proliferation/programmed cell death occurs in closure of the ductus arteriosus (Slomp et al., 1997), and reduction in lumen size of infraumbilical arteries after birth (Cho and Langille, 1993; Cho et al., 1995). Surgical reduction in flow also results in compensatory VSMC apoptosis (Cho et al., 1997; Kumar and Lindner, 1997). Remodelling also occurs in primary atherosclerosis, after angioplasty and in angioplasty restenosis. Although apoptosis undoubtedly occurs in all of these conditions (see below), the role of VSMC apoptosis in determining the outcome of remodelling is unclear.

Arterial injury

Acute arterial injury, such as that occurring at angioplasty, is followed by rapid induction of medial cell apoptosis, at least in animal models. Thus, in rat or rabbit vessels, balloon overstretch injury results in medial cell apoptosis from 30 min to 4 h after injury (Perlman et al., 1997; Pollman et al., 1998, 1999). In pigs, apoptotic cells occur within the media at 6 h with peaks in the media, adventitia and neointima at 18 h. 6 h and 7 days after balloon injury, respectively (Malik et al., 1998). Although we have no direct evidence, the consistency of this response in animal models suggests that human vessels may behave similarly. Repair of the vessel after injury is also associated with VSMC apoptosis, both in the media and in the intima, and in the rat occurs 8–21 days after injury (Bochaton-Piallat et al., 1995). In humans, restenosis after angioplasty has been reported to be associated with either an increase (Isner et al., 1995) or decrease (Bauriedel et al., 1998) in VSMC apoptosis. The role of VSMC apoptosis in either the initial injury or the remodelling process in restenosis is still unclear in human vessels.

Aneurysm formation

The commonest form of arterial aneurysm in humans is associated with advanced atherosclerosis, and is characterized by a loss of VSMCs from the vessel media, with fragmentation of elastin and matrix degradation, leading to progressive dilatation and eventually rupture. Apoptosis of VSMCs is increased in aortic aneurysms (Thompson et al., 1997; LopezCandales et al., 1997; Henderson et al., 1999) compared with normal aorta, associated with an increase in expression of a number of proapoptotic molecules, such as death receptors and p53 (Lopez-Candales et al., 1997; Henderson et al., 1999). Macrophages and T-lymphocytes are found in aneurysmal lesions, suggesting that inflammatory mediators released by these cells may promote VSMC apoptosis. Morever, the production of tissue metalloproteinases by macrophages may accelerate cell death by degrading the extracellular matrix from which VSMCs derive survival signals (see below).

Atherosclerosis

Rupture of atherosclerotic plaques is associated with a thinning of the VSMC-rich fibrous cap overlying the core. Rupture occurs particularly at the shoulder regions of plaques, which are noted for their lack of VSMCs and the presence of macrophages and other inflammatory cells. Apoptotic VSMCs are evident in advanced human plaques (Geng and Libby, 1995; Han et al., 1995; Isner et al., 1995), including the shoulder regions, prompting the suggestions that VSMC apoptosis may hasten plaque rupture. Indeed, increased VSMC apoptosis occurs in unstable versus stable angina lesions (Bauriedel et al., 1998).

Although loss of VSMCs would be expected to promote plaque rupture, there is no direct evidence of the effect of apoptosis per se in advanced human atherosclerosis. Most apoptotic cells in histological sections are found in advanced lesions next to the lipid core (Kockx, 1998), and most of these apoptotic cells are macrophages, not VSMCs. Loss of macrophages from atherosclerotic lesions is likely to promote plaque stability rather than rupture, since macrophages can promote VSMC apoptosis by both direct interactions (Boyle et al., 1998) and by release of cytokines (Geng et al., 1996). Of interest, apoptosis also occurs in early stages of atherosclerosis induced by cholesterol feeding in animals, at the fatty streak stage or before morphological evidence of lesion formation (Hasdai et al.,

1999). Again, the effect of apoptosis at this early stage of lesion development is unknown.

Effect of VSMC apoptosis

The effect of VSMC apoptosis is clearly context-dependent. Thus, VSMC apoptosis in advanced atherosclerotic plaques would be expected to promote plaque rupture, and medial atrophy in aneurysm formation. In neointima formation postinjury, VSMC apoptosis of both the intima and media can limit neointimal formation (Pollman et al., 1998, 1999; Sata et al., 1998) at a defined time point, although long-term studies have not been performed to ensure that the neointima is not simply delayed. It is not yet known whether such inhibition of neointimal formation in an animal model can translate into suppression of restenosis following angioplasty or stenting.

Therapeutic induction of apoptosis in the vessel wall may also be limited by important sequelae. In contrast to the dogma that apoptosis is silent (that is, it does not elicit an immune response), a number of deleterious effects of apoptotic cells have emerged within the vasculature. In particular, exposure of phosphatidylserine on the surface of apoptotic cells, which normally marks the condemned cell as ready for phagocytosis, provides a potent substrate for the generation of thrombin and activation of the coagulation cascade (Bombeli et al., 1997; Flynn et al., 1997). Whether or not this is the result of delayed phagocytosis due to a disruption of phagocytic signals by molecules within the plaque is not yet clear. Apoptotic cells can also release membrane-bound microparticles into the circulation; these remain procoagulant and are increased in patients with unstable versus stable coronary syndromes (Mallat et al., 1998, 1999). Although apoptotic cells are not the only source of circulating microparticles, such microparticles may contribute to the increased procoagulant state in these syndromes.

Regulation of VSMC apoptosis

Apoptosis via death receptors

Many stimuli can trigger apoptosis in cells, but in vascular disease it is likely that specific alterations within the VSMC itself elicit sensitivity to a particular stimulus that is disease-associated. Thus, remodelling may trigger apoptosis following reduction in blood flow, and the major stimulus may therefore be flow-dependent stimuli such as nitric oxide or shear stress. In contrast, apoptosis in atherosclerosis or aneurysm formation may be due to the surrounding influences of inflammatory cells that express death ligands on their surface or secrete proapoptotic cytokines. Whatever the stimulus, many of the downstream pathways by which the apoptotic stimuli are transmitted are similar.

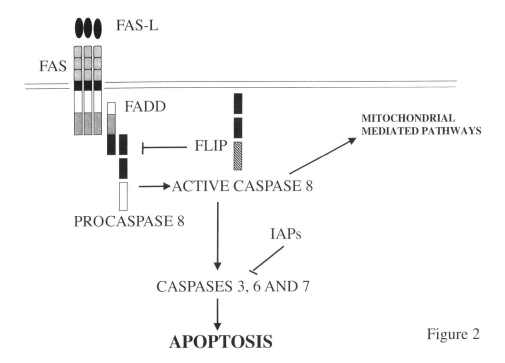

Figure 6.2   Schematic of Fas death-signalling pathways. Fas, the prototypic member of the tumour necrosis factor death receptor family, binds to its cognate ligand. Recruitment of the adapter molecule FADD and procaspase 8 results in activation of the latter. Caspase 8 activation directly activates downstream caspases (3, 6 and 7), resulting in DNA fragmentation and cleavage of cellular proteins. This pathway is thought to occur in type I cells and does not involve mitochondrial pathways. Alternatively, caspase 8 activation also results in cleavage of Bid, which translocates and interacts with other Bcl-2 family members (Figure 6.3).

The regulation of apoptosis within the cell can be simplified into two major pathways (Figures 6.2 and 6.3). First, membrane-bound death receptors of the tumour necrosis receptor family (TNF-R), such as Fas (CD95), TNF-R1, death receptor (DR)-3 DR4 and DR5 bind their trimerized ligands causing receptor aggregation, and subsequent recruitment of a number of adapter proteins through protein–protein interactions (Ashkenazi and Dixit, 1998; Figure 6.2). For example, binding of agonistic anti-Fas monoclonal antibody or its natural ligand, Fas-ligand, to its cognate receptor induces receptor trimerization, with subsequent recruitment of adapter molecules such as FADD and RIP to the receptor complex (Chinnaiyan et al., 1995, 1996; Stanger et al., 1995). In turn, FADD and RIP can recruit cell death cysteine proteases (caspases) such as caspase 8 (FLICE) and caspase 2 to the complex (Cohen, 1997). Within the complex of Fas, FADD and

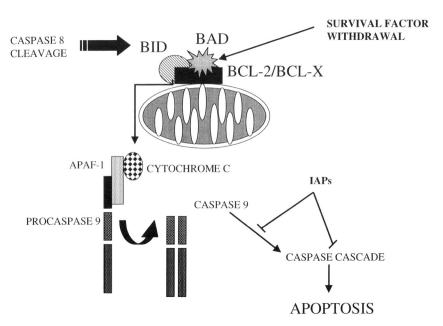

Figure 6.3 Schematic of mitochondrial death-signalling pathways. Antiapoptotic members of the Bcl-2 family, such as Bcl-2 and Bcl-X$_L$, are located on the mitochondrial outer membrane. Here they act to prevent the release of apoptogenic factors from the inner mitochondrial space. Binding of the proapoptotic proteins Bid (after cleavage by caspase 8) or Bad (after dephosphorylation) to Bcl-2 mitigates the protective effect of Bcl-2 and triggers release of cytochrome C. Cytochrome C, in concert with the adapter protein apaf-1 and caspase 9, activates caspase 3 and the downstream caspase cascade. Stimuli such as growth factor withdrawal or activation of p53 and Fas activation in type II cells act through this mitochondrial pathway.

caspase 8 (known as the death-inducing signalling complex a DISC), caspase 8 becomes proteolytically activated by oligomerization (Muzio et al., 1996). This facilitates the subsequent activation of terminal effector caspases such as caspases 3, 6 and 7 (Fernandes-Alnemri et al., 1995; Enari et al., 1996; Srinivasula et al., 1996; Muzio et al., 1997; Takahashi et al., 1997) responsible for cleavage of intracellular substrates required for cellular survival, architecture and metabolic function (Dixit, 1996; Krammer, 1996). Caspase activation is also responsible for many of the hallmarks of apoptosis, such as DNA fragmentation, chromatin condensation and apoptotic body formation (Enari et al., 1998; Hirata et al., 1998; Janicke et al., 1998). The major active caspases in Fas-mediated apoptosis are caspases 8, 3, 6 and 7 (Hirata et al., 1998), with stepwise appearance of active caspases suggesting a caspase cascade. Cells in which caspase 8 is expressed in abundance, recently termed type I cells, use this pathway of direct caspase 3 activation. Moreover, in these cells, Fas-mediated cell death cannot be inhibited by antiapoptotic factors such as Bcl-2 and Bcl-X_L since the pathway does not require amplification by proapoptotic factors released by mitochrondria (Scaffidi et al., 1998).

Apoptosis via mitochondrial amplification

In contrast, cells in which caspase 8 is not abundantly expressed cannot activate caspase 3 and other downstream caspases directly. Instead, in these cells termed type II cells (Scaffidi et al., 1998), caspase 8 activation causes cleavage of proteins of the *bcl-2* family such as *bid* [Li et al., 1998) (see Figure 6.3). Bcl-2 family members are characterized as either proapoptotic (Bax, Bid, Bik, Bak) or anti-apoptotic (Bcl-2, Bcl-X_L). Activation of proapoptotic Bcl-2 family members causes their translocation to mitochondria, where they interact with antiapoptotic members that are anchored at the mitochondrial membrane. This interaction is thought to cause changes in voltage-dependent mitochondrial channels and release of mitochondrial mediators of apoptosis such as cytochrome c (Shimizu et al., 1999). In turn the association of cytochrome c with an adapter molecule apaf-1 and caspase 9 activates caspase 3, and the caspase cascade. The amplification of death signals via the mitochondrial route also occurs in response to many other physiological and nonphysiological death triggers that do not involve activation of the death receptors.

Death induced by Fas signalling may or may not be inhibitable by Bcl-2 family members, suggesting that high levels of expression of antiapoptotic Bcl-2 family members do not automatically correlate with suppression of cell death. The classification of human VSMCs into type I or type II cells has yet to be made; however, the kinetics of cell death in response to anti-Fas antibodies suggests that they are type II cells.

Inhibition of death receptor-induced apoptosis

Fas-induced apoptosis can also be blocked by expression of several intracellular proteins, including FLIPs (FLICE-inhibitory protein) and IAPs (inhibitors of apoptosis; Figure 6.2). FLIPs are similar to caspase molecules, having the same prodomain structure as caspase 8, but not the active caspase site within the C-terminus. The prodomain of caspase 8 has two protein–protein interaction motifs called death effector domains (DEDs) that are also found in FADD. These DEDs facilitate the binding of FADD to caspase 8 and the binding of FLIP to FADD. Caspase 8 is activated upon binding to FADD via a series of cleavage reactions. FLIP undergoes the first of these cleavages, but not the second, preventing the activation of caspase 8 (Irmler et al., 1997). In contrast, IAPs can inhibit the enzymatic activity of downstream caspases (Liston et al., 1996; Deveraux et al.,

1997, see below), or they can mediate antiapoptotic signalling pathways through the activation of nuclear transcription factor B (NF-$\kappa\beta$).

How important is death receptor-induced apoptosis in VSCMs?

Human VSMCs express both Fas and TNF-R1 (Geng et al., 1997) and, given the widespread occurrence of TRAIL-receptors, are also likely to express these receptors. T lymphocytes and macrophages within the atherosclerotic plaque express Fas ligand and TNF-α, and interaction between membrane-bound ligands on T cells and receptors on VSMC may induce the death of VSMC. VSMCs can also express Fas-L and TNF-α, which exist as membrane-bound or soluble forms. The soluble forms are cleaved from the cell membrane by a metalloproteinase of the A disintegrin and metalloproteinase (ADAM) family. Interestingly, a recent study of the tissue inhibitors of metalloproteinases (TIMPs), indicates that TIMP-3 can induce VSMC apoptosis in vitro and in vivo (Baker et al., 1998). How TIMP-3 induces apoptosis has yet to be elucidated.

Interestingly, soluble ligand binding to death receptors is a very weak inducer of apoptosis in VSMCs (Geng et al., 1996; Bennett et al., 1998), although the death receptor machinery is present, since overexpression of FADD can induce VSMC apoptosis in vitro and in vivo (Schaub et al., 1998). Soluble ligand binding does not induce apoptosis in the absence of 'priming' of the cell, usually with cycloheximide. Some of this resistance can be explained by the observation that death receptors are sequestered intracellularly in VSMCs (Bennett et al., 1998), and priming of the cell is required for increased surface expression. Physiologically, increased death receptor expression can be achieved via combination of cytokines such as interleukin-1β, interferon-γ and TNF-α (Fukuo et al., 1997; Geng et al., 1997; Hoffmann et al., 1998), possibly via nitric oxide and subsequent p53 stabilization (Fukuo et al., 1996; Geng et al., 1996; Hoffmann et al., 1998; Boyle et al., 1999), or via other mechanisms that activate p53 (Bennett et al., 1998). Free radicals and nitric oxide can also induce apoptosis which may be independent of p53 stabilization and death receptor signalling, but associated with caspase 3 activation (Pollman et al., 1996; Li et al., 1997; Nishio and Watanabe, 1997; Zhao et al., 1997; Iwashina et al., 1998; Wang and Keiser, 1998). Thus, DNA damage induced by nitric oxide, anoxia or free radical formation may stabilize p53, effectively priming VSMCs to death receptor-mediated apoptosis. In contrast, efficient death receptor-mediated apoptosis of VSMCs can also be achieved directly by ectopic expression of death ligands such as Fas-L on populations of VSMCs in vitro and in vivo (Sata et al., 1998), possibly by increasing expression of membrane-bound forms of these ligands.

Irrespective of the local environment, VSMCs derived from atherosclerotic plaques show increased rates of apoptosis in culture compared with cells from normal vessels, reflecting an intrinsic sensitivity to apoptosis (Bennett et al., 1995). This appears to be a stable property, and is part of the phenotype of plaque VSMCs that includes slow proliferation and early senescence. Heterogeneity of sensitivity to apoptosis within VSMCs in the vessel wall has also been demonstrated in animal vessels after injury (Bochaton-Piallat et al., 1996), and in medial VSMCs from normal human arteries (Chan et al., 1998). This is likely to reflect differences in expression of pro- and antiapoptotic molecules, specifically those regulating signalling from survival cytokines, cell–cell and cell–matrix interactions and members of the *bcl-2* family. Indeed, insulin-like growth factor 1 (IGF-1) is a potent survival factor for normal VSMCs, although IGF-1 cannot completely inhibit plaque VSMC apoptosis in vitro after serum withdrawal (Bennett et al., 1995). Similarly, inhibition of basic fibroblast growth factor binding induces VSMC apoptosis both in vitro (Fox and Shanley, 1996; Miyamoto et al., 1998) and in vivo (Neschis et al., 1998). Basic fibroblast growth factor may protect against apoptosis by induction of the oncogene *mdm2*, which inactivates p53 (Shaulian et al., 1997).

Bcl-2 family members and VSMC apoptosis

Evidence suggesting the critical role of *bcl-2* family members in regulating VSMC apoptosis has come from both in vitro and in vivo studies. Human VSMCs express low levels of Bcl-2 (Bennett et al., 1995; Konstadoulakis et al., 1998), but Bax expression is seen particularly in atherosclerotic plaques, both in human and animal models of atherosclerosis and injury (Kockx, 1998; Konstadoulakis et al., 1998; Igase et al., 1999). In addition, spontaneous and growth factor withdrawal-induced apoptosis can be inhibited by overexpression of *bcl-2* (Bennett et al., 1995). In vivo, rat VSMCs express minimal Bcl-2, but high levels of Bcl-X$_L$ can be found after injury (Igase et al., 1999). Indeed, inhibition of Bcl-X$_L$ can dramatically induce apoptosis of VSMCs after balloon injury (Pollman et al., 1998) and differences in expression of Bcl-X$_L$ may account for differences in sensitivity to apoptosis after injury of intimal versus medial VSMCs (Pollman et al., 1999). The reduced levels of VSMC apoptosis seen after cholesterol lowering in rabbit models of atherosclerosis are also associated with a loss of Bax immunoreactivity (Kockx et al., 1998), arguing for a proapoptotic role of this protein in VSMC apoptosis. However, it should be noted that excessive reliance on immunocytochemistry of one member of the bcl-2 family to ascertain a role for that protein in vivo should be avoided. Although Bcl-X is upregulated after injury, in rats it is the short Bcl-X$_s$ or proapoptotic form that appears to predominate (Igase et al., 1999).

Regulation of sensitivity to apoptosis in VSMCs is also mediated by expression of IAP proteins (Erl et al., 1999) and individual caspases (Krajewska et al., 1997; Chan et al., 1998), and it is likely that there are marked differences in expression of multiple proteins which regulate apoptosis of individual VSMCs in response to specific stimuli. This may underlie observations that despite (apparently) the same stimulus for apoptosis, VSMC apoptosis in either the normal or diseased vessel wall is highly localized.

Summary

VSMC apoptosis occurs in the vasculature in both physiological and pathological contexts. Specific proteins that serve either to induce or protect against apoptosis regulate these deaths. We are now beginning to understand the complex biology observed in lesions such as atherosclerosis and to identify potential proapoptotic factors that may lead to the loss of cells from the vasculature. Sensitivity to apoptosis is determined by expression of cell death receptors and ligands, and by multiple protein species below receptor level. In addition, sensitivity to apoptosis is determined by the presence and response to survival cytokines, mitogens, and local cell and matrix interactions, and by the growth status of the cell. Although much of this research has been carried out in vitro, future studies in animal models should help to identify which of the pro- and antiapoptotic factors that are effective in vitro are also relevant in vivo. Moreover, a closer examination of the population dynamics of vascular cells within the vessel wall will aid the understanding of the timing and triggers of VSMC apoptosis in disease.

REFERENCES

Ashkenazi, A. & Dixit, V. (1998). Death receptors: signalling and modulation. *Science*, **281**, 1305–8.

Baker, A.H., Zaltsman, A.B., George, S.J. & Newby, A.C. (1998). Divergent effects of tissue inhibitor of metalloproteinase-1, -2, or -3 overexpression on rat vascular smooth muscle cell invasion, proliferation, and death in vitro – TIMP-3 promotes apoptosis. *J. Clin. Invest.*, **101**, 1478–87.

Bauriedel, G., Schluckebier, S., Hutter, S. et al. (1998). Apoptosis in restenosis versus stable-angina atherosclerosis. *Arterioscler. Thromb. Vasc. Biol.*, **18**, 1132–9.

Bennett, M.R., Evans, G.I. & Schwartz, S.M. (1995). Apoptosis of human vascular smooth muscle cells derived from normal vessels and coronary atherosclerotic plaques. *J. Clin. Invest.*, **95**, 2266–74.

Bennett, M., Macdonald, K., Chan, S.-W. et al. (1998). Cell surface trafficking of Fas: a rapid mechanism of p53-mediated apoptosis. *Science*, **282**, 290–3.

Bochaton-Piallat, M., Gabbiani, F., Redard, M., Desmouliere, A. & Gabbiani, G. (1995). Apoptosis participates in cellularity regulation during rat aortic intimal thickening. *Am. J. Pathol.*, **146**, 1059–64.

Bochaton-Piallat, M.-L., Ropraz, P., Gabbiani, F. & Gabbiani, G. (1996). Phenotypic heterogeneity of rat aortic smooth muscle cell clones. *Arterioscler. Thromb. Vasc. Biol.*, **16**, 815–20.

Bombeli, T., Karsan, A., Tait, J.F. & Harlan, J.M. (1997). Apoptotic vascular endothelial cells become procoagulant. *Blood*, **89**, 2429–42.

Boyle, J., Bennett, M., Proudfoot, D., Bowyer, D. & Weissberg, P. (1998). Human monocyte/macrophages induce human vascular smooth muscle cell apoptosis in culture. *J. Pathol.*, **184**, A13 (abstract).

Boyle, J.J., Bowyer, D.E., Weissberg, P.L. & Bennett, M.R. (1999). Interactions between TNF alpha and nitric oxide in human macrophage-induced vascular smooth muscle cell apoptosis. *J. Pathol.*, **187**, A12.

Chan, S., Weissberg, P. & Bennett, M. (1998). Heterogeneity of caspase regulation of human vascular smooth muscle cell apoptosis. *Heart*, **71**, 12 (abstract).

Chinnaiyan, A., O'Rourke, K., Tewari, M. & Dixit, V. (1995). FADD, a novel death domain-containing protein, interacts with the death domain of fas and initiates apoptosis. *Cell*, **81**, 505.

Chinnaiyan, A., Tepper, C., Seldin, M. et al. (1996). FADD/mort1 is a common mediator of CD95 (Fas/Apo-1) and tumor necrosis factor receptor induced apoptosis. *J. Biol. Chem.*, **271**, 4961–5.

Cho, A. & Langille, B.L. (1993). Arterial smooth-muscle cell turnover during the postnatal period in lambs. *Faseb J.*, **7**, A756.

Cho, A., Courtman, D. & Langille, L. (1995). Apoptosis (programmed cell death) in arteries of the neonatal lamb. *Circ. Res.*, **76**, 168–75.

Cho, A., Mitchell, L., Koopmans, D. & Langille, B.L. (1997). Effects of changes in blood flow rate on cell death and cell proliferation in carotid arteries of immature rabbits. *Circ. Res.*, **81**, 328–37.

Cohen, G.M. (1997). Caspases: the executioners of apoptosis. *Biochem. J.*, **326**, 1–16.

Deveraux, Q.L., Takahashi, R., Salvesen, G.S. & Reed, J.C. (1997). X-linked IAP is a direct inhibitor of cell-death proteases. *Nature*, **388**, 300–4.

Deveraux, Q.L., Roy, N., Stennicke, H.R. et al. (1998). IAPs block apoptotic events induced by caspase-8 and cytochrome c by direct inhibition of distinct caspases. *EMBO J.*, **17**, 2215–23.

Dixit, V. (1996). The cell-death machine. *Curr. Biol.*, **6**, 555–62.

Enari, M., Talanian, R., Wong, W. & Nagata, S. (1996). Sequential activation of ICE-like and CPP32-like proteases during Fas-mediated apoptosis. *Nature*, **380**, 723–6.

Enari, M., Sakahira, H., Yokoyama, H. et al. (1998). A caspase-activated DNase that degrades DNA during apoptosis and its inhibitor ICAD. *Nature*, **391**, 43–50.

Erl, W., Hansson, G., de Martin, R. et al. (1999). Nuclear factor-$\kappa\beta$ regulates induction of apoptosis and inhibitor of apoptosis protein-1 expression in vascular smooth muscle cells. *Circ. Res.*, **84**, 668–77.

Fernandes-Alnemri, T., Litwack, G. & Alnemri, E. (1995). Mch2, a new member of the apoptotic ced-3/ice cysteine protease gene family. *Cancer Res.*, **55**, 2737–42.

Flynn, P., Byrne, C., Baglin, T., Weissberg, P. & Bennett, M. (1997). Thrombin generation by apoptotic vascular smooth muscle cells. *Blood*, **89**, 4373–84.

Fox, J. & Shanley, J. (1996). Antisense inhibition of basic fibroblast growth factor induces apoptosis in vascular smooth muscle cells. *J. Biol. Chem.*, **271**, 12578–84.

Fukuo, K., Hata, S., Suhara, T. et al. (1996). Nitric oxide induces up regulation of fas and apoptosis in vascular smooth muscle. *Hypertension*, **27**, 823–6.

Fukuo, K., Nakahashi, T., Nomura, S. et al. (1997). Possible participation of Fas-mediated apoptosis in the mechanism of atherosclerosis. *Gerontology*, **43**, 35–42.

Geng, Y. & Libby, P. (1995). Evidence for apoptosis in advanced human atheroma: colocalization with interleukin-1β converting enzyme. *Am. J. Pathol.*, **147**, 251–66.

Geng, Y., Wu, Q., Muszynski, M., Hansson, G. & Libby, P. (1996). Apoptosis of vascular smooth-muscle cells induced by in vitro stimulation with interferon-gamma, tumor necrosis factor-alpha, and interleukin-1-beta. *Arterioscler. Thromb. Vasc. Biol.*, **16**, 19–27.

Geng, Y.J., Henderson, L.E., Levesque, E.B., Muszynski, M. & Libby, P. (1997). Fas is expressed in human atherosclerotic intima and promotes apoptosis of cytokine-primed human vascular smooth muscle cells. *Arterioscler. Thromb. Vasc. Biol.*, **17**, 2200–8.

Gordon, D., Reidy, M.A., Benditt, E.P. & Schwartz, S.M. (1990). Cell proliferation in human coronary arteries. *Proc. Natl Acad. Sci. USA*, **87**, 4600–4.

Han, D., Haudenschild, C., Hong, M. et al. (1995). Evidence for apoptosis in human atherosclerosis and in a rat vascular injury model. *Am. J. Pathol.*, **147**, 267–77.

Hasdai, D., Sangiorgi, G., Spagnoli, L.G. et al. (1999). Coronary artery apoptosis in experimental hypercholesterolemia. *Atherosclerosis*, **142**, 317–25.

Henderson, E.L., Gang, Y.J., Sukhova, G.K. et al. (1999). Death of smooth muscle cells and expression of mediators of apoptosis by T lymphocytes in human abdominal aortic aneurysms. *Circulation*, **99**, 96–104.

Hirata, H., Takahashi, A., Kobayashi, S. et al. (1998). Caspases are activated in a branched protease cascade and control distinct downstream processes in Fas-induced apoptosis. *J. Exp. Med.*, **187**, 587–600.

Hoffmann, G., Kenn, S., Wirleitner, B. et al. (1998). Neopterin induces nitric oxide-dependent apoptosis in rat vascular smooth muscle cells. *Immunobiology*, **199**, 63–73.

Igase, M., Okura, T., Kitami, Y. & Hiwada, K. (1999). Apoptosis and Bcl-xs in the intimal thickening of balloon-injured carotid arteries. *Clin. Sci.*, **96**, 605–12.

Irmler, M., Thome, M., Hahne, M. et al. (1997). Inhibition of death receptor signals by cellular FLIP. *Nature*, **388**, 190–5.

Isner, J., Kearney, M., Bortman, S. & Passeri, J. (1995). Apoptosis in human atherosclerosis and restenosis. *Circulation*, **91**, 2703–11.

Iwashina, M., Shichiri, M., Marumo, F. & Hirata, Y. (1998). Transfection of inducible nitric oxide synthase gene causes apoptosis in vascular smooth muscle cells. *Circulation*, **98**, 1212–18.

Janicke, R.U., Sprengart, M.L., Wati, M.R. & Porter, A.G. (1998). Caspase-3 is required for DNA fragmentation and morphological changes associated with apoptosis. *J. Biol. Chem.*, **273**, 9357–60.

Kerr, J.F., Wyllie, A.H. & Currie, A.R. (1972). Apoptosis: a basic biological phenomenon with wide-ranging implications in tissue kinetics. *Br. J. Cancer*, **26**, 239–57.

Kockx, M.M. (1998). Apoptosis in the atherosclerotic plaque – quantitative and qualitative aspects. *Arterioscler. Thromb. Vasc. Biol.*, **18**, 1519–22.

Kockx, M.M., DeMeyer, G.Y., Buyssens, N. et al. (1998). Cell composition, replication, and apoptosis in atherosclerotic plaques after 6 months of cholesterol withdrawal. *Circ. Res.*, **83**, 378–87.

Konstadoulakis, M.M., Kymionis, G.D., Karagiani, M. et al. (1998). Evidence of apoptosis in human carotid atheroma. *J. Vasc. Surg.*, **27**, 733–9.

Krajewska, M., Wang, H.G., Krajewski, S. et al. (1997). Immunohistochemical analysis of in vivo patterns of expression of CPP32 (caspase-3), a cell death protease. *Cancer Res.*, **57**, 1605–13.

Krammer, P. (1996). The CD95 (Apo-1/Fas) receptor/ligand system – death signals and diseases. *Cell Death Differ.*, **3**, 159–60.

Kumar, A. & Lindner, V. (1997). Remodeling with neointima formation in the mouse carotid artery after cessation of blood flow. *Arterioscler. Thromb. Vasc. Biol.*, **17**, 2238–44.

Li, P.F., Dietz, R. & vonHarsdorf, R. (1997). Differential effect of hydrogen peroxide and superoxide anion on apoptosis and proliferation of vascular smooth muscle cells. *Circulation*, **96**, 3602–9.

Li, H.L., Zhu, H., Xu, C.J. & Yuan, J.Y. (1998). Cleavage of BID by caspase 8 mediates the mitochondrial damage in the Fas pathway of apoptosis. *Cell*, **94**, 491–501.

Liston, P., Roy, N., Tamai, K. et al. (1996). Suppression of apoptosis in mammalian cells by NAIP and a related family of IAP genes. *Nature*, **379**, 349–53.

LopezCandales, A., Holmes, D.R., Liao, S.X. et al. (1997). Decreased vascular smooth muscle cell density in medial degeneration of human abdominal aortic aneurysms. *Am. J. Pathol.*, **150**, 993–1007.

Malik, N., Francis, S.E., Holt, C.M. et al. (1998). Apoptosis and cell proliferation after porcine coronary angioplasty. *Circulation*, **98**, 1657–65.

Mallat, Z., Benamer, H., Hugel, B. et al. (1998). Elevated plasma levels of shed membrane microparticles in patients with acute coronary syndromes. *Circulation*, **98**, I-172 (abstract).

Mallat, Z., Hugel, B., Ohan, J. et al. (1999). Shed membrane microparticles with procoagulant potential in human atherosclerotic plaques – a role for apoptosis in plaque thrombogenicity. *Circulation*, **99**, 348–53.

Miyamoto, T., Leconte, I., Swain, J.L. et al. (1998). Autocrine FGF signaling is required for vascular smooth muscle cell survival in vitro. *J. Cell Physiol.*, **177**, 58–67.

Muzio, M., Chinnaiyan, A., Kischkel, F. et al. (1996). FLICE, a novel FADD-homologous ice/ced-3-like protease, is recruited to the CD95 (Fas/Apo-1) death-inducing signaling complex. *Cell*, **85**, 817–27.

Muzio, M., Salvesen, G.S. & Dixit, V.M. (1997). FLICE induced apoptosis in a cell-free system – cleavage of caspase zymogens. *J. Biol. Chem.*, **272**, 2952–6.

Nishio, E. & Watanabe, Y. (1997). NO induced apoptosis accompanying the change of onco-protein expression and the activation of CPP32 protease. *Life Sci.*, **62**, 239–45.

Neschis, D.G., Safford, S.D., Hanna, A.K., Fox, J.C. & Golden, M.A. (1998). Antisense basic fibroblast growth factor gene transfer reduces early intimal thickening in a rabbit femoral artery balloon injury model. *J. Vasc. Surg.*, **27**, 126–34.

Perlman, H., Maillard, L., Krasinski, K. & Walsh, K. (1997). Evidence for the rapid onset of apoptosis in medial smooth muscle cells after balloon injury. *Circulation*, **95**, 981–7.

Pollman, M.J., Yamada, T., Horiuchi, M. & Gibbons, G.H. (1996). Vasoactive substances regulate vascular smooth-muscle cell apoptosis – countervailing influences of nitric-oxide and angiotensin-Ii. *Circ. Res.*, **79**, 748–56.

Pollman, M.J., Hall, J.L., Mann, M.J., Zhang, L.N. & Gibbons, G.H. (1998). Inhibition of neointimal cell bcl-x expression induces apoptosis and regression of vascular disease. *Nature Med.*, **4**, 222–7.

Pollman, M.J., Hall, J.L. & Gibbons, G.H. (1999). Determinants of vascular smooth muscle cell apoptosis after balloon angioplasty injury – influence of redox state and cell phenotype. *Circ. Res.*, **84**, 113–21.

Sata, M., Perlman, H.R., Muruve, D.A. et al. (1998). Fas ligand gene transfer to the vessel wall inhibits neointima formation and overrides the adenovirus-mediated T cell response. *Proc. Natl Acad. Sci. USA*, **95**, 1213–17.

Scaffidi, C., Fulda, S., Srinivasan, A. et al. (1998). Two CD95 (APO-1/Fas) signaling pathways. *EMBO J.*, **17**, 1675–87.

Schaub, F., Coats, S., Seifert, R. et al. (1998). Regulated overexpression of the Fas-associated death domain (FADD) protein in seeded vascular smooth muscle cells causes apoptosis followed by recruitment of macrophages. *Circulation*, **98**, I-597 (abstract).

Shaulian, E., Resnitzky, D., Shifman, O. et al. (1997). Induction of Mdm2 and enhancement of cell survival by bFGF. *Oncogene*, **15**, 2717–25.

Shimizu, S., Narita, M. & Tsujimoto, Y. (1999). Bcl-2 family proteins regulate the release of apoptogenic cytochrome c by the mitochondrial channel VDAC. *Nature*, **399**, 483–7.

Slomp, J., GittenbergerdeGroot, A.C., Glukhova, M.A. et al. (1997). Differentiation, dedifferentiation, and apoptosis of smooth muscle cells during the development of the human ductus arteriosus. *Arterioscler. Thromb. Vasc. Biol.*, **17**, 1003–9.

Srinivasula, S., Ahmad, M., Fermandes-Alnemri, T., Litwack, G. & Alnemri, E. (1996). Molecular ordering of the fas-apoptotic pathway: the fas/APO-1 protease mch-5 is a CrmA-inhibitable protease that activates multiple Ced-3/ICE-like cysteine proteases. *Proc. Natl Acad. Sci. USA*, **93**, 14486–91.

Stanger, B.Z., Leder, P., Lee, T.H., Kim, E. & Seed, B. (1995). Rip – a novel protein containing a death domain that interacts with Fas/Apo-1 (Cd95) in yeast and causes cell-death. *Cell*, **81**, 513–23.

Takahashi, A., Hirata, H., Yonehara, S. et al. (1997). Affinity labeling displays the stepwise activation of ICE-related proteases by Fas, staurosporine, and CrmA-sensitive caspase-8. *Oncogene*, **14**, 2741–52.

Thompson, R.W., Liao, S.X. & Curci, J.A. (1997). Vascular smooth muscle cell apoptosis in abdominal aortic aneurysms. *Coron. Artery Dis.*, **8**, 623–31.

Wang, H. & Keiser, J.A. (1998). Molecular characterization of rabbit CPP32 and its function in vascular smooth muscle cell apoptosis. *Am. J. Physiol.*, **43**, H1132–40.

Zhao, Z.H., Francis, C.E., Welch, G., Loscalzo, J. & Ravid, K. (1997). Reduced glutathione prevents nitric oxide-induced apoptosis in vascular smooth muscle cells. *Biochim. et Biophys. Acta*, **1359**, 143–52.

7

Wound healing: laboratory investigation and modulating agents

Nick L. Occleston, Julie T. Daniels and Peng T. Khaw

Department of Pathology, Moorfields Eye Hospital, London

In recent years our understanding of the cellular and molecular mechanisms underlying the wound-healing process has increased considerably. As we enter the postgenomic era the potential to investigate the role and regulation of this vital response to injury at the gene level will elucidate the process further. Tissue repair is a series of interactive events between different cell types, the extracellular matrix (ECM) and a number of chemical mediators and has been the subject of many excellent reviews. As the field of wound-healing research has become too large to cover in depth in a single chapter, in the following chapter we will try to highlight crucial components of the wound-healing process, methods of investigating these components and, finally, ways in which the healing process can be modulated.

Wound healing: an overview

The repair of lost or damaged adult tissue is achieved by the production of scar tissue. The healing response generally consists of a series of ordered events, some of which occur concurrently, involving several cell types, regulators of cell function and ultimately the production and remodelling of new tissue (Figure 7.1). Variations in the processes involved in this response can result in inadequate or excessive healing, both of which may result in the impairment or loss of tissue or organ function. Excessive healing in particular is a major cause of clinical morbidity, for example in atherosclerosis, restenosis following angioplasty and vein graft disease; following thermal, chemical or radiation burns; following injury or surgery, e.g. internal adhesions, intestinal blockage and keloids; and scarring due to disease, e.g. cirrhosis and scleroderma. In addition to this, the scarring response plays an extremely important role in the pathogenesis or failure of

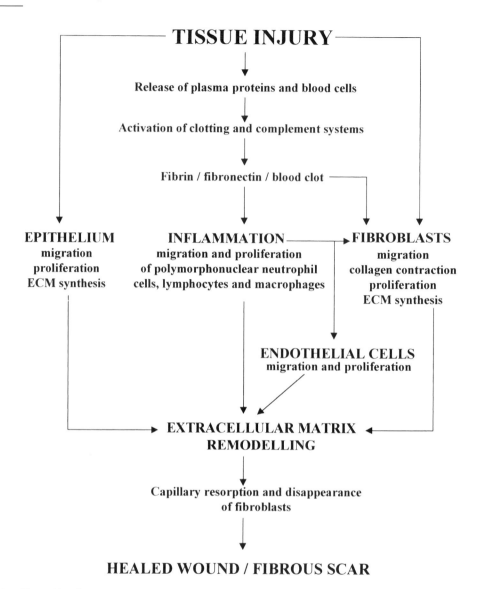

Figure 7.1   Wound healing response.

treatment of many visually disabling or blinding conditions in the world today including cataracts, trachoma, glaucoma, burns, proliferative vitreoretinopathy (following retinal detachment or diabetes) and age-related macular degeneration.

For simplicity and discussion in the following chapter, the multistage healing process has been arbitrarily divided into early, central and late events.

Wound healing: early events

Role of the blood and clotting systems

Activation of the coagulation system is one of the earliest repair events. Following vascular damage fibrin (derived from plasma fibrinogen) and a variety of coagulation factors cross-link clots to fill the wound site (Clark et al., 1983). Fibronectin then covalently cross-links to fibrin, forming a fibrin-fibronectin matrix (Kurkinen et al., 1980; Grinnell, 1984), probably serving as a framework for later collagen deposition (McDonald et al., 1982; Grinnell, 1984). Platelets and extravascular coagulation-promoting factors (Maynard et al., 1975; Dvorak et al., 1985) promote rapid clotting of trapped plasma and blood proteins. Platelets aggregate and attach, via interactions with collagen fibrils and von Willebrand factor (factor VIII), to damaged blood vessels and then degranulate (Samuelsson et al., 1978) releasing a variety of factors. These include platelet-derived growth factor (PDGF), epidermal growth factor (EGF), and transforming growth factor-β ((TGF-β); Ross et al., 1986), which have been reported to stimulate the chemotaxis of monocytes (Deuel et al., 1982), fibroblasts (Seppa et al., 1982) and vascular smooth muscle cells (Heldin and Westermark 1984; Ross, 1989). Interleukin-7 (IL-7), stem cell factor (SCF), and the transcription factor NFE2 have also been detected in platelets at the messenger RNA level (Soslau et al., 1997). During interaction with the injured vessel wall platelets also release vascular endothelial growth factor (VEGF), required for survival of microvascular endothelial cells (Weltermann et al., 1999). Unlike other sites in the body, following injury in the cornea no haemorrhage occurs at the wound site. However, haemostatic factors still play a significant role as plasmin is responsible for fibrinolysis preventing an adverse inflammatory response to prolonged fibrin and fibrinogen deposition (Kao et al., 1998).

Role of inflammatory cells

The first inflammatory cells entering the wound site are granulocytes, appearing within 24 h postinjury (Burger et al., 1983). Following this, neutrophils enter the site via the chemotactic effects of various factors released from platelets and the complement cascade. Adhesion molecules (selectins) expressed on activated endothelium and platelets are also required for inflammatory cell recruitment (Subramaniam et al., 1997). Monocytes are the next cells to appear in the wound site (Issekutz et al., 1981), and these then differentiate into macrophages. Once at the wound site, macrophages (which do not differentiate into fibroblasts) not only produce a whole range of regulatory factors which influence the control of the following healing process (Riches, 1988; Knighton and Fiegel, 1989), but also phagacytose and break down cellular debris and bacteria.

Wound healing: central events

Roles of the fibroblast

The fibroblast is the key player in the wound-healing process, carrying out a number of crucial functions including migration, wound contraction, proliferation, synthesis of new ECM and remodelling of this new matrix. As such, work in our and many other laboratories has concentrated on understanding the mechanisms underlying the regulation of fibroblast function. In a few specialized parts of the body other cells carry out this pivotal part of the healing function, e.g. retinal pigmented epithelial cells in the retina, glia in the central nervous system and vascular smooth muscle cells in the vasculature.

Migration

The movement of fibroblasts to the wound site is mediated by various polypeptides, including inflammatory cell products (Postlethwaite et al., 1976; Sobel and Gallin, 1979; Postlethwaite and Kang, 1980), complement (Postlethwaite et al., 1979), PDGF (Seppa et al., 1982), TGF-β (Postlethwaite et al., 1987) and ECM components including collagen (Postlethwaite et al., 1978), elastin (Senior et al., 1984), fibrinogen derivatives (Senior et al., 1986) and fibronectin (Joseph et al., 1987) which provides a conduit for fibroblast transmigration from collagenous stroma into the provisional matrix of the fibrin clot (Greiling and Clark, 1997). These polypeptides (termed chemoattractants) are regarded as stimulating migration through the process of chemotaxis. Chemotaxis has been defined as the directed migration of cells in response to a concentration gradient of a soluble chemoattractant (McCarthy et al., 1988) and is regarded as the major mechanism by which cellular migration is controlled. In addition to chemotaxis, the movement of cells independently of the chemoattractant gradient (termed chemokinesis: Zigmond and Hirsch, 1973), haptotaxis (the movement of cells via a substratum-bound gradient of a particular matrix constituent: Harris, 1973), and contact guidance (the tendency of cells to align and move along discontinuities in the ECM: Weiss, 1945, 1958) may also contribute to the migration of cells into the wound site. In the eye, following injury to the cornea the fibroblasts immediately beneath the wound site disappear, possibly by the mechanism of cell death termed apoptosis (Wilson and Kim, 1998). Once epithelial cells cover the wound fibroblasts return to take part in the healing process. Our work has demonstrated a potential paracrine interaction between the newly forming epithelium and the returning fibroblasts. We have found, in vitro, that as corneal epithelium differentiates it produces increasing amounts of factors chemotactic to fibroblasts, including PDGF. However, once the epithelium reaches maturity and achieves homeostasis these factors are significantly

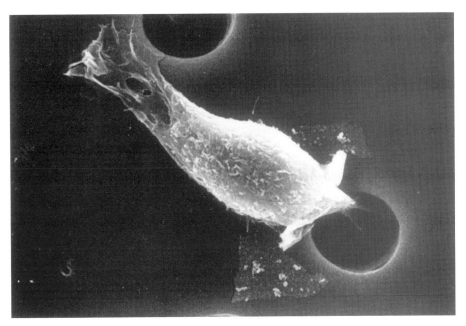

Figure 7.2   Cell migration assay. Photograph shows an ocular fibroblast migrating through a Transwell pore, by scanning electron microscopy.

reduced. In support of our findings the PDGF system has now been reported to operate in the cornea (Kim et al., 1999).

A number of in vitro assay systems have been used to study cellular migration including Boyden migration chambers (Boyden, 1962), two-compartment Boyden chambers (Zigmond and Hirsch, 1973), orientation chambers (Zigmond, 1977), under agarose (Nelson et al., 1978) and modified 48-microwell two-tiered blindwell Boyden migration chambers. We use 48-microwell modified Boyden chambers to study the effects of varying concentrations of growth factors, including TGF-β_1, EGF, PDGF, basic fibroblast growth factor (bFGF) and insulin-like growth factor-1 (IGF-1) on ocular fibroblast migration. In addition to Boyden chambers, we have also found 24-well Transwell tissue culture inserts (Figure 7.2) a useful way of studying cellular migration (Occleston et al., 1997; Daniels et al., 1999), as have other studies investigating vascular smooth muscle cell migration (Noda Heiny and Sobel, 1995; Okada et al., 1995). Although the use of Transwells reduces the technical difficulty of the migration assay, the volume of chemoattractant required is approximately 20 times greater than used in the modified Boyden chamber. When using any of the above assay systems to study migration, it should be borne in mind that, although they allow quantitation of cellular migration and the study of individual chemoattractants, the conditions are obviously very different to those in vivo. In the in vivo situation, not only are cells moving through their surrounding ECM during migration, but also this process is probably under the control of not one but several regulatory signals acting in concert.

Extracellular matrix contraction

The contraction of collagen-containing tissues is fundamental not only to the wound-healing process (Grinnell, 1994) but also morphogenesis (Stopak and Harris, 1982; Lewis, 1984) and development (Brenner et al., 1989). The mechanism of ECM contraction is controversial and hotly debated. It was first proposed that specialized cells, myofibroblasts, exhibiting smooth muscle cell characteristics such as expression of α smooth muscle actin are required for ECM contraction (Gabbiani et al., 1972). It is been suggested that fibroblasts differentiate into myofibroblasts for this purpose (Jester et al., 1995) as 'regular' fibroblasts are not thought to exert enough force by movement alone to contract matrix (Jester et al., 1995; Roy et al., 1997, 1999). These studies were however performed with fibroblasts seeded upon the matrix rather than within it. Indeed, biopsies of incisional wounds in humans demonstrated that myofibroblasts did not appear until day 11 and, unlike observations made in laboratory animals, myofibroblasts only comprised 10% of the total cell population (Berry et al., 1998). An alternative theory suggests that fibroblasts may contract wound matrix by cell locomotion or migration (Harris et al., 1981; Ehrlich and Rajaratnam, 1990; Eastwood et al., 1996). In support of the migration theory a rat wound-healing model, devoid of myofibroblasts, proceeded to heal normally with a more orderly arrangement of collagen bundles, suggesting that myofibroblasts are not required for wound contraction (Ehrlich et al., 1999).

Many groups, including ours, have used an in vitro model of contraction based upon fibroblast-populated collagen matrices originally described by Bell et al. (1979). The cells within this matrix reorganize and subsequently contract the matrix over several days by the forces of cellular locomotion (Figure 7.3a). The morphological characteristics of these cells resemble those in vivo (Tomasek and Hay, 1984). We have used fluorescence confocal microscopy to observe the morphology of fibroblasts seeded within collagen matrix and as a result hypothesize that cell–cell contact may be an important feature in matrix contraction (Figure 7.3b). This matrix contraction is dependent upon collagen concentration and cell number (Bell et al., 1979; Allen and Schor, 1983; Buttle and Ehrlich, 1983; Occleston et al., 1994), an intact cytoskeleton (Bell et al., 1979; Guidry and Grinnell, 1985), attachment of cells to their surrounding matrix (Klein et al., 1991; Schiro et al., 1991), and protein synthesis (Guidry and Grinnell, 1985). In addition to this, the contraction of collagen has been shown to be stimulated by a variety of growth factors, including EGF, TGF-β, IGF-1, PDGF and inhibited by bFGF (Ono et al., 1999), and to involve intracellular signalling involving protein

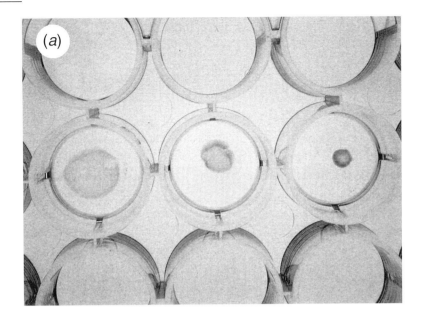

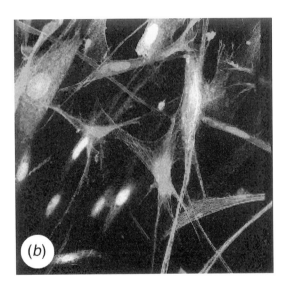

Figure 7.3   Model of in vitro Contraction. (*a*) Fibroblasts seeded within three-dimensional collagen matrices reorganize and subsequently contract their surrounding matrix over several days. (*b*) Fluorescence confocal microsopy showing fibroblasts within a 4-day-old contracting collagen matrix. The nucleus (red) is stained with propidium iodide and the actin cytoskeleton is labelled with fluorescein isothiocyanate (FITC) conjugated to phalloidin.

kinase C and the nitrogen-activated protein (MAP) kinases ERK1 and ERK2 (Guidry, 1993; Cheresh et al., 1999).

Although much research into the process of collagen contraction has been carried out, the exact mechanisms underlying this process are currently unclear. Such mechanisms include the elucidation of how fibroblasts within a three-dimensional matrix migrate, are signalled to start and stop contraction, and how these cells respond to changes in biophysical forces within granulation tissue. Studies in our laboratory have suggested that the matrix metalloproteinases (MMPs) play an essential role in the contraction of collagen lattices in vitro. We have demonstrated that fibroblasts markedly increase their production of MMPs both at the mRNA level, using a quantitative competitive reverse transcriptase polymerase chain reaction (QCRT-PCR) technique developed by our colleagues at the Institute for Wound Research, University of Florida (Tarnuzzer et al., 1996), and at the protein level. This QCRT-PCR technique is extremely powerful as we are able to quantitate the levels of mRNA in cells or tissue for a variety of MMPs, ECM components, growth factors and growth factor receptors (Tarnuzzer et al., 1996; Figure 7.4) from the same sample and using only small amounts of RNA. From further experiments in our laboratory, it appears that the MMPs allow fibroblasts to penetrate/invade their surrounding collagen matrix and then move through this matrix. It is this penetration of the matrix and subsequent movement through the matrix which ultimately result in its contraction. We and others have demonstrated a reduction in fibroblast-mediated collagen matrix contraction using a synthetic broad-spectrum inhibitor of MMP activity (Scott et al., 1998). Impaired wound contraction has also been observed in mice deficient in stromelysin-1, a member of the MMP family (Bullard et al., 1999). In addition to the above techniques, our colleagues at the Phoenix Tissue Repair Unit, University College London, have developed a novel system for studying fibroblast behaviour in ECM – the culture force monitor (CFM; Figure 7.5). The original prototype of the CFM allowed accurate, sensitive and reproducible measurement of the contractile forces generated by cells within a collagen matrix (Eastwood et al., 1994). Using fibronectin strands within the collagen matrix to provide contact guidance cues for fibroblasts, perpendicular to the axis of loading by the CFM, cells were placed in their most sensitive configuration. The fibroblasts in the nonaligned zone demonstrated an increase in MMP expression at the mRNA, suggesting that cells unable to align to applied loads remodel their matrix more rapidly than oriented cells (Mudera et al., 2000). Other instruments have now been developed at the Phoenix Tissue Repair Unit to investigate the effects of biophysical forces on cellular behaviour in ECM (tension CFM) and the formation of adhesions between tissue interfaces in vitro (adhesion CFM; Cacou et al., 1996).

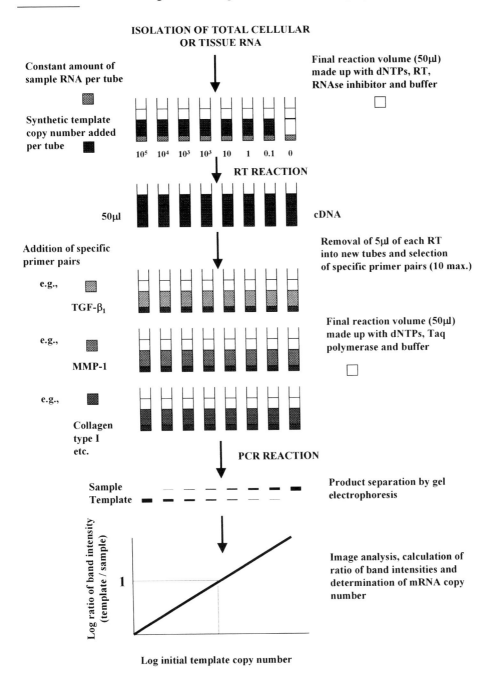

Figure 7.4   Quantitative competitive reverse transcriptase polymerase chain reaction (QCRT-PCR)
technique. This technique allows the quantitation of mRNA levels from cells or tissues for a
variety of growth factors, growth factor receptors, extracellular matrix (ECM) components,
ECM-degrading enzymes and their inhibitors.

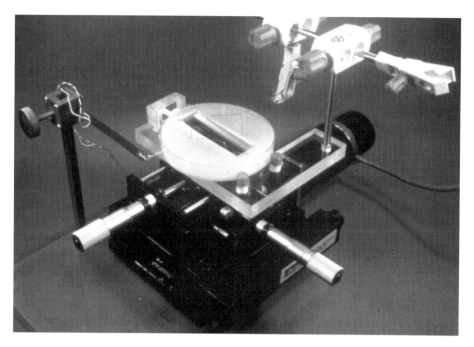

Figure 7.5   Culture force monitor (CFM).

Proliferation

Following the migration of fibroblasts to the wound site and the resultant contraction of the ECM, they then proliferate, reaching maximal numbers within 1–2 weeks postinjury (Ross and Odland, 1968). The proliferation of fibroblasts at the wound site is important in order for the cell number to be sufficient to allow adequate healing. As for fibroblast migration and ECM contraction, the proliferation of these cells is stimulated by a number of growth factors, including EGF, TGF-β, IGF-1, PDGF and bFGF. However, these growth factors also have inhibitory as well as stimulatory effects on cellular functions related to wound healing, depending upon the cell type studied (Table 7.1). The quantitation of proliferation in response to a variety of stimuli has been achieved using several methods, including ^{3}H-thymidine assays (Freshney, 1987), counted cell number, e.g. haemocytometer, Coulter counter and colorimetric assays, e.g. 3-[4,5-dimethyl-thiazol-2-yl]-2,5-diphenyl tetrazolium bromide (MTT) and 4-[3-(4-iodophenyl)-2-(4-nitrophenyl)-^{2}H-5-tetrazodo]-1,3-benzeme disulphonate (WST) assays based upon cellular metabolic activity (Kawase et al., 1995), and the methylene blue assay based upon dye binding to the cell monolayer (Finlay et al., 1984).

Role of endothelial cells

Neovascularization of the wound occurs simultaneously with the migration into and the proliferation of fibroblasts at the wound site. The process of formation of capillary beds via the influx of microvessel buds from the surrounding tissue vasculature (angiogenesis) is a central component of the wound-healing process. Angiogenesis is a complex process and is thought to involve several stages, including migration, growth and capillary tube formation. As for the other stages of wound healing, angiogenesis is regulated by several factors, including chemical mediators, and the reader is referred to other chapters within this book for a more extensive review of this process. Interestingly, recent work has suggested a role for the MMPs in angiogenesis (Galardy et al., 1994; Reed et al., 2000), and the modulation of this process and other inhibitors of angiogenesis are highlighted later in this chapter.

Role of epithelial cells

Reepithelialization is an important factor in the closure of wounds. Depending upon body site and injury, the timing of this event can vary. For example, in large skin wounds such as burns, reepithelialization may not be complete until the late stages of wound repair whereas in the cornea reepithelialization occurs before fibroblasts arrive in large numbers at the wound site. Two different mechanisms have been reported to be involved in the reepithelialization of wounds. Studies have suggested a purse string closure mechanism involving the formation of an actin cable in fetal epithelial healing and gastrointestinal epithelial healing (Martin and Lewis, 1992; Bement et al., 1993). In addition, it is also thought that basal epithelial cells migrate directionally across the wound defect pulling the upper layers of the epidermis passively along, followed by proliferation and finally deposition of a new basement membrane and restratification of the epidermis (Mackenzie and Fusenig, 1983). In the cornea following a short lag phase reepithelialization begins, independently of proliferation, with cell slide from the wound edge. Cell numbers are subsequently replaced by division and centripetal migration of cells derived from the stem cell population located at the edge of the cornea in the limbus (Tuft et al., 1993). Recently, this migration of epithelial cells across a wound defect has been shown to involve and require the action of MMPs (Woodley et al. 1986; Saarialho Kere et al., 1993, 1995; Iwasaki et al., 1994; Agren, 1999). Interestingly, the induction of electric fields following the disruption of cell–cell connections may induce components of the repair process incuding cell orientation, migration and clustering of growth factor receptors (Zhao et al., 1999). Once reepithelialization has occurred, the remodelling and maturation phases of the healing process begin (see below).

We have used an established colony dispersion assay (Pilcher et al., 1997) to

Table 7.1 Role of growth factors in wound healing

Growth factor	Molecular weight (kDa)	Found in:	Reported effects on cellular functions related to wound healing			
			Fibroblasts	Endothelial cells	Epithelial cells	Vascular smooth muscle cells
EGF	6	Almost all body fluids, platelets	Stimulates migration, ECM contraction, proliferation and ECM synthesis	Stimulates proliferation and angiogenesis	Stimulates migration and proliferation	Stimulates proliferation
TGF-α	5–20	Macrophages Eosinophils Keratinocytes	See effects of EGF above			
TGF-β	25	Platelets Macrophages Lymphocytes Fibroblasts Keratinocytes	Stimulates migration, ECM contraction, proliferation and ECM synthesis	Inhibits proliferation and migration Stimulates angiogenesis	Inhibits proliferation and migration Stimulates differentiation and ECM synthesis	Stimulates proliferation (normal cells) Stimulates ECM proliferation and ECM synthesis (cells from vascular lesions)
IGF-1	7.5	Most tissues Macrophages Fibroblasts	Stimulates migration, ECM contraction, proliferation and ECM synthesis	Stimulates migration and proliferation	Stimulates migration and proliferation	
PDGF	28–35	Platelets Macrophages Fibroblasts Endothelial cells	Stimulates migration and proliferation	Stimulates migration and proliferation	Stimulates proliferation	Stimulates migration and proliferation

Factor	MW (kDa)	Source cells		
VEGF	45	Pituitary cells; Vascular smooth muscle cells	Stimulates proliferation and angiogenesis	Stimulates migration and Stimulates migration and proliferation
FGF-α and β	16–18	Fibroblasts; Endothelial cells	Stimulates migration, ECM contraction, proliferation and ECM synthesis	Stimulates migration, proliferation, ECM synthesis and angiogenesis	Stimulates migration and ECM synthesis
KGF	28	Fibroblasts		Stimulates migration and proliferation
HGF	62	Fibroblasts		Stimulates migration and proliferation

EGF, epidermal growth factor; TGF, transforming growth factor; IGF-1, insulin-like growth factor-1; PDGF, platelet-derived growth factor; VEGF, vascular endothelial growth factor; FGF, fibroblast growth factor; KGF, keratinocyte growth factor; HGF, hepatocyte growth factor.

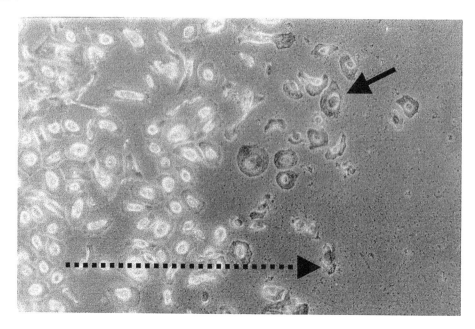

Figure 7.6   MMP expression by migrating corneal epithelial cells. Corneal epithelial cells migrating in
the direction of the arrow in a colony dispersion assay. The darkly stained cells at the
leading edge are expressing matrix metalloproteinase-1 as detected by
immunocytochemistry, indicated by the solid arrow. The dotted arrow shows the direction
of cell migration.

study the interaction between extracellular matrix and corneal epithelial cell
migration in response to growth factors such as hepatocyte growth factor (HGF)
and EGF. For this assay, cells are initially seeded and cultured to confluence within
cloning rings upon ECM-coated wells. The cells are growth-arrested with hy-
droxyurea overnight to negate the influence of proliferation on the distance the
cells migrate. With time the cells migrate outwards and at intervals the cells are
fixed and stained with haematoxylin to indicate the area of cell dispersion.
Alternatively the cells are stained using immunocytochemistry to detect MMP
expression. Our findings demonstrate that when human corneal epithelial cells are
cultured upon type I collagen, the cells at the leading migratory front are positive
for MMP-1 whereas those further back are not (Figure 7.6). This probably
indicates an important role for MMP-1 during reepithelialization in vivo.

To study the influence of growth factors or other agents upon reepithelialization in vitro we have developed a wound model. Epithelial cells are cultured to
confluence and then stimulated to undergo terminal differentiation as previously
described (Rheinwald and Green, 1975). After about 14 days in culture a mature
multilayered epithelium develops with expression of cytokeratins typical of

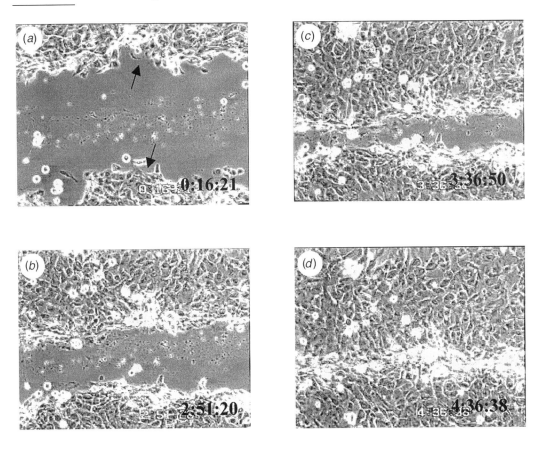

Figure 7.7   In vitro model of reepithelialization. The series of photographs shows the advancing edges of the repairing epithelium with time. By 4 h the wound had closed completely. (*a*) Time: 16 min 21 s; (*b*) 2 h 51 min 20 s; (*c*) 3 h 36 min 50 s; (*d*) 4 h 36 min 38 s.

differentiated epithelium in vivo. The epithelium is then wounded by scoring with a pipette tip and the healing process is recorded microscopically by time-lapse video recording. Photographs from a typical epithelial wound closure sequence are shown in Figure 7.7.

Wound healing: late events

ECM production and remodelling

The reformation of the ECM begins simultaneously with the formation of granulation tissue by inflammatory cells, fibroblasts and endothelial cells. Initially high levels of fibronectin and hyaluronic acid are deposited at the wound site, disappearing as the matrix matures over several weeks with increasing wound collagen and proteoglycan content. In addition to repairing the ECM damage, the production of collagen types I and III as well as fibronectin and fibrin provides support for epithelial cell migration (Clark et al., 1982a; Woodley et al., 1985) and thus reepithelialization of the wound. The production of new ECM at the wound site involves several cell types involved in the healing process. For example, fibronectin is derived from macrophages, endothelial cells, fibroblasts and some epithelial cells (Oh et al., 1981; Clark et al., 1982b), while proteoglycans have been shown to be produced by fibroblasts, smooth muscle and endothelial cells (Lane et al., 1986; Paulsson et al., 1986).

However it is the fibroblast which is the major producer of new ECM; these cells secrete a number of ECM molecules including fibronectin, glycosaminoglycans, hyaluronic acid and collagen types I and III (Barnes et al., 1976; Williams et al., 1984). Collagen is the major component of the wound matrix and, as such, two members of this large family of proteins, collagen types I and III, are highlighted here since the roles of these in wound healing is best defined. The first collagen to be laid down at the wound site is collagen type III (Gabbiani et al., 1976; Guber and Rudolph, 1978) in close association with preexisting fibrin networks, and subsequently stabilized by mucopolysaccharides (Ross and Odland, 1968). Following the regression of both fibroblasts and endothelial cells, collagen type III is replaced by collagen type I (Dvorak et al., 1985). The procollagen molecule, consisting of three helical polypeptides (Gabbiani and Montandon, 1977), is secreted into the extracellular space forming the collagen precursor tropocollagen, via the loss of NH_2 and COOH domains (Gabbiani and Montandon, 1977). This tropocollagen molecule is then cross-linked by lysyl oxidase; the degree of cross-linking reflects the strength of the healed tissue (Chvapil and Koopman, 1984). A number of growth factors have been shown to stimulate ECM synthesis including PDGF (Grotendorst et al., 1985), TGF-β (Sporn et al., 1983; Ignotz and Massague, 1986), EGF, IGF-1 and bFGF (also see Table 7.1).

Several degradative enzymes play crucial roles in the remodelling of the existing and newly synthesized ECM throughout the healing process. For discussion, these enzymes have been divided into two groups: plasminogen activators (PAs) and MMPs. The PAs include urokinase (uPA) and tissue-type (tPA) and are capable of activating plasminogen to plasmin, which has been shown to be involved in the degradation of fibrin clots (Robbins et al., 1981). uPA has been shown to be produced by inflammatory cells (Gordon et al., 1974) and it is thought that, in conjunction with tPA derived from vessel disruption, it leads to the degradation of the fibrin clot. In addition to this, plasmin has been shown to degrade fibronectin (Werb et al., 1980) and to activate the latent forms of MMPs. PAs have also been implicated in the migration of fibroblasts and endothelial cells, although the exact mechanisms of this process are unclear, as well as the proliferative process during arterial repair (Wysocki et al., 1996).

The other major group of ECM degrading enzymes are the MMPs, which are involved in the degradation of collagens (types I–V and VII–XI), gelatin (denatured collagen), fibronectin, laminin, elastin and proteoglycan core protein (for reviews see Birkedal Hansen, 1995; Shapiro, 1998; Nagase and Woessner, 1999). To date more than 20 members of this family have been identified. Several members of the MMP family share a number of structural and functional features, including a Zn^{2+}-binding site, and may be regarded as derivatives (formed by deletion or addition of domains) of the modular structure of collagenases and stromelysins. Members of this family include MMP-1 (collagenase), MMP-2 (72-kDa gelatinase), MMP-3 (stromelysin), MMP-7 (PUMP-1, putative metalloproteinase-1), MMP-8 (neutrophil collagenase), MMP-9 (92 kDa gelatinase), MMP-10 (stromelysin-2), MMP-11 (stromelysin-3) and MMP-12 (metalloelastase). Individual MMPs tend to cleave specific ECM substrates, although there is some overlap in the substrate specificity of these enzymes. These enzymes are initially secreted in an inactive or proform, and are subsequently activated extracellularly. MMPs have been reported to be produced by a variety of cells involved in the wound-healing process including neutrophils, macrophages, fibroblasts, endothelial cells, keratinocytes and vascular smooth muscle cells (Birkedal Hansen et al., 1993; Pauly et al., 1994), their production being regulated by a number of external stimuli including growth factors. Another characteristic of these enzymes is that their activity is regulated by TIMPs, of which four forms have currently been reported (TIMP 1–4). The degree of degradation of the ECM is dependent upon the balance between the ratio of MMPs to TIMPs – a relative increase in MMPs or a decrease in TIMPs results in an overall increase in degradation and vice versa. An example of the importance of the balance of these two systems in ECM turnover has been highlighted in restenosis, where an increase in ECM production and a decrease in MMP activity compared to normal artery has been found (Tyagi et al., 1995). Studies have also suggested that the MMPs may be involved in the proliferation and outgrowth of vascular smooth muscle cells in atherosclerosis (Newby et al., 1994). Delayed wound healing may also result from an imbalance of MMP and TIMP (Vaalamo et al., 1999). Our work has demonstrated that patients with sterile corneal ulcers have large amounts of MMP-9 in their tears and that this may contribute to the tissue 'melting' that can occur (Geerling et al., 1998).

In addition to these secreted MMPs, members of a novel subclass of the MMP family, membrane type-matrix metalloproteinases (MT-MMPs), have recently been reported (Sato et al., 1994; Takino et al., 1995). Evidence suggests that the MT-MMPs play a role in MMP activation at the cell surface. For example, MMP-14 and 16 activate MMP-2 (Lewalle et al., 1995; Strongin et al., 1995; Takino et al., 1995; Cowell et al., 1998).

We have successfully used a variety of techniques for studying ECM production and MMP/TIMP expression. These include QCRT-PCR, zymography, reverse zymography, Western blotting, enzyme-linked immunosorbent assays (ELISAs) and immunocytochemistry.

What determines when the wound-healing process is complete and indicates to the cells that synthesis of new tissue is no longer required is currently receiving much attention. The process of apoptosis or programmed cell death has been indicated in the 'switching-off' process. Apoptosis has been shown to participate in the transition between granulation tissue and development of a scar (Desmouliere et al., 1995). When the apoptotic profiles of fibroblasts from normal and keloid skin (which shows excessive scarring) were compared it was found that keloid fibroblasts showed decreased expression of apoptosis-associated genes (Messadi et al., 1999). The application of pressure treatment to hypertrophic scars results in decreased cellularity which is thought to be a consequence of induced apoptosis and improved matrix organization (Costa et al., 1999). This evidence strongly suggests an important role for apoptosis in the cessation of the healing response.

Role of growth factors in wound healing

Several growth factors have been implicated in the wound-healing process, including members of the EGF, TGF-β, IGF, PDGF, HGF and FGF families. These growth factors are thought to play many key roles not only in the initiation but also in sustaining the wound-healing process, the properties and molecular biology of these factors being the subject of several reviews (Clark and Henson, 1988; Bennett and Schultz, 1993a, b; Imanishi et al., 2000). The roles of growth factors include the stimulation or inhibition of several cellular functions including proliferation, migration, ECM contraction and ECM synthesis. The effects of these growth factors on cell function regulation relating to wound healing are summarized in Table 7.1, and the reader is referred to the above references for a more comprehensive treatise. Although the effects and roles of individual growth factors have been extensively studied in vitro, their interactions and roles in vivo during the wound-healing process are obviously extremely complex and as yet are incompletely elucidated.

A number of techniques have been used in our laboratory to quantitate growth factor and growth factor receptor expression. These include QCRT-PCR for quantitation at the mRNA level, and ELISAs, radioreceptor assays and immunocytochemistry at the protein levels for members of the EGF, TGF-β, IGF, PDGF and FGF families.

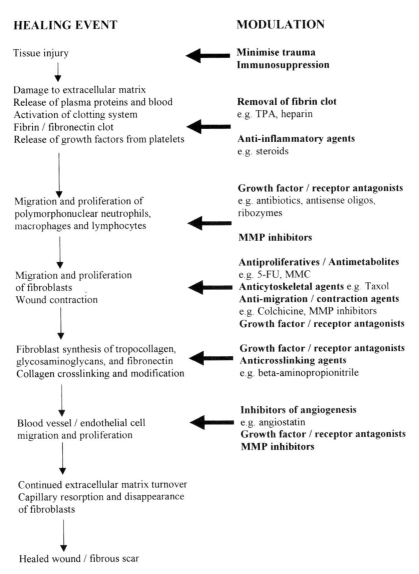

HEALING EVENT

MODULATION

Tissue injury

Minimise trauma
Immunosuppression

Damage to extracellular matrix
Release of plasma proteins and blood
Activation of clotting system
Fibrin / fibronectin clot
Release of growth factors from platelets

Removal of fibrin clot
e.g. TPA, heparin

Anti-inflammatory agents
e.g. steroids

Migration and proliferation of
polymorphonuclear neutrophils,
macrophages and lymphocytes

Growth factor / receptor antagonists
e.g. antibiotics, antisense oligos,
ribozymes

MMP inhibitors

Migration and proliferation
of fibroblasts
Wound contraction

Antiproliferatives / Antimetabolites
e.g. 5-FU, MMC
Anticytoskeletal agents e.g. Taxol
Anti-migration / contraction agents
e.g. Colchicine, MMP inhibitors
Growth factor / receptor antagonists

Fibroblast synthesis of tropocollagen,
glycosaminoglycans, and fibronectin
Collagen crosslinking and modification

Growth factor / receptor antagonists
Anticrosslinking agents
e.g. beta-aminopropionitrile

Blood vessel / endothelial cell
migration and proliferation

Inhibitors of angiogenesis
e.g. angiostatin
Growth factor / receptor antagonists
MMP inhibitors

Continued extracellular matrix turnover
Capillary resorption and disappearance
of fibroblasts

Healed wound / fibrous scar

Figure 7.8   Modulation of wound healing. TPA, tissue plasminogen activator; 5-FU, 5-fluorouracil; MMC, mitomycin-C; MMP, matrix metalloproteinase.

Modulation of wound healing

The wound-healing process as illustrated above is a complex array of cellular, ECM and chemical mediator interactions. As a result, wound healing can be modulated at various stages, as shown in Figure 7.8. Many antiscarring therapies have been available for several years, but it is only recently that our increase in knowledge of the mechanisms underlying the healing process in both adult and fetal tissue (which does not scar), that therapy refinement and the development of potential therapies have been achieved. In addition to this, the application of both basic science and therapeutic findings from different fields of wound-healing research may prove not only essential but also successful. Some of the recent advances in our understanding of the healing process, agents available for modifying healing (and their modes of action) and new/potential methods for modulating healing are outlined below.

Attempts have been made particularly to target specific cell functions during the wound-healing process. Many of the agents used have effects on several cell functions and types. For simplicity of discussion, these agents have been divided into immunosuppressives/antiinflammatories, antimigration/anticytoskeletal agents, antiproliferative/antimetabolic agents, inhibitors of angiogenesis, agents affecting ECM synthesis and degradation and agents affecting growth factors and growth factor receptors.

Immunosuppressives/antiinflammatories

These agents affect the early phases of the wound-healing process. As the influx of inflammatory cells into the wound site is thought to play a role in the stimulation of later healing events, the use of corticosteroids and other immunosuppressives has been shown not only to impair inflammatory cell chemotaxis but also subsequent angiogenesis, fibroblast proliferation and matrix synthesis (Wahl, 1989), resulting in reduced scarring in tissues such as the conjunctiva (Roth et al., 1991). Therapies involving combined treatment of antibiotic with antiinflammatory agents have been found to reduce scarring in patients with idiopathic pulmonary fibrosis (Ziesche et al., 1999) and also in rats with pyelonephritis (Huang et al., 1999). Recently, the extravasation of inflammatory cells both in vitro and in vivo (Gijbels et al., 1994; Leppert et al., 1995) has been shown to involve the MMPs, suggesting a potential role for potent, broad-spectrum MMP inhibitors in the modulation of the inflammatory response and subsequent scarring (also see below).

Antimigration/anticytoskeletal agents

Examples of these agents include colchicine, cytochalasin b and particularly taxol, which has been shown to inhibit the ability of fibroblasts to migrate towards a chemical stimulus (Metcalfe and Weetman, 1994). Colchicine has been shown to inhibit vascular smooth muscle cell proliferation in vitro (Voisard et al., 1995), while taxol has also been shown to inhibit fibroblast proliferation and to reduce scarring in an aggressive in vivo model (Jampel et al., 1990), as well as restenosis following angioplasty (Sollott et al., 1995). As described earlier, the ability of cells to contract the ECM appears to be dependent upon the migration of these cells, as it is the subsequent generation of tractional forces upon their substratum via cell movement which ultimately results in contraction of the ECM. We have been using collagen type I matrices populated with fibroblasts as an in vitro model of wound contraction. Upon stimulation with serum or growth factors, the fibroblasts contract these matrices. We have demonstrated that the degree of collagen contraction can be significantly inhibited upon single 5-minute exposures to the antiproliferative/antimetabolic agents 5-fluorouracil (5-FU) and mitomycin-C (MMC), without cell death (Occleston et al., 1994). Observations made during this study suggested that the MMPs might play a major role in the process of collagen contraction. Subsequent work in our laboratory has shown that the MMPs are essential to the process of collagen contraction and that this process can be significantly inhibited using specific MMP inhibitors. In addition, we have found that the requirement of MMPs for contraction may be a ubiquitous mechanism, not only throughout different tissue sites (cornea, conjunctiva, dermis, synovial sheath and endotendon) but also species (human, rabbit and rat). These findings may have important therapeutic implications as we have also demonstrated that the effects of MMP inhibitors on collagen contraction are specific, nontoxic and can be applied to or removed from tissue constructs to control the degree of contraction. MMPs may also be an important prognostic factor in certain types of scarring (Kon et al., 1998).

MMPs have also been implicated in the migration of a variety of other cell types through basement membrane in vitro, including inflammatory cells, endothelial cells and vascular smooth muscle cells (Pauly et al., 1994; Leppert et al., 1995; Taraboletti et al., 1995). The inhibition of these enzymes also reduces angiogenesis in vivo (Galardy et al., 1994; Taraboletti et al., 1995), suggesting a potential role for MMP inhibitors in the modulation of these healing-related processes.

Antiproliferative/antimetabolic agents

Much of the antiscarring research in ophthalmology has concentrated on the use of these agents, primarily to reduce cell division. Blumenkranz and colleagues established that 5-FU inhibited the proliferation of fibroblasts in vitro and ocular scarring in vivo (Blumenkranz et al., 1982, 1984). Following these findings, an antiscarring regimen involving subconjunctival 5-FU injections after glaucoma filtration surgery was developed in Miami, Florida, USA, resulting in a multicentre trial (The Fluorouracil Filtering Surgery Group, 1989). Largely unnoticed for more than a decade was the use of single applications of the agent MMC (Chen, 1983; Chen et al., 1990). Further research in our laboratory demonstrated that single exposures to β-radiation, 5-FU and MMC had long-term antiproliferative effects on fibroblasts, with single exposures as short as 5 min (Khaw et al., 1991, 1992a; Constable et al., 1998). We subsequently showed that effective suppression

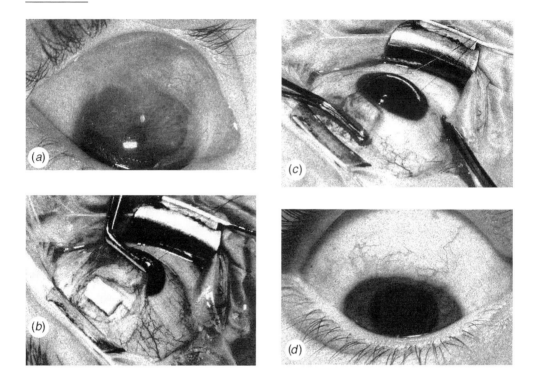

Figure 7.9   Reduction of postoperative scarring using short, single applications of antiproliferatives. (*a*)
Scarring and tissue contraction following unsuccessful glaucoma filtration surgery. (*b/c*)
Intraoperative application of a sponge soaked in antiproliferative/antimetabolite. (*d*)
Reduction in scarring following a short, single application of antiproliferative/
antimetabolite, resulting in successful filtration surgery.

of proliferation in excess of 36 days, without cell necrosis, could be achieved
(Khaw et al., 1992b,c). These single 5-min treatments were also found to be
effective in vivo, being titratable in terms of length of action (Doyle et al., 1993;
Khaw et al., 1993b) and focal (Khaw et al., 1992b, 1993a). These single intraoperative 5-min exposures to 5-FU and MMC are now the standard treatment
for patients undergoing glaucoma filtration surgery at Moorfields Eye Hospital
(Figure 7.9), and are currently the subject of a 5-year Medical Research Council
clinical trial. We are also carrying out a long-term trial of a single exposure to
β-radiation from a strontium-90 probe in Africa.

The main advantage of these agents is that they can be applied relatively focally
and then washed out. The use of 5-FU has also been shown by our collaborators to
have potential for reducing contractile scarring in injured tendon (Khan et al.,
1997). Recently we showed that clinically relevant doses of MMC and 5-FU
induced apoptosis, rather than necrosis, in treated fibroblasts (Crowston et al.,

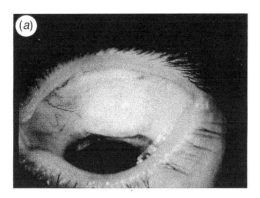
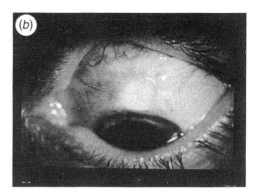
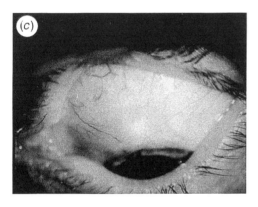

Figure 7.10 Glaucoma filtration surgery failure due to scarring. This series of photographs was taken of the same patient at (*a*) 2 weeks, (*b*), 4 weeks and (*c*) 3 months post-filtration surgery. With time the bleb size decreases as scar tissue forms around it, blocking drainage. Figure adapted with the kind permission of Microscopy and Research Technique. Daniels, J.T., Occleston, N.L., Crowston, J.G. et al. (1998). Understanding and controlling the scarring response: the contribution of histology and microscopy. *Microsc. Res. Tech.*, **42**: 317–33.

1998). This may provide another novel target for antiscarring therapy and our aim in the laboratory is always to identify new antiscarring targets. Whilst the application of antimetabolites during filtration surgery suppresses the scarring response for most patients, unfortunately a small number of patients still scar, causing surgical failure (Figure 7.10). Our laboratory work has demonstrated that, as the antimetabolite-treated fibroblasts recover from growth arrest, they produce a number of growth factors. These may be produced by the cells to overcome growth arrest (Occleston et al., 1997). We have also shown in vitro that growth-arrested fibroblasts produce factors that can stimulate wound-healing activity in nontreated cells, perhaps indicating a mechanism where scarring activity is

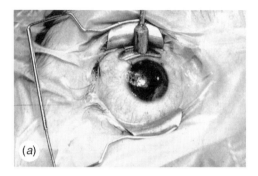
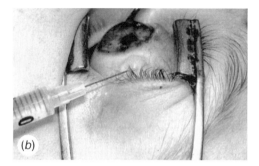
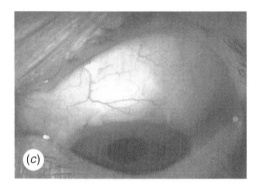

Figure 7.11   New approaches to antiscarring therapy. (*a*) The application of β-radiation to the eye during glaucoma filtration surgery. (*b*) Post surgical injection of a novel antibody to transforming growth factor-β_2 (TGF-β_2). (*c*) Filtering bleb following injection of antibody to TGF-β_2.

induced peripherally to the area of antimetabolite application (Daniels et al., 1999). MMC has also been shown to inhibit vascular smooth muscle cell migration and proliferation in vitro (Tanaka et al., 1994), perhaps suggesting a role for these agents in the modulation of restenosis. Additionally, we have demonstrated that applications of β-radiation (Figure 7.11*a*) have similar antiproliferative effects as the agents above in vitro (Khaw et al., 1991; Constable et al., 1998) and focal applications result in reduced scarring in vivo (Miller and Rice, 1991). These findings are similar to the reported effects of β-radiation on restenosis in animal models (Verin et al., 1995; Waksman et al., 1995; Laird et al., 1996). Interestingly, recent clinical trials have shown that doses of β-radiation can reduce long-term stenosis following coronary angioplasty (Teirstein et al., 2000).

Ultimately, combination of these agents with others may offer the best therapeutic index. We have recently combined heparin with 5-FU in patients at high risk of developing blinding retinal scarring in a randomized masked placebo-controlled trial and shown a reduction in scarring from 26.1% to 12.8% (Asaria et al., 2001).

Inhibitors of angiogenesis

As highlighted earlier, angiogenesis plays a crucial role in the formation of granulation tissue during wound healing. Although several studies have revealed important targets for the inhibition of angiogenesis and subsequent inhibitors, e.g. inhibitors of VEGF/FGF, angiostatin, urokinase receptor antagonists and scatter factor inhibitors, their use in modulating the wound-healing response is still unclear. In addition to this, MMPs have been implicated in endothelial cell migration in vitro and subsequently the inhibition of MMP activity has been shown to reduce angiogenesis in vivo (Galardy et al., 1994).

Agents affecting ECM synthesis and degradation

Examples of agents which affect ECM synthesis include the lathyrogenic agent β-aminopropionitrile, which is thought to have its clinical effect (McGuigan et al., 1986, 1987; Moorhead et al., 1990) by inhibiting the enzyme lysyl oxidase and thus preventing collagen cross-linking (Siegel, 1977). As discussed above, the ECM present in wounds is the product of both synthesis and degradative processes. Major players in the degradation of the ECM are the MMPs and their inhibitors (TIMPs). As such, interfering with either of these families of molecules may have profound effects on the healing process. Potential modulating agents include chemical inhibitors of the MMPs, MMP/TIMP neutralizing antibodies, antisense oligonucleotides or ribozymes to MMPs or TIMPs (see below), which may have future uses in healing modulation. These molecules (MMPs/TIMPs) are of particular importance in the modulation of wound healing since they appear to play crucial roles throughout the healing response, as shown in earlier sections, and as such are receiving considerable attention.

Agents affecting growth factors and growth factor receptors

As highlighted earlier, growth factors and their receptors play a central regulatory role in the wound-healing process. Consequently, the growth factors, the receptors through which they elicit their effects, and the intracellular signalling cascades involved are extremely good candidates for therapeutic intervention. In the following paragraph the modulation of one of the pivotal growth factor families in wound healing at many tissue sites, TGF-β, will be used as an example.

We have shown that all three isoforms of TGF-β stimulate a conjunctival scarring response (Cordeiro et al., 1999a). Several approaches to the modulation of TGF-β have been or are currently being investigated. These include the neutralization of TGF-β activity using antibodies or TGF-β_3, which have been shown to reduce scarring in vivo (Shah et al., 1992, 1994, 1995; Logan et al., 1999). In fact, our group has successfully developed a new mouse model of conjunctival scarring (Reichel et al., 1998) and applied a novel antibody to TGF-β_2 capable of significantly reducing scarring (Cordeiro et al., 1999b) which has now entered multicentre clinical trials in the United Kingdom. Studies to date have suggested that the antibody is clinically safe, nontoxic and well tolerated when injected following glaucoma surgery (Figure 7.11b and c). In addition to this, there is a potential antiscarring role for TGF-β receptor antagonists. Studies have shown that the sugar mannose-6-phosphate (which competitively binds to the mannose-6-phosphate/IGF-II receptor) reduces cutaneous scarring by inhibiting the activation of latent TGF-β. Recently it was shown that inhibition of ras proteins (which are key players in the transduction of growth factor signals from the cell surface to the nucleus) prevents smooth muscle cell proliferation in vivo following vascular injury (Indolfi et al., 1995). Another possible approach to interfering with TGF-β protein production at the wound site would be the local application of specific antisense oligonucleotides to TGF-β mRNA, although their use is still clearly in the early stages. A related, potential way of modulating TGF-β would be the use of ribozymes. These are RNA molecules that have been shown to cleave other RNA molecules (Bartel and Szostak, 1993; Moore, 1995; Wilson and Szostak, 1995). Like antisense oligonuleotides, ribozymes can be designed to attach to a specific mRNA of choice. There are, however, significant advantages of ribozymes over antisense. Once the ribozyme has attached to the 'target' mRNA, it cleaves the mRNA and then is free to attach to and cleave another 'target' mRNA. So, theoretically, the actions of ribozymes, unlike antisense oligonucleotides, should not be concentration- or time-dependent. The use of ribozymes as RNA-directed gene therapies has been shown (Altman, 1993; Dorai et al., 1994) although their use as antiscarring agents has still to be fully investigated. Current work in our laboratory, in conjunction with our colleagues at the University of Florida, is investigating the use of ribozymes directed against TGF-β_1 and the TGF-β type II receptor in the modulation of ocular scarring.

In summary, we now have a variety of techniques available to investigate the basic science of the cellular and molecular mechanisms underlying the wound-healing process. Our recent advances in understanding have directly led to methods to modulate healing, several of which are now in clinical trial or are used routinely in the clinic (e.g. TGF-β antibody and single, short exposures to 5-FU or MMC). It is only by gaining a deeper understanding of the basic cellular and molecular biology of the healing response throughout the body that we will be able to achieve our ultimate goal: safe, effective control of healing with retention of both function and aesthetics.

REFERENCES

Agren, M.S. (1999). Matrix metalloproteinases (MMPs) are required for re-epithelialisation of cutaneous wounds. *Arch. Dermatol. Res.*, **291**, 583–90.

Allen, T.D. & Schor, S.L. (1983). The contraction of collagen matrices by dermal fibroblasts. *J. Ultrastruct. Res.*, **83**, 205–19.

Altman, S. (1993). RNA enzyme-directed gene therapy [comment]. *Proc. Natl Acad. Sci. U.S.A.*, **90**, 10898–900.

Asaria, R.H.Y., Kon, C.H., Bunce, K. et al. (2001). Adjuvant therapy with 5-fluorouracil and low molecular weight heparin prevents post operative proliferative retinopathy: results from a randomised controlled clinical trial. *Ophthalmology* (in press).

Barnes, M.J., Morton, L.F., Bennett, R.C., Bailey, A.J. & Sims, T.J. (1976). Presence of type III collagen in guinea-pig dermal scar. *Biochem. J.*, **157**, 263–6.

Bartel, D.P. & Szostak, J.W. (1993). Isolation of new ribozymes from a large pool of random sequences [see comment]. *Science*, **261**, 1411–18.

Bell, E., Ivarsson, B. & Merrill, C. (1979). Production of a tissue-like structure by contraction of collagen lattices by human fibroblasts of different proliferative potential in vitro. *Proc. Natl Acad. Sci. U.S.A.*, **76**, 1274–8.

Bement, W.M., Forscher, P. & Mooseker, M.S. (1993). A novel cytoskeletal structure involved in purse string wound closure and cell polarity maintenance. *J. Cell Biol.*, **121**, 565–78.

Bennett, N.T. & Schultz, G.S. (1993a). Growth factors and wound healing: biochemical properties of growth factors and their receptors. *Am. J. Surg.*, **165**, 728–37.

Bennett, N.T. & Schultz, G.S. (1993b). Growth factors and wound healing: part II. Role in normal and chronic wound healing. *Am. J. Surg.*, **166**, 74–81.

Berry, D.P., Harding, K.G., Stanton, M.R., Jasani, B. & Ehrlich, H.P. (1998). Human wound contraction: collagen organization, fibroblasts, and myofibroblasts. *Plast. Reconstr. Surg.*, **102**, 124–31.

Birkedal Hansen, H. (1995). Proteolytic remodeling of extracellular matrix. *Curr. Opin. Cell Biol.*, **7**, 728–35.

Birkedal Hansen, H., Moore, W.G., Bodden, M.K. et al. (1993). Matrix metalloproteinases: a review. *Crit. Rev. Oral Biol. Med.*, **4**, 197–250.

Blumenkranz, M.S., Ophir, A., Claflin, A.J. & Hajek, A. (1982). Fluorouracil for the treatment of massive periretinal proliferation. *Am. J. Ophthalmol.*, **94**, 458–67.

Blumenkranz, M.S., Claflin, A. & Hajek, A.S. (1984). Selection of therapeutic agents for intraocular proliferative disease. Cell culture evaluation. *Arch. Ophthalmol.*, **102**, 598–604.

Boyden, S. (1962). The chemotactic effect of mixtures of antibody and antigen on polymorphonuclear leucocytes. *J. Exp. Med.*, **115**, 453–66.

Brenner, C.A., Adler, R.R., Rappolee, D.A., Pedersen, R.A. & Werb, Z. (1989). Genes for extracellular-matrix-degrading metalloproteinases and their inhibitor, TIMP, are expressed during early mammalian development. *Genes Dev.*, **3**, 848–59.

Bullard, K.M., Lund, L., Mudgett, J.S. et al. (1999). Impaired wound contraction in stromelysin-1-deficient mice. *Ann. Surg.*, **230**, 260–5.

Burger, P.C., Chandler, D.B. & Klintworth, G.K. (1983). Corneal neovascularization as studied by scanning electron microscopy of vascular casts. *Lab. Invest.*, **48**, 169–80.

Buttle, D.J. & Ehrlich, H.P. (1983). Comparative studies of collagen lattice contraction utilizing a normal and a transformed cell line. *J. Cell Physiol.*, **116**, 159–66.

Cacou, C., Eastwood, M., McGrouther, D.A. & Brown, R.A. (1996). Culture force monitor or investigating the formation of adhesions between tissue interfaces in vitro. *Cell. Engineering*, **1**, 109–14.

Chen, C.W. (1983). Enhanced intraocular pressure controlling effectiveness of trabeculectomy by local application of mitomycin *C. Trans. Asia Pacific Acad. Ophthalmol.*, **9**, 172–7.

Chen, C.W., Huang, H.T., Bair, J.S. & Lee, C.C. (1990). Trabeculectomy with simultaneous topical application of mitomycin-C in refractory glaucoma. *J. Ocul. Pharmacol.*, **6**, 175–82.

Cheresh, D.A., Leng, J. & Klemke, R.L. (1999). Regulation of cell contraction and membrane ruffling by distinct signals in migratory cells. *J. Cell. Biol.*, **146**, 1107–16.

Chvapil, M. & Koopman, C.F. (1984). Scar formation: physiology and pathology states. *Otolaryng. Clin. North Am.*, **17**, 265–72.

Clark, R.A.F. & Henson, P.M. (1988). *The Molecular and Cellular Biology of Wound Repair.* New York: Plenum Press.

Clark, R.A., Lanigan, J.M., DellaPelle, P. et al. (1982a). Fibronectin and fibrin provide a provisional matrix for epidermal cell migration during wound reepithelialization. *J. Invest. Dermatol.*, **79**, 264–9.

Clark, R.A., DellaPelle, P., Manseau, E. et al. (1982b). Blood vessel fibronectin increases in conjunction with endothelial cell proliferation and capillary ingrowth during wound healing. *J. Invest. Dermatol.*, **79**, 269–76.

Clark, J.G., Kuhn, C.D., McDonald, J.A. & Mecham, R.P. (1983). Lung connective tissue. *Int. Rev. Connect. Tissue Res.*, **10**, 249–331.

Constable, P.H., Crowston, J.G., Occleston, N.L., Cordeiro, M.F. & Khaw, P.T. (1998). Long term growth arrest of human Tenon's fibroblasts following single applications of beta radiation. *Br. J. Ophthalmol.*, **82**, 448–52.

Cordeiro, M.F., Reichel, M.B., Gay, J.A. et al. (1999a). Transforming growth factor-beta1, -beta2, and -beta3 in vivo: effects on normal and mitomycin C-modulated conjunctival scarring. *Invest. Ophthalmol. Vis. Sci.*, **40**, 1975–82.

Cordeiro, M.F., Gay, J.A. & Khaw, P.T. (1999b). Human anti-transforming growth factor-beta2 antibody: a new glaucoma anti-scarring agent. *Invest. Ophthalmol. Vis. Sci.*, **40**, 2225–34.

Costa, A.M., Peyrol, S., Porto, L.C. et al. (1999). Mechanical forces induce scar remodelling. Study in non-pressure-treated versus pressure-treated hypertrophic scars. *Am. J. Pathol.*, **155**, 1671–9.

Cowell, S., Knauper, V., Stewart, M.L. et al. (1998). Induction of matrix metalloproteinase activation cascades based on membrane-type 1 matrix metalloproteinase: associated activation of gelatinase A, gelatinase B and collagenase 3. *Biochem. J.*, **331**, 453–8.

Crowston, J.G., Akbar, A.N., Constable, P.H. et al. (1998). Antimetabolite-induced apoptosis in Tenon's capsule fibroblasts. *Invest. Ophthalmol. Vis. Sci.*, **39**, 449–54.

Daniels, J.T., Occleston, N.L., Crowston, J.G. & Khaw, P.T. (1999). Effects of antimetabolite induced cellular growth arrest on fibroblast-fibroblast interactions. *Exp. Eye Res.*, **69**, 117–27.

Desmouliere, A., Redard, M., Darby, I. & Gabbiani, G. (1995). Apoptosis mediates the decrease in cellularity during the transition between granulation tissue and scar. *Am. J. Pathol.*, **146**, 56–66.

Deuel, T.F., Senior, R.M., Huang, J.S. & Griffin, G.L. (1982). Chemotaxis of monocytes and neutrophils to platelet-derived growth factor. *J. Clin. Invest.*, **69**, 1046–9.

Dorai, T., Kobayashi, H., Holland, J.F. & Ohnuma, T. (1994). Modulation of platelet-derived growth factor-beta mRNA expression and cell growth in a human mesothelioma cell line by a hammerhead ribozyme. *Mol. Pharmacol.*, **46**, 437–44.

Doyle, J.W., Sherwood, M.B., Khaw, P.T., McGrory, S. & Smith, M.F. (1993). Intraoperative 5-fluorouracil for filtration surgery in the rabbit. *Invest. Ophthalmol. Vis. Sci.*, **34**, 3313–19.

Dvorak, H.F., Senger, D.R., Dvorak, A.M., Harvey, V.S. & McDonagh, J. (1985). Regulation of extravascular coagulation by microvascular permeability. *Science*, **227**, 1059–61.

Eastwood, M., McGrouther, D.A. & Brown, R.A. (1994). A culture force monitor for measurement of contraction forces generated in human dermal fibroblast cultures: evidence for cell-matrix mechanical signalling. *Biochim. Biophys. Acta*, **1201**, 186–92.

Eastwood, M., Porter, R., Khan, U., McGrouther, G. & Brown, R. (1996). Quantitative analysis of collagen gel contractile forces generated by dermal fibroblasts and the relationship to cell morphology. *J. Cell Physiol.*, **166**, 33–42.

Ehrlich, H.P. & Rajaratnam, J.B. (1990). Cell locomotion forces versus cell contraction forces for collagen lattice contraction: an in vitro model of wound contraction. *Tissue Cell*, **22**, 407–17.

Ehrlich, H.P., Keefer, K.A., Myers, R.L. & Passaniti, A. (1999). Vanadate and the absence of myofibroblasts in wound contraction. *Arch. Surg.*, **134**, 494–501.

Finlay, G.J., Baguley, B.C. & Wilson, W.R. (1984). A semiautomated microculture method for investigating growth inhibitory effects of cytotoxic compounds on exponentially growing carcinoma cells. *Anal. Biochem.*, **139**, 272–7.

Fluorouracil Filtering Surgery Group (1989). Fluorouracil filtering surgery study one-year follow-up. *Am. J. Ophthalmol.*, **108**, 625–35.

Freshney, R.I. (1987). *Culture of Animal Cells. A Manual of Basic Technique.* New York: A.R. Liss.

Gabbiani, G. & Montandon, D. (1977). Reparative processes in mammalian wound healing: the role of contractile phenomena. *Int. Rev. Cytol.*, **48**, 187–219.

Gabbiani, G., Hirschel, B.J., Ryan, G.B., Statkov, P.R. & Majno, G. (1972). Granulation tissue as a contractile organ. A study of structure and function. *J. Exp. Med.*, **135**, 719–34.

Gabbiani, G., Le Lous, M., Bailey, A.J., Bazin, S. & Delaunay, A. (1976). Collagen and myofibroblasts of granulation tissue. A chemical, ultrastructural and immunologic study. *Virchows Arch. B Cell Pathol.*, **21**, 133–45.

Galardy, R.E., Grobelny, D., Foellmer, H.G. & Fernandez, L.A. (1994). Inhibition of angiogenesis by the matrix metalloprotease inhibitor N-[2R-2-(hydroxamidocarbonymethyl)-4-methylpentanoyl)]-L-tryptophan methylamide. *Cancer Res.*, **54**, 4715–18.

Geerling, G., Joussen, A., Daniels, J., Khaw, P. & Dart, J. (1998). Matrix metalloproteinases in sterile corneal melts. *Ann. N.Y. Acad, Sci.*, **878**, 571–4.

Gijbels, K., Galardy, R.E. & Steinman, L. (1994). Reversal of experimental autoimmune encephalomyelitis with a hydroxamate inhibitor of matrix metalloproteases. *J. Clin. Invest.*, **94**, 2177–82.

Gordon, S., Unkeless, J.C. & Cohn, Z.A. (1974). Induction of macrophage plasminogen activator by endotoxin stimulation and phagocytosis: evidence for a two-stage process. *J. Exp. Med.*, **140**, 995–1010.

Greiling, D. & Clark, R.A. (1997). Fibronectin provides a conduit for fibroblast transmigration from collagenous stroma into fibrin clot provisional matrix. *J. Cell Sci.*, **110**, 861–70.

Grinnell, F. (1984). Fibronectin and wound healing. *J. Cell Biochem.*, **26**, 107–16.

Grinnell, F. (1994). Mini-review of the cellular mechanisms of disease: fibroblasts, myofibroblasts and wound contraction. *J. Cell Biol.*, **124**, 401–4.

Grotendorst, G.R., Martin, G.R., Pencev, D., Sodek, J. & Harvey, A.K. (1985). Stimulation of granulation tissue formation by platelet-derived growth factor in normal and diabetic rats. *J. Clin. Invest.*, **76**, 2323–9.

Guber, S. & Rudolph, R. (1978). The myofibroblast. *Surg. Gynecol. Obstet.*, **146**, 641–9.

Guidry, C. (1993). Fibroblast contraction of collagen gels requires activation of protein kinase C. *J. Cell Physiol.*, **155**, 358–67.

Guidry, C. & Grinnell, F. (1985). Studies on the mechanism of hydrated collagen gel reorganization by human skin fibroblasts. *J. Cell Sci.*, **79**, 67–81.

Harris, A.K. (1973). The behaviour of cultured cells on substrata of variable adhesiveness. *Exp. Cell Res.*, **77**, 285–97.

Harris, A.K., Stopak, D. & Wild, P. (1981). Fibroblast traction as a mechanism for collagen morphogenesis. *Nature*, **290**, 249–51.

Heldin, C.H. & Westermark, B. (1984). Growth factors: mechanism of action and relation to oncogenes. *Cell*, **37**, 9–20.

Huang, A., Palmer, L.S., Hom, D. et al. (1999). Ibuprofen combined with antibiotics suppresses renal scarring due to ascending pyelonephritis. *J. Urol.*, **162**, 1396–8.

Ignotz, R. & Massague, J. (1986). Transforming growth factor beta stimulates the expression of fibronectin and their incorporation into the extracellular matrix. *J. Biol. Chem.*, **261**, 4337–45.

Imanishi, J., Kamiyama, K., Iguchi, I. et al. (2000). Growth factors: importance in wound healing and maintenance of transparency of the cornea. *Prog. Retin. Eye Res.*, **19**, 113–29.

Indolfi, C., Avvedimento, E.V., Rapacciuolo, A. et al. (1995). Inhibition of cellular ras prevents smooth muscle cell proliferation after vascular injury in vivo [see comments]. *Nature Med.*, **1**, 541–5.

Issekutz, T.B., Issekutz, A.C. & Movat, H.Z. (1981). The in vivo quantitation and kinetics of monocyte migration into acute inflammatory tissue. *Am. J. Pathol.*, **103**, 47–55.

Iwasaki, T., Chen, J.D., Kim, J.P., Wynn, K.C. & Woodley, D.T. (1994). Dibutyryl cyclic AMP modulates keratinocyte migration without alteration of integrin expression. *J. Invest. Dermatol.*, **102**, 891–7.

Jampel, H.D., Leong, K.W., Koya, P. & Quigley, H.A. (1990). The use of hydrophobic drugs incorporated into polyanhydrides in experimental glaucoma surgery. *Invest. Ophthalmol. Vis. Sci.*, **31S**, 2.

Jester, J.V., Petroll, W.M., Barry, P.A. & Cavanagh, H.D. (1995). Temporal, 3-dimensional, cellular anatomy of corneal wound tissue. *J. Anat.*, **186**, 301–11.

Joseph, J.P., Grierson, I. & Hitchings, R.A. (1987). Normal rabbit aqueous humour, fibronectin, and fibroblast conditioned medium are chemoattractant to Tenon's capsule fibroblasts. *Eye*,

1, 585–92.

Kao, W.W., Kao, C.W., Kaufman, A.H. et al. (1998). Healing of corneal epithelial defects in plasminogen- and fibrinogen-deficient mice. *Invest. Ophthalmol. Vis. Sci.*, **39**, 502–8.

Kawase, T., Ogata, S., Orikasa, M. & Burns, D.M. (1995). 1,25-Dihydroxyvitamin D$_3$ promotes prostaglandin E$_1$-induced differentiation of HL-60 cells. *Calcif. Tissue Int.*, **57**, 359–66.

Khan, U., Occleston, N.L., Khaw, P.T. & McGrouther, D.A. (1997). Single exposures to 5-fluorouracil: a possible mode of targeted therapy to reduce contractile scarring in the injured tendon. *Plast. Reconstr. Surg.*, **99**, 465–71.

Khaw, P.T., Ward, S., Grierson, I. & Rice, N.S. (1991). Effect of beta radiation on proliferating human Tenon's capsule fibroblasts. *Br. J. Ophthalmol.*, **75**, 580–3.

Khaw, P.T., Sherwood, M.B., MacKay, S.L., Rossi, M.J. & Schultz, G. (1992a). Five-minute treatments with fluorouracil, floxuridine, and mitomycin have long-term effects on human Tenon's capsule fibroblasts. *Arch. Ophthalmol.*, **110**, 1150–4.

Khaw, P.T., Sherwood, M.B., Doyle, J.W. et al. (1992b). Intraoperative and post operative treatment with 5-fluorouracil and mitomycin-C: long term effects in vivo on subconjunctival and scleral fibroblasts. *Int. Ophthalmol.*, **16**, 381–5.

Khaw, P.T., Ward, S., Porter, A. et al. (1992c). The long-term effects of 5-fluorouracil and sodium butyrate on human Tenon's fibroblasts. *Invest. Ophthalmol. Vis. Sci.*, **33**, 2043–52.

Khaw, P.T., Doyle, J.W., Sherwood, M.B. et al. (1993a). Prolonged localized tissue effects from 5-minute exposures to fluorouracil and mitomycin C. *Arch. Ophthalmol.*, **111**, 263–7.

Khaw, P.T., Doyle, J.W., Sherwood, M.B., Smith, M.F. & McGorray, S. (1993b). Effects of intraoperative 5-fluorouracil or mitomycin C on glaucoma filtration surgery in the rabbit. *Ophthalmology*, **100**, 367–72.

Kim, W.J., Mohan, R.R. & Wilson, S.E. (1999). Effect of PDGF, IL-1alpha, and BMP2/4 on corneal fibroblast chemotaxis: expression of the platelet-derived growth factor system in the cornea. *Invest. Ophthalmol. Vis. Sci.*, **40**, 1364–72.

Klein, C.E., Dressel, D., Steinmayer, T. et al. (1991). Integrin alpha 2 beta 1 is upregulated in fibroblasts and highly aggressive melanoma cells in three-dimensional collagen lattices and mediates the reorganization of collagen I fibrils. *J. Cell Biol.*, **115**, 1427–36.

Knighton, D.R. & Fiegel, V.D. (1989). The macrophages: effector cell wound repair. *Prog. Clin. Biol. Res.*, **299**, 217–26.

Kon, C.H., Occleston, N.L., Daniels, J. et al. (1998). Expression of MMP-2 and MMP-9 in retinal wound healing: a prospective analysis of vitreous in patients with retinal detachment and proliferative vitreoretinopathy. *Invest. Ophthalmol. Vis. Sci.*, **39**, 1524–9.

Kurkinen, M., Vaheri, A., Roberts, P.J. & Stenman, S. (1980). Sequential appearance of fibronectin and collagen in experimental granulation tissue. *Lab. Invest.*, **43**, 47–51.

Laird, J.R., Carter, A.J., Kufs, W.M. et al. (1996). Inhibition of neointimal proliferation with low-dose irradiation from a beta-particle-emitting stent. *Circulation*, **93**, 529–36.

Lane, D.A., Pejler, G., Flynn, A.M., Thompson, E.A. & Lindahl, U. (1986). Neutralization of heparin-related saccharides by histidine-rich glycoprotein and platelet factor 4 [published erratum appears in *J. Biol. Chem.* (1986) **261**: 13387]. *J. Biol. Chem.*, **261**, 3980–6.

Leppert, D., Waubant, E., Galardy, R., Bunnett, N.W. & Hauser, S.L. (1995). T cell gelatinases mediate basement membrane transmigration in vitro. *J. Immunol.*, **154**, 4379–89.

Lewalle, J.M., Munaut, C., Pichot, B. et al. (1995). Plasma membrane-dependent activation of gelatinase A in human vascular endothelial cells. *J. Cell Physiol.*, **165**, 475–83.

Lewis, J. (1984). Morphogenesis by fibroblast traction [news]. *Nature*, **307**, 413–14.

Logan, A., Green, J., Hunter, A., Jackson, R. & Berry, M. (1999). Inhibition of glial scarring in the injured rat brain by a recombinant human monoclonal antibody to transforming growth factor-beta2. *Eur. J. Neurosci.*, **11**, 2367–74.

Mackenzie, I.C. & Fusenig, N.E. (1983). Regeneration of organized epithelial structure. *J. Invest. Dermatol.*, **81**, 189s–94s.

Martin, P. & Lewis, J. (1992). Actin cables and epidermal movement in embryonic wound healing. *Nature*, **360**, 179–83.

Maynard, J.R., Heckman, C.A., Pitlick, F.A. & Nemerson, Y. (1975). Association of tissue factor activity with the surface of cultured cells. *J. Clin. Invest.*, **55**, 814–24.

McCarthy, J.B., Sas, D.F. & Furcht, L.T. (1988). Mechanisms of parenchymal cell migration into wounds. In: *The Molecular and Cellular Biology of Wound Repair*, ed. Clark, R.A.F. & Henson, P.M., pp. 281–319. New York: Plenum Press.

McDonald, J.A., Kelley, D.G. & Broekelmann, T.J. (1982). Role of fibronectin in collagen deposition: Fab' to the gelatin-binding domain of fibronectin inhibits both fibronectin and collagen organization in fibroblast extracellular matrix. *J. Cell Biol.*, **92**, 485–92.

McGuigan, L.J., Cook, D.J. & Yablonski, M.E. (1986). Dexamethasone, D-penicillamine, and glaucoma filter surgery in rabbits. *Invest. Ophthalmol. Vis. Sci.*, **27**, 1755–7.

McGuigan, L.J., Mason, R.P., Sanchez, R. & Quigley, H.A. (1987). D-penicillamine and beta-aminopropionitrile effects on experimental filtering surgery. *Invest. Ophthalmol. Vis. Sci.*, **28**, 1625–9.

Messadi, D.V., Le, A., Berg, S. et al. (1999). Expression of apoptosis-associated genes by human dermal scar fibroblasts. *Wound Repair Regen.*, **7**, 511–17.

Metcalfe, R.A. & Weetman, A.P. (1994). Stimulation of extraocular muscle fibroblasts by cytokines and hypoxia: possible role in thyroid-associated ophthalmopathy. *Clin. Endocrinol. Oxf.*, **40**, 67–72.

Miller, M. & Rice, N. (1991). Trabeculectomy combined with B radiation for congential glaucoma. *Br. J. Ophthalmol.*, **75**, 584–90.

Moore, M.J. (1995). Ribozymes. Exploration by lamp light [news; comment]. *Nature*, **374**, 766–7.

Moorhead, L.C., Stewart, R.H., Kimbrough, P.L. et al. (1990). Use of beta-aminopropiono-nitrile following glaucoma filtration surgery. *Invest. Ophthalmol. Vis. Sci.*, **31S**, 3.

Mudera, V.C., Pleass, R., Eastwood, M. et al. (2000). Molecular responses of human dermal fibroblasts to dual cues: contact guidance and mechnical load. *Cell Motil. Cytoskeleton*, **45**, 1–9.

Nagase, H. & Woessner, F. (1999). Matrix metalloproteinases. *J. Biol. Chem.*, **274**, 21491–4.

Nelson, R.D., McCormack, R.T. & Fiegel, V.D. (1978). Chemotaxis of human leukocytes under agarose. In: *Leukocyte Chemotaxis*, vol. 690, ed. Gallin, J.I. & Quie, P.G., pp. 25–42. New York: Raven Press.

Newby, A.C., Southgate, K.M. & Davies, M. (1994). Extracellular matrix degrading metallop-roteinases in the pathogenesis of arteriosclerosis. *Basic Res. Cardiol.*, **89** (suppl. 1), 59–70.

Noda Heiny, H. & Sobel, B.E. (1995). Vascular smooth muscle cell migration mediated by thrombin and urokinase receptor. *Am. J. Physiol.*, **268**, C1195–201.

Occleston, N.L., Alexander, R.A., Mazure, A., Larkin, G. & Khaw, P.T. (1994). Effects of single exposures to antiproliferative agents on ocular fibroblast-mediated collagen contraction. *Invest. Ophthalmol. Vis. Sci.*, **35**, 3681–90.

Occleston, N.L., Daniels, J.T., Tarnuzzer, R.W. et al. (1997). Single exposures to anti-proliferatives: long-term effects on ocular fibroblast wound-healing behavior. *Invest. Ophthalmol. Vis. Sci.*, **38**, 1998–2007.

Oh, E., Pierschbacher, M. & Ruoslahti, E. (1981). Deposition of plasma fibronectin in tissues. *Proc. Natl Acad. Sci. U.S.A.*, **78**, 3218–21.

Okada, S.S., Kuo, A., Muttreja, M.R. et al. (1995). Inhibition of human vascular smooth muscle cell migration and proliferation by beta-cyclodextrin tetradecasulfate. *J. Pharmacol. Exp. Ther.*, **273**, 948–54.

Ono, I., Tateshita, T. & Inoue, M. (1999). Effects of a collagen matrix containing basic fibroblast growth factor on wound contraction. *J. Biomed. Mater. Res.*, **48**, 621–30.

Paulsson, M., Fujiwara, S., Dziadek, M. et al. (1986). Structure and function of basement membrane proteoglycans. *Ciba Found. Symp.*, **124**, 189–203.

Pauly, R.R., Passaniti, A., Bilato, C. et al. (1994). Migration of cultured vascular smooth muscle cells through a basement membrane barrier requires type IV collagenase activity and is inhibited by cellular differentiation. *Circ. Res.*, **75**, 41–54.

Pilcher, B.K., Dumin, J.A., Sudbeck, B.D. et al. (1997). The activity of collagenase-1 is required for keratinocyte migration on a type I collagen matrix. *J. Cell Biol.*, **137**, 1445–57.

Postlethwaite, A.E. & Kang, A.H. (1980). Characterization of guinea pig lymphocyte-derived chemotactic factor for fibroblasts. *J. Immunol.*, **124**, 1462–6.

Postlethwaite, A.E., Snyderman, R. & Kang, A.H. (1976). The chemotactic attraction of human fibroblasts to a lymphocyte-derived factor. *J. Exp. Med.*, **144**, 1188–203.

Postlethwaite, A.E., Seyer, J.M. & Kang, A.H. (1978). Chemotactic attraction of human fibro-blasts to type I, II and III collagen-derived peptides. *Proc. Natl Acad. Sci. U.S.A.*, **75**, 871–5.

Postlethwaite, A.E., Snyderman, R.K. & Kang, A.H. (1979). Generation of a fibroblast chemotactic factor in serum by activation of complement. *J. Clin. Invest.*, **64**, 1379–85.

Postlethwaite, A.E., Keski-Oja, J., Moses, H.L. & Kang, A.H. (1987). Stimulation of the chemotactic migration of human fibroblasts by transforming growth factor beta. *J. Exp. Med.*, **165**, 251–6.

Reed, M.J., Corsa, A.C., Kudravi, S.A., McCormick, R.S. & Arthur, W.T. (2000). A deficit in collagenase activity contributes to impaired migration of aged microvascular endothelial cells. *J. Cell. Biochem.*, **77**, 116–26.

Reichel, M.B., Cordeiro, M.F., Alexander, R.A. et al. (1998). New model of conjunctival scarring in the mouse eye. *Br. J. Ophthalmol.*, **82**, 1072–7.

Rheinwald, J.G. & Green, H. (1975). Serial cultivation of strains of human epidermal keratinocytes: the formation of keratinizing colonies from single cells. *Cell*, **6**, 331–43.

Riches, D.W. (1988). The multiple roles of macrophages in wound healing. In: *The Molecular and Cellular Biology of Wound Repair*. ed. Clark, R.A.F. & Henson, P.M., pp. 213–33. New York: Plenum Press.

Robbins, K.C., Summaria, L. & Wohl, R. (1981). Human plasmin. *Methods Enzymol.*, **80**, 379–87.

Ross, R. (1989). Platelet-derived growth factor. *Lancet*, **i**, 1179–82.

Ross, R. & Odland, G. (1968). Human wound repair.II. Inflammatory cells, epithelial mesen-chymal interrelations and fibrinogenesis. *J. Cell Biol.*, **39**, 152–68.

Ross, R., Raines, E.W. & Bowen Pope, D.F. (1986). The biology of platelet-derived growth factor. *Cell*, **46**, 155–69.

Roth, S.M., Spaeth, G.L., Starita, R.J., Birbillis, E.M. & Steinmann, W.C. (1991). The effects of postoperative corticosteroids on trabeculectomy and the clinical course of glaucoma: five-year follow-up study. *Ophthalmic Surg.*, **22**, 724–9.

Roy, P., Petroll, W.M., Cavanagh, H.D., Chuong, C.J. & Jester, J.V. (1997). An in vitro force measurement assay to study the early mechanical interaction between corneal fibroblasts and collagen matrix. *Exp. Cell Res.*, **232**, 106–17.

Roy, P., Petroll, W.M., Choung, C.J., Cavanagh, H.D. & Jester, J.V. (1999). Effect of cell migration on the maintenance of tension on a collagen matrix. *Ann. Biomed Eng.*, **27**, 721–30.

Saarialho Kere, U.K., Kovacs, S.O., Pentland, A.P. et al. (1993). Cell–matrix interactions modulate interstitial collagenase expression by human keratinocytes actively involved in wound healing. *J. Clin. Invest.*, **92**, 2858–66.

Saarialho Kere, U.K., Vaalamo, M., Airola, K. et al. (1995). Interstitial collagenase is expressed by keratinocytes that are actively involved in reepithelialization in blistering skin disease. *J. Invest. Dermatol.*, **104**, 982–8.

Samuelsson, B., Goldyne, M., Granstrom, E. et al. (1978). Prostaglandins and thromboxanes. *Annu. Rev. Biochem.*, **47**, 997–1029.

Sato, H., Takino, T., Okada, Y. et al. (1994). A matrix metalloproteinase expressed on the surface of invasive tumour cells [see comments]. *Nature*, **370**, 61–5.

Schiro, J.A., Chan, B.M., Roswit, W.T. et al. (1991). Integrin alpha 2 beta 1 (VLA-2) mediates reorganization and contraction of collagen matrices by human cells. *Cell*, **67**, 403–10.

Scott, K.A., Wood, E.J. & Karran, E.H. (1998). A matrix metalloproteinase inhibitor which prevents fibroblast-mediated collagen lattice contraction. *FEBS Lett.*, **441**, 137–40.

Senior, R.M., Griffin, G.L., Mecham, R.P. et al. (1984). Val-Gly-Val-Ala-Pro-Gly, a repeating peptide in elastin, is chemotactic for fibroblasts and monocytes. *J. Cell Biol.*, **99**, 870–4.

Senior, R.M., Skogen, W.F., Griffin, G.L. & Wilner, G.D. (1986). Effects of fibrinogen derivatives upon the inflammatory response. Studies with human fibrinopeptide B. *J. Clin. Invest.*, **77**, 1014–19.

Seppa, H.E.J., Grotendorst, G.R., Seppa, S.I., Schiffmann, E. & Martin, G.R. (1982). Platelet-derived growth factor is chemotactic for fibroblasts. *J. Cell Biol.*, **92**, 584–8.

Shah, M., Foreman, D.M. & Ferguson, M.W. (1992). Control of scarring in adult wounds by neutralising antibody to transforming growth factor beta. *Lancet*, **339**, 213–14.

Shah, M., Foreman, D.M. & Ferguson, M.W. (1994). Neutralising antibody to TGF-beta 1,2 reduces cutaneous scarring in adult rodents. *J. Cell Sci.*, **107**, 1137–57.

Shah, M., Foreman, D.M. & Ferguson, M.W. (1995). Neutralisation of TGF-beta 1 and TGF-beta 2 or exogenous addition of TGF-beta 3 to cutaneous rat wounds reduces scarring. *J. Cell Sci.*, **108**, 985–1002.

Shapiro, S.D. (1998). Matrix metalloproteinase degradation of extracellular matrix: biological consequences. *Curr. Opin. Cell Biol.*, **10**, 602–8.

Siegel, R.C. (1977). Collagen cross-linking. Effect of D-penicillamine on cross-linking in vitro. *J. Biol. Chem.*, **252**, 254–9.

Sobel, J.D. & Gallin, J.I. (1979). Polymorphonuclear leukocyte and monocyte chemoattractants produced by human fibroblasts. *J. Clin. Invest.*, **63**, 609–18.

Sollott, S.J., Cheng, L., Pauly, R.R. et al. (1995). Taxol inhibits neointimal smooth muscle cell accumulation after angioplasty in the rat. *J. Clin. Invest.*, **95**, 1869–76.

Soslau, G., Morgan, D.A., Jaffe, J.S., Brodsky, I. & Wang, Y. (1997). Cytokine mRNA expression in human platelets and a megakaryocytic cell line and cytokine modulation of platelet function. *Cytokine*, **9**, 405–11.

Sporn, M.B., Roberts, A.B., Shull, J.H. et al. (1983). Polypeptide transforming growth factors isolated from bovine sources and used for wound healing in vivo. *Science*, **219**, 1329–31.

Stopak, D. & Harris, A.K. (1982). Connective tissue morphogenesis by fibroblast traction. I. Tissue culture observations. *Dev. Biol.*, **90**, 383–98.

Strongin, A.Y., Collier, I., Bannikov, G. et al. (1995). Mechanism of cell surface activation of 72-kDa type IV collagenase. Isolation of the activated form of the membrane metalloprotease. *J. Biol. Chem.*, **270**, 5331–8.

Subramaniam, M., Saffaripour, S., Van De Water, L. et al. (1997). Role of endothelial selectins in wound repair. *Am. J. Pathol.*, **150**, 1701–9.

Takino, T., Sato, H., Shinagawa, A. & Seiki, M. (1995). Identification of the second membrane-type matrix metalloproteinase (MT-MMP-2) gene from a human placenta cDNA library. MT-MMPs form a unique membrane-type subclass in the MMP family. *J. Biol. Chem.*, **270**, 23013–20.

Tanaka, K., Honda, M., Kuramochi, T. & Morioka, S. (1994). Prominent inhibitory effects of tranilast on migration and proliferation of and collagen synthesis by vascular smooth muscle cells. *Atherosclerosis*, **107**, 179–85.

Taraboletti, G., Garofalo, A., Belotti, D. et al. (1995). Inhibition of angiogenesis and murine hemangioma growth by batimastat, a synthetic inhibitor of matrix metalloproteinases. *J. Natl Cancer Inst.*, **87**, 293–8.

Tarnuzzer, R.W., Macauley, S.P., Farmerie, W.G. et al. (1996). Competitive RNA templates for detection and quantitation of growth factors, cytokines, extracellular matrix components and matrix metalloproteinases. *Biotechniques*, **20**, 670–4.

Teirstein, P.S., Massullo, V., Jani, S. et al. (2000). Three-year clinical and angiographic follow-up after intracoronary radiation: results of a randomised clinical trial. *Clin. Invest. Rep.*, **101**, 360–5.

Tomasek, J.J. & Hay, E.D. (1984). Analysis of the role of microfilaments and microtubules in acquisition of bipolarity and elongation of fibroblasts in hydrated collagen gels. *J. Cell Biol.*, **99**, 536–49.

Tuft, S.J., Gartry, D.S., Rawe, I.M. & Meek, K.M. (1993). Photorefractive keratectomy: implications of corneal wound healing. *Br. J. Ophthalmol.*, **77**, 243–7.

Tyagi, S.C., Meyer, L., Schmaltz, R.A., Reddy, H.K. & Voelker, D.J. (1995). Proteinases and restenosis in the human coronary artery: extracellular matrix production exceeds the expression of proteolytic activity. *Atherosclerosis*, **116**, 43–57.

Vaalamo, M., Leivo, T. & Saarialho Kere, U. (1999). Differential expression of tissue inhibitors of metalloproteinases (TIMP-1, -2, -3, and -4) in normal and aberrant wound healing. *Hum. Pathol.*, **30**, 795–802.

Verin, V., Popowski, Y., Urban, P. et al. (1995). Intra-arterial beta irradiation prevents neointimal hyperplasia in a hypercholesterolemic rabbit restenosis model. *Circulation*, **92**, 2284–90.

Voisard, R., Seitzer, U., Baur, R. et al. (1995). A prescreening system for potential antiproliferative agents: implications for local treatment strategies of postangioplasty restenosis. *Int. J. Cardiol.*, **51**, 15–28.

Wahl, S.M. (1989). Glucocorticoids and wound healing. In: *Antiinflammatory Steroid Action: Basic and Clinical Aspects*, ed. Scleimer, R.P. & Claman, E., pp. 280–302. New York: Academic Press.

Waksman, R., Robinson, K.A., Crocker, I.R. et al. (1995). Intracoronary low-dose beta-irradiation inhibits neointima formation after coronary artery balloon injury in the swine restenosis model. *Circulation*, **92**, 3025–31.

Weiss, P. (1945). The problem of specificity in growth and development. *Yale J. Biol. Med.*, **19**, 239–78.

Weiss, P. (1958). Cell contact. *Int. Rev. Cytol.*, **7**, 391–423.

Weltermann, A., Wolzt, M., Petersmann, K. et al. (1999). Large amounts of vascular endothelial growth factor at the site of hemostatic plug formation in vivo. *Arterioscler. Thromb. Vasc. Biol.*, **19**, 1757–60.

Werb, Z., Banda, M.J. & Jones, P.A. (1980). Degradation of connective tissue matrices by macrophages. I. Proteolysis of elastin, glycoproteins, and collagen by proteinases isolated from macrophages. *J. Exp. Med.*, **152**, 1340–57.

Williams, I.F., McCullagh, K.G. & Silver, I.A. (1984). The distribution of types I and III collagen and fibronectin in the healing equine tendon. *Connect. Tissue Res.*, **12**, 211–27.

Wilson, C. & Szostak, J.W. (1995). In vitro evolution of a self-alkylating ribozyme [see comments]. *Nature*, **374**, 777–82.

Wilson, S.E. & Kim, W.J. (1998). Keratocyte apoptosis: implications on corneal wound healing, tissue organization, and disease. *Invest. Ophthalmol. Vis. Sci.*, **39**, 220–6.

Woodley, D.T., O'Keefe, E.J. & Prunieras, M. (1985). Cutaneous wound healing: a model for cell–matrix interactions. *J. Am. Acad. Dermatol.*, **12**, 420–33.

Woodley, D.T., Kalebec, T., Banes, A.J. et al. (1986). Adult human keratinocytes migrating over nonviable dermal collagen produce collagenolytic enzymes that degrade type I and type IV collagen. *J. Invest. Dermatol.*, **86**, 418–23.

Wysocki, S.J., Zheng, M.H., Fan, Y. et al. (1996). Expression of transforming growth factor-beta1 (TGF-beta1) and urokinase-type plasminogen activator (u-PA) genes during arterial repair in the pig. *Cardiovasc. Res.*, **31**, 28–36.

Zhao, M., Forrester, J.V. & McCraig, C.D. (1999). A small, physiological electric field orients cell division. *Proc. Natl Acad. Sci. U.S.A.*, **96**, 4942–6.

Ziesche, R., Hofbauer, E., Wittman, K., Petkov, V. & Block, L.H. (1999). A preliminary study of long-term treatment with interferon gamma-1b and low-dose prednisolone in patients with idiopathic pulmonary fibrosis. *N. Engl. J. Med.*, **341**, 1264–9.

Zigmond, S.H. (1977). Ability of polymorphonuclear leukocytes to orient in gradients of chemotactic factors. *J. Cell Biol.*, **75**, 606–16.

Zigmond, S.H. & Hirsch, J.G. (1973). Leukocyte locomotion and chemotaxis. New methods for evaluation, and demonstration of a cell-derived chemotactic factor. *J. Exp. Med.*, **137**, 387–410.

Part II

Pathophysiology: mechanisms and imaging

8

Genes for hypertension

Mark Caulfield, Joanne Knight, Suzanne O'Shea, Gerard Gardner and Patricia Munroe

Department of Clinical Pharmacology, St Bartholomew's and The Royal London School of Medicine and Dentistry, London

Earlier this century researchers became intrigued by the frequent presence of a positive family history for hypertension in patients and this generated an intense debate between Pickering and Platt regarding genetic influences upon blood pressure. The former pointed to the observation of a normal distribution of blood pressure in the population as argument for a multigenic influence upon blood pressure variation and thus hypertension (Pickering, 1965). The latter suggested that hypertension was under the influence of a single gene which, through an autosomal dominant mode of Mendelian inheritance, led to the hypertensive phenotype (Platt, 1963). Nowadays, many accept the view that several genes are probably involved in elevating blood pressure. However, some of the greatest advances in understanding genetic influences upon blood pressure have been made in a series of rare hypertensive traits where anomalies within single genes have a profound effect upon blood pressure.

Patterns of inheritance in essential hypertension

In single-gene disorders such as cystic fibrosis it is possible to demonstrate Mendelian patterns of inheritance and it becomes easier to categorize a family member as affected or unaffected (Lander and Schork, 1994). Although there are rare hypertensive traits which exhibit Mendelian patterns of inheritance, this is frequently not so easy to define amongst patients with essential hypertension (White, 1996). Since hypertension is a disorder with variable age of onset defined by a threshold at which intervention with treatment reduces cardiovascular risk, it may not be possible to assert at a fixed point in time that a family member is never going to be hypertensive. This is illustrated by the family pedigree shown in Figure 8.1 where the pattern of hypertension shown in (*a*) would conform to an autosomal-dominant trait, with one in two individuals diagnosed as hypertensive.

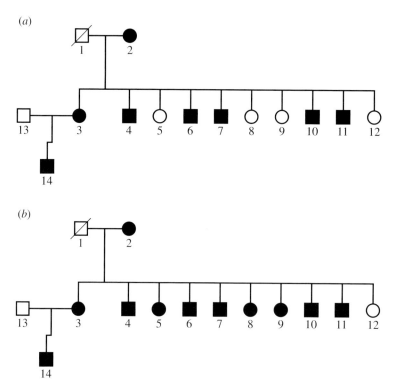

Figure 8.1   Inheritance pattern of hypertension. A white European family pedigree with the phenotype of hypertension is shown. Affected individuals are shown as solid circles or squares; white circles or squares denote individuals who are unaffected at this time. The pedigree in (*a*) implies an autosomal-dominant mode of inheritance. However, 3 years later, as shown in (*b*), the condition no longer exhibits a Mendelian pattern of inheritance as almost all of the offspring are now defined as hypertensive.

However, 3 years later several new family members had developed raised blood pressure requiring therapy and this pedigree no longer exhibits a clear Mendelian pattern of inheritance (Figure 8.1*b*).

Genetic susceptibility to raised blood pressure

This departure from Mendelian patterns of inheritance may be explained by the requirement for coinheritance of several susceptibility variants for raised blood pressure to be present in an individual (Lander and Schork, 1994). This genetic interplay might result in a synergistic or epistatic interaction, where the blood pressure is greatly augmented by two genetic susceptibility variants operating in concert. Alternatively, the effect of two or more genetic variants might be to add a modest increment to the blood pressure.

Environmental factors for raised blood pressure

It is probable that some susceptibility genes require the presence of specific environmental triggers to elevate blood pressure. These may include a high sodium salt diet, ingestion of alcohol or the presence of excess weight (Whelton, 1994). Indeed, in some hypertensive families resemblance in blood pressure may be entirely due to common environmental factors (Lander and Schork, 1994).

Family study designs used in hypertension

Affected sibling pair methods

The central feature of affected sibling pair analysis is the demonstration of an excess sharing of alleles above that expected by Mendelian inheritance in a family (Lander and Schork, 1994). At a genetic locus each parent will have two versions of a genetic marker or alleles (one derived from each chromosome). Thus an offspring may inherit any one of four alleles from the parents. This means that a random group of siblings would be expected to share none, one or two alleles transmitted from their parents at a frequency of 25%, 50% or 25% respectively. If instead we select hypertensive sibling pairs, we can measure whether the observed allelic sharing amongst the pairs deviates from the expected frequency of 25%, 50% or 25%. In the event that the observed distribution of allele sharing conforms to that expected then there is no support for linkage (Lander and Schork, 1994). These analyses can either be employed to test known candidates for hypertension, or in genomic screening and require no specification of model of inheritance for analysis.

Extreme discordant sib pairs

An alternative form of sibling pair analysis can be used in quantitative traits like blood pressure where genotypes of siblings with extremely discordant blood pressures are compared after adjustment for age, body mass index and alcohol consumption (Risch and Zhang, 1995). Some have suggested that if extreme discordant sibling pairs can be found they may offer considerable power to detect loci for quantitative traits, with 250 pairs offering similar power to much larger numbers of affected sibling pairs (Risch and Zhang, 1995).

Transmission disequilibrium testing

Family-based association studies, preferably based upon two parents and an affected offspring, have been advocated to avoid selection bias, or latent ethnic admixture, which may occur in case-control association studies (Spielman and Ewens, 1996). This uses the transmission disequilibrium test, which relies upon a comparison between those alleles transmitted from heterozygous parents to an affected offspring with those that are not. The untransmitted alleles offer an ethnically matched 'control' within the family. This protects against problems of occult ethnic admixture and selection bias. This could be used to fine-map regions of interest and has been employed in insulin-dependent diabetes to clarify the role of the insulin gene locus (Spielman et al., 1993). As hypertension has a late age of onset it can be difficult to obtain access to parental genotype. In this situation it is still possible to apply this approach as long as parental genotype can be accurately inferred by recruiting several additional siblings to the index case (Sham and Curtis, 1995).

Population association or case-control studies

Association of a genetic variation with hypertension relies upon the genetic variant under study being in close proximity to the susceptibility variant. Such studies employ the principle of linkage disequilibrium, whereby a few ancestral variations are transmitted together on the same piece of DNA over time (Lander and Schork, 1994). This means that association of genetic marker with the trait of interest implies that the true aetiological variation and the marker under study (assuming it is not the functional variant itself) do not become separated by recombination during meiosis.

A problem with some studies is that they explore genetic hypotheses in case-control studies, using highly selected clinic populations and without representative controls (Lander and Schork, 1994). Even when population-based studies are drawn from the general population using sound epidemiological approaches it is not possible to exclude hidden population substructures which may create spurious associations in genetic studies.

It is possible that the power of association studies may be reduced by the traditional comparison of hypertensive cases versus the rest of blood pressure distribution, or 'normotension'. Raised blood pressure is not an all-or-none phenomenon and depends upon interaction of susceptibility genes with environmental factors. It would be possible to possess a susceptibility variant but never manifest the trait, because of the absence of other factors. Such an individual may well have blood pressure in the upper half of the blood pressure distribution and, in a comparison of the upper decile, or quintile, with the rest of the populus could dilute or obliterate an association. It may be preferable to adopt a comparison of the upper and lower deciles, or quintiles, of the blood pressure distribution from a population. In such a comparison we must take account of those in the lower section, who receive treatment, which may influence blood pressure (Jeunemaitre et al., 1992a).

Rare hypertensive phenotypes: clues for essential hypertension

Several researchers have focused upon rare hypertensive phenotypes where a constellation of clinical or biochemical features and clear patterns of Mendelian inheritance distinguish these syndromes from essential hypertension (Table 8.1). The motivation to identify the genetic influences in such traits is that more subtle susceptibility variants within the same genes may contribute to essential hypertension (Lifton et al., 1992; White, 1996).

Epithelial sodium channel, Liddle's syndrome and hypertension

The importance of sodium handling by the kidney is demonstrated by Liddle's syndrome, which is characterized by hypertension with a suppressed renin–angiotensin system and aldosterone secretion with hypokalaemia (Liddle et al., 1963). These features, coupled with response of blood pressure to triamterene, suggested that the epithelial sodium channel expressed within the distal tubule and regulated by aldosterone might be important. This sodium channel comprises an α subunit that supports sodium conductance and β and γ subunits, which greatly enhance the activity of the α subunit but only support very low levels of sodium transport. Mutations which lead to constitutive overactivity, by inhibition of degradation of this channel, have been discovered within the genes encoding the β and γ subunits located on human chromosome 16 (Shimkets et al., 1994; Hansson et al., 1995) in patients with Liddle's syndrome.

These findings are of particular interest because the features of low renin, hypertension and suppressed aldosterone levels, are analogous to that seen in some people of African origin with essential hypertension (Cooper and Rotini, 1994). A study in African American families implies that there are heritable components to salt-responsive blood pressure (Svetkey et al., 1996a). These observations led to a small exploratory study using genetic markers flanking the epithelial sodium channel subunits in 63 African Caribbean sibling pairs with essential hypertension (Munroe et al., 1998). In our limited study we did not find support for linkage of any of the subunits to hypertension. However, it was not possible to characterize our African Caribbean families for blood pressure response to sodium loading, or depletion. Therefore we cannot evaluate our data according to salt sensitivity, or exclude a role for this channel in hypertension (Munroe et al., 1998).

There have been several studies of the epithelial sodium channel subunits in the hypertensive rat models that have not demonstrated linkage of any subunits of the epithelial sodium channel to hypertension (Grunder et al., 1997; Kreutz et al., 1997). Sequencing of β and γ subunits in rat models has only detected polymorphisms within the γ subunit which do not affect the sodium channel activity when expressed in *Xenopus* oocytes (Kreutz et al., 1997).

Table 8.1 Rare monogenic forms of hypertension

Syndrome	Phenotype		Gene	Reference
Glucocorticoid remediable aldosteronism (GRA)	Autosomal-dominant		Chimeric 11β Hydroxylase/aldosterone Synthase	Lifton et al. (1992)
	Aldosterone	↑		
	Potassium	→		
	RAAS	↓		
Apparent mineralocorticoid excess (AME)	Autosomal-recessive		11β-hydroxysteroid Dehydrogenase type II	Mune et al. (1995)
	Aldosterone	→		
	Potassium	→		
	RAAS	→		
	Sodium	↑		
Liddle's syndrome	Autosomal-dominant		Epithelial sodium channel	Shimkets et al. (1994); Hansson et al. (1995)
	Aldosterone	→		
	Potassium	→		
	RAAS	→		
	Sodium	↑		
Gordon's syndrome	Autosomal-dominant		1q31–q42 17p11–q21	Mansfield et al. (1997)
	Potassium	↑		
	RAAS	→		

RAAS, renin–angiotensin–aldosterone system.

The existence of more subtle variations within the subunits has been explored by single-stranded conformational polymorphism analysis and using direct sequencing in human essential hypertension. In a case-control study of UK-based people of West African ancestry a variant exchanging threonine at position 594 for methionine was associated with hypertension (Baker et al., 1998); this association will need to be confirmed in other populations.

Genetic clues from hypertensive models

Some of the strongest support for a genetic basis to hypertension arises from animal models such as the spontaneously hypertensive rat (Kurtz, 1994). An important advantage of animal models is that we can completely control the environment in terms of dietary and other influences. Furthermore, recent advances in blood pressure measurement, such as remote telemetry, have been employed and offer greater precision over tail cuff measurement (Clark et al., 1996).

Comparative mapping: rat hypertensive loci translated to humans

In the early 1990s, two groups concurrently reported linkage of a region on rat chromosome 10 to blood pressure in hypertensive models. This locus was estimated to account for 20% of the blood pressure variance when the animals were sodium-loaded (Hilbert et al., 1991; Jacob et al., 1991). This was of particular interest because the corresponding region in humans is located on chromosome 17 and contains the gene encoding angiotensin-converting enzyme (ACE). An early exploratory study of the ACE gene locus in affected sibling pairs with essential hypertension did not support a role for this gene in hypertension (Jeunemaitre et al., 1992b). However, this study did not offer the power to exclude either the ACE gene or chromosome 17 as a locus for hypertension. Subsequent mapping studies on rat chromosome 10 suggest that there are two blood pressure-elevating loci: one that is close to the ACE gene and one about 26 cM proximal to the ACE gene (Kreutz et al., 1995).

Recently, comparative mapping of rat chromosome 10 and human chromosome 17 has revealed that these regions are highly conserved between species. The density of the human genome map facilitated the identification of 21 highly polymorphic markers extending over 110 million bases from the short arm of chromosome 17 to a region approximately 20 million bases below the ACE gene locus on the long arm of that chromosome (Julier et al., 1997).

These genetic markers were then genotyped in 357 French and UK families with strict hypertensive criteria conforming to the upper 1–5% of the blood pressure distribution (Julier et al., 1997). The families included a mixture of affected hypertensive sibling pairs from France, families recruited based upon an hypertensive index case from Oxford and some families with type 1 and type 2 diabetes who also had at least one hypertensive member. After genotyping, linkage analysis with several different methods indicated support for linkage to hypertension of an interval of 13 million bases proximal to the ACE gene at 17q23 between the growth hormone gene and a dinucleotide repeat (D17S934). Although this report does not specify a precise candidate gene or variant as a cause for raised blood pressure, it emphasizes the benefit of comparative mapping between hypertensive models and humans in appropriately large family numbers. It has been proposed that selecting families based upon severity of blood pressure phenotype may strengthen the power of a study (Lander and Schork, 1994; Julier et al., 1997). Interestingly, in this study the support for linkage did increase by an order of magnitude when affected siblings were selected based upon blood pressures in the upper 1% of the distribution when compared with those in the upper 5%. Subsequently, Baima et al. (1999) reported further support for this region of chromosome 17 in a smaller study of white European families but not African Americans. The inclusion in both studies of diabetic hypertensives who could represent a different phenotype for raised blood pressure, or even have secondary hypertension due to renal damage, could be a source of concern.

Candidate genes in rats guide studies in humans

Studies in Milan hypertensive and normotensive rats suggested that genetic influence on renal tubular sodium reabsorption may be due to mutations within the gene encoding a component of the cellular skeleton known as α adducin (Bianchi et al., 1994; Tripodi et al., 1996). In the Milan model, point mutations within the α adducin gene were thought to account for as much as 50% of the difference in blood pressure level between hypertensive and normotensive strains (Tripodi et al., 1996). There is marked conservation of the α adducin gene between rodents and humans and thus human studies in 86 hypertensive families were undertaken using genetic markers adjacent and at increasing distance from the α adducin gene located on human chromosome 4 (Cusi et al., 1997). There was support for linkage of this locus to hypertension in humans. Importantly, the evidence in favour of linkage diminished when genetic markers at increasing distance from locus were tested. This implies that the α adducin gene is the most likely candidate in that area. In addition, these researchers have associated a polymorphism within this candidate gene with hypertension. The variant involves exchange of tryptophan for glycine at position 460 in the final adducin molecule.

In further, smaller studies, they presented evidence suggesting that this polymorphism altered response of blood pressure to sodium loading, or depletion and chronic response to therapy with a thiazide diuretic (Cusi et al., 1997). Those subjects who were heterozygous for the polymorphism exhibited a greater blood pressure response to sodium depletion and chronic therapy with a diuretic than those who were homozygous for the glycine variant. Recently, the initial group to report on adducin have studied two case-control populations from Italy with conflicting results regarding association with hypertension (Glorioso et al., 1999). However, response to thiazide diuretics by genotype illustrated a consistent relationship with the glycine variant.

Candidates for human hypertension

Rare single-gene disorders have suggested that it will be possible to identify genes which play a part in raised blood pressure in rigorously phenotyped individuals. However, several candidate genes have been evaluated in essential hypertension, with some interesting and sometimes conflicting results.

The angiotensinogen gene locus: analysis in humans

The angiotensinogen gene locus emerged as a candidate for hypertension because studies indicate that plasma angiotensinogen is elevated with raised blood pressure and tracks with hypertension through families (Walker et al., 1979; Watt et al., 1992). In addition, the cleavage of angiotensinogen by renin is a rate-limiting step within the renin–angiotensin system and the kinetics of this reaction indicate that there is considerable reserve capability of renin to process angiotensinogen (Menard et al., 1993). In animal models, transgenic mice with overexpression of a rat angiotensinogen gene develop hypertension (Kimura et al., 1992).

In 1992, Jeunemaitre et al. reported linkage of the angiotensinogen gene locus to hypertension in 215 sibships from Paris and Utah. By employing mutation detection techniques, 15 polymorphisms were identified within the gene. Of great interest was the observation that a variant encoding threonine rather than methionine at position 235 (*M235T*) was associated with hypertension and plasma angiotensinogen level. Subsequently, studies in white Europeans, Mexican Americans and African Caribbeans have supported linkage of angiotensinogen locus to raised blood pressure (Caulfield et al., 1994, 1995; Atwood et al., 1997). Several studies both confirming and disputing the association of *M235T* with hypertension have been published in different ethnic groups (Hata et al., 1994; Rotimi et al., 1994; Iwai et al., 1995). A recent metaanalysis of the literature on *M235T* in white Europeans suggests methodological flaws in several studies, with selection bias, differing definitions of phenotype and failure to match cases and controls

(Kunz et al., 1997). In spite of these problems the metaanalysis suggested a small but significant relationship between *M235T* and hypertension.

The mechanism by which *M235T* could alter plasma angiotensinogen or blood pressure level remains obscure. The variant is remote from angiotensin peptide cleavage sites and regulatory sequences. Thus it is important to consider other variations within the angiotensinogen gene that might alter the level of gene product and play a role in hypertension.

Recent evidence in Japanese populations suggests that a functional variant which swaps a guanine for adenine at position −6 bp upstream of the transcription start site is in complete linkage disequilibrium with *M235T* (Inoue et al., 1997; Ishigami et al., 1997). Studies of in vitro angiotensinogen promoter activity indicate that the −6 bp variant alters basal transcription rate, which might explain higher levels of angiotensinogen and a relationship with blood pressure (Inoue et al., 1997; Ishigami et al., 1997). If this is borne out in further studies, then it will emphasize the need to consider that an associated variant is not necessarily the cause. Indeed, it may well prove that several variants of angiotensinogen gene contribute to altered expression of gene product and that specific combinations of these variations or haplotypes may be needed to elevate blood pressure.

Gene targeting and angiotensinogen: the synthetic experiments

In an elegant series of experiments using gene targeting in mouse models, Oliver Smithies' group have evaluated the effect of up to four copies of the angiotensinogen gene on blood pressure and gene product (Kim et al., 1995; Smithies, 1997). In the angiotensinogen knockout mice models, gene disruption leads to much lower blood pressure than normal mice and absence of gene product. As Smithies (1997) points out, it is more interesting to evaluate the influence of a polymorphism on plasma level of angiotensinogen and blood pressure. Ideally, such experiments would start by introducing a known functional mutation. However, detailed data are frequently inadequate on the regulatory regions of genes and it was more practical to consider the influence of reducing to one copy instead of the normal two copies of the angiotensinogen gene. Then, by a series of experimental crosses, mice with up to four copies of the gene could be evaluated. The results indicate that each extra copy of the gene adds approximately 8 mmHg to the mouse blood pressure and about a 20% increment of angiotensinogen (Kim et al., 1995; Smithies, 1997). In fact these experiments show a remarkable dose–response curve for both gene product and blood pressure, which provides important evidence that genetic manipulation of angiotensinogen could elevate blood pressure. Furthermore, they underscore the value of such models in the testing of genetic hypotheses.

Angiotensinogen: a definitive cause for hypertension or false positive?

The evidence for a role for functional variation within angiotensinogen influencing blood pressure looks encouraging but not watertight. In the context of the evidence above it is worth tempering enthusiasm with the knowledge that there are a number of negative studies on this gene. A large European affected sib pair study, involving 350 European families and studies in Chinese families, has not supported a role of this gene in hypertension (Brand et al., 1998; Niu et al., 1999). Nevertheless, at this time we suspect that angiotensinogen will probably prove to have some genetic influence on blood pressure in some populations.

G protein variant alters sodium exchange

There is some evidence suggesting that sodium hydrogen exchange activity is enhanced in 50% of hypertensives (Siffert and Dusing, 1995). The persistence of this feature in cell lines and concomitant increased intracellular calcium mobilization and DNA synthesis implies that altered signal transduction may be the cause. An intriguing series of experiments points to anomalies within the guanine nucleotide-binding regulatory proteins linked to the sodium hydrogen exchanger as a potential mechanism for this link with hypertension. These so-called G proteins are a family of heterotrimeric α, β and γ subunits, which are linked to a variety of second messenger systems. They are triggered through the α subunit by stimulation of seven transmembrane domain receptors. Activation of the α subunit leads to dissociation of the β and γ subunits releasing cyclic guanine monophosphate which in turn activates the second messenger systems.

Within the gene encoding a specific β subunit known as *GNB3*, a base change where cytosine is changed to thymidine at position 825 creates an alternate splice site leading to a 123 bp in frame deletion (Siffert et al., 1998). Surprisingly, in spite of this variation truncating the final *GNB3* protein, the activity of the downstream sodium exchanger is not attenuated. On the contrary, when expressed in cell lines, those homozygous for the thymidine variant with the deletion exhibit considerable gain in sodium hydrogen exchange.

The same workers followed this up by showing association of the thymidine allele with hypertension in a large case-control study (Siffert et al., 1998). However, the source of these cases or controls is not revealed in the paper so it is difficult to evaluate the possibility of selection bias. In the same vein as studies on angiotensinogen there are now positive and negative associations of the *GNB3* subunit with hypertension (Benjafield et al., 1998; Kato et al., 1998; Tsai et al., 2000). In spite of this, if subsequent research confirms the association, this will demonstrate that an intermediary measure such as sodium hydrogen exchange may be applied to delineate susceptibility variants for hypertension.

Candidates from the sympathetic nervous system

The sympathetic nervous system adjusts cardiac output, vascular tone, renal sodium reabsorption and renin release and could be implicated in enhanced vascular responsiveness observed in some hypertensives (Victor and Mark, 1995). This might arise from genetic variants which affect agonist response of α_1 or α_2-adrenoceptors, leading to augmented vasoconstriction or attenuated β_2-adrenoceptor-mediated vasodilatation. There is some evidence of a blunted vasodilator response to the β-agonist isoprenaline in African Americans (Lang et al., 1995). A variation of the β_2-adrenoceptor gene which encodes glycine, rather than arginine, at position 16 (Arg16 → Gly), has been found to enhance receptor downregulation which could attenuate vasodilation (Kotanko et al., 1997). There have been several studies which have suggested a role for polymorphisms within the β_2-adrenoceptor gene in people of African ancestry but further studies are needed (Svetkey et al., 1996b, 1997). There are also studies on the gene encoding the α_2-adrenoceptor, which is located on presynaptic neurons and reduces release of noradrenaline (norepinephrine), but these are difficult to interpret at this time (Lockette et al., 1995).

Genome-wide screens in human hypertension

Attempts to screen the human genome in family studies of common complex traits are now being undertaken. This approach uses markers spread at even distances throughout the genome in the hope of identifying segments of the genome as large as 30 million bases. These segments offer the basis for fine-mapping, or positional cloning to identify genes of interest. At present, there are several inconclusive genome screens for human hypertension within the public domain (Table 8.2). In a survey of 200 000 people from the Anquing Province, 200 Chinese families, based upon hypertensive affected sib pairs and 200 discordant sib pairs, were identified. A genome screen of these individuals has provided a number of interesting areas for further study (Xu et al., 1999). A screen on 55 discordant sib pairs from the Rochester Family Heart Study has given several regions of suggestive linkage to hypertension and one region on chromosome 6 that reaches significance at a genome-wide screen level (Krushkal et al., 1999). Recently a British genome screen has identified a potential area of interest on chromosome 11 (Sharma et al., 2000). The preliminary results of a genome screen by the Family Blood Pressure Program are available on their internet site http://www.hypertensiongenetics.org. However, there are no loci within the screen that reach significance.

Hypertension genetics: quo vadis?

The substantial worldwide research on genetics of hypertension is only

Table 8.2 Blood pressure quantitative trait loci detected in genome-wide screens in humans

Human populations	Chromosome	P value	Marker	Reference
Caucasian[a]	2	0.0089	D2S1788	Krushkal et al. (1999)
	5	0.0076	D5S1471	
	6	< 0.0001	D6S1009	
	15	0.0033	D15S652	
Caucasian[b]	11	0.004	D11S934	Sharma et al. (2000)
Chinese[c]	3	0.0011	D3S2387	Xu et al. (1999)
	11	0.001	D11S2019	
	16	0.0002	D16S3396	
	17	0.0008	D17S1303	
	15	0.0002	D15S657	

[a] Only loci with significant P values from the study are listed, all are linked with systolic blood pressure (SBP).

[b] No P values of a genome-wide screen level of significance were obtained. The locus highlighted is in the region that was most suggestive of linkage.

[c] No P values of a genome-wide screen level of significance were obtained. The loci with unadjusted $P < 0.001$ or logarithmic odds ratio scores > 2.0 are listed. Regions on chromosomes 3, 11, 16 and 17 gave suggestive evidence of linkage with SBP, the region on chromosome 15 gave suggestive evidence of linkage with diastolic blood pressure.

summarized herein; many groups are establishing large-scale family studies to evaluate known candidates and screen the genome. The scale of family resources required and the early difficulties experienced during genome screens have prompted some expressions of scepticism about hypertension genetics research (Bell and Lathrop, 1996).

At this time we can draw upon several strands of evidence which encourage optimism. Firstly, it has been possible to demonstrate clear genetic causes for rare hypertensive phenotypes. Secondly, we are beginning to realize the potential of comparative mapping between rodent and human hypertension. Finally, and perhaps most importantly, we know we can take information from analytical human studies of candidate genes and test in synthetic gene-targeted animal models whether the hypothesis holds true.

These developments are further boosted by the availability of the human genome sequence (http://www.gdb.org). The importance of additional sequence variation data has been recognized by the Pharmaceutical Industry and the Wellcome Trust who have formed a partnership known as the Single Nucleotide Polymorphism (SNP) Consortium to define 300 000 novel SNPs by 2001. Like the human genome project, the SNP Consortium releases data on to the world wide web at http://snp.well.ox.ac.uk. Alongside new high-throughput technologies, such as microarray, chip-based or mass spectrometry genotyping, these advances offer the possibility of testing many candidates in an efficient and comprehensive manner (Chipping Forecast, 1999).

If these labours bear fruit (or even genes), then we may be able to identify specific hypertensive phenotypes, tailor therapy appropriately for our patients, develop novel therapeutic agents and spot individuals who have specific risks for end-organ damage and intervene to minimize their risks.

Acknowledgements

Mark Caulfield coordinates the MRC British Genetics of Hypertension Study and is supported by the Medical Research Council, the British Heart Foundation and the Joint Research Board and the Special Trustees of St Bartholomew's Hospital. Joanne Knight is funded by the joint research board of St Bartholomew's Hospital. Suzanne O'Shea is supported by the Wellcome Trust. Gerard Gardener was supported by the British Heart Foundation. Patricia Munroe is supported by the Special Trustees of St Bartholomew's Hospital.

REFERENCES

Atwood, L.D., Kammerer, C.M., Samollow, P.B. et al. (1997). Linkage of essential hypertension to the angiotensinogen locus in Mexican Americans. *Hypertension*, **30**, 326–30.

Baima, J., Nicolaou, M., Schwartz, F. et al. (1999). Evidence for linkage between essential hypertension and a putative locus on human chromosome 17. *Hypertension*, **34**, 4–7.

Baker, E.H., Dong, Y.B., Sagnella, G.A. et al. (1998). Association of hypertension with T594M mutation in beta subunit of epithelial sodium channels in black people resident in London. *Lancet*, **351**, 1388–92.

Bell, J.I. & Lathrop, G.M. (1996). Multiple loci for multiple sclerosis. *Nat. Genet.*, **13**, 377–8.

Benjafield, A.V., Jeyasingam, C.L., Nyholt, D.R., Griffiths, L.R. & Morris, B.J. (1998). G-protein beta₃ subunit gene (GNB3) variant in causation of essential hypertension. *Hypertension*, **32**, 1094–7.

Bianchi, G., Tripodi, G., Casari, G. et al. (1994). Two point mutations within the adducin genes are involved in blood pressure variation. *Proc. Natl Acad. Sci. U.S.A.*, **91**, 3999–4003.

Brand, E., Chatelain, N., Keavney, B. et al. (1998). Evaluation of the angiotensinogen locus in human essential hypertension: a European study. *Hypertension*, **31**, 725–9.

Caulfield, M., Lavender, P., Farrall, M. et al. (1994). Linkage of the angiotensinogen gene to essential hypertension. *N. Engl. J. Med.*, **330**, 1629–33.

Caulfield, M., Lavender, P., Newell-Price, J. et al. (1995). Linkage of the angiotensinogen gene locus to human essential hypertension in African Caribbeans. *J. Clin. Invest.*, **96**, 687–92.

Clark, J.S., Jeffs, B., Davidson, A.O. et al. (1996). Quantitative trait loci in genetically hypertensive rats. Possible sex specificity. *Hypertension*, **28**, 898–906.

Cooper, R. & Rotini, C. (1994). Hypertension in populations of West African origin: is there a genetic predisposition? *J. Hypertens.*, **12**, 215–27.

Cusi, D., Barlassina, C., Azzani, T. et al. (1997). Polymorphisms of alpha-adducin and salt sensitivity in patients with essential hypertension. *Lancet*, **349**, 1353–7.

Glorioso, N., Manunta, P., Filigheddu, F. et al. (1999). The role of alpha-adducin polymorphism in blood pressure and sodium handling regulation may not be excluded by a negative association study. *Hypertension*, **34**, 649–54.

Grunder, S., Zagato, L., Yagil, C. et al. (1997). Polymorphisms in the carboxy-terminus of the epithelial sodium channel in rat models for hypertension. *J. Hypertens.*, **15**, 173–9.

Hansson, J.H., Nelson-Williams, C., Suzuki, H. et al. (1995). Hypertension caused by a truncated epithelial sodium channel gamma subunit: genetic heterogeneity of Liddle syndrome. *Nat. Genet.*, **11**, 76–82.

Hata, A., Namikawa, C., Sasaki, M. et al. (1994). Angiotensinogen as a risk factor for essential hypertension in Japan. *J. Clin. Invest.*, **93**, 1285–7.

Hilbert, P., Lindpaintner, K., Beckmann, J.S. et al. (1991). Chromosomal mapping of two genetic loci associated with blood-pressure regulation in hereditary hypertensive rats. *Nature*, **353**, 521–9.

Inoue, I., Nakajima, T., Williams, C.S. et al. (1997). A nucleotide substitution in the promoter of human angiotensinogen is associated with essential hypertension and affects basal transcription in vitro. *J. Clin. Invest.*, **99**, 1786–97.

Ishigami, T., Umemura, S., Tamura, K. et al. (1997). Essential hypertension and 5' upstream core promoter region of human angiotensinogen gene. *Hypertension*, **30**, 1325–30.

Iwai, N., Shimoike, H., Ohmichi, N. & Kinoshita, M. (1995). Angiotensinogen gene and blood pressure in the Japanese population. *Hypertension*, **25**, 688–93.

Jacob, H.J., Lindpaintner, K., Lincoln, S.E. et al. (1991). Genetic mapping of a gene causing hypertension in the stroke-prone spontaneously hypertensive rat. *Cell*, **67**, 213–24.

Jeunemaitre, X., Soubrier, F., Kotelevtsev, Y.V. et al. (1992a). Molecular basis of human hypertension: role of angiotensinogen. *Cell*, **71**, 169–80.

Jeunemaitre, X., Lifton, R.P., Hunt, S.C., Williams, R.R. & Lalouel, J.M. (1992b). Absence of linkage between the angiotensin converting enzyme locus and human essential hypertension. *Nat. Genet.*, **1**, 72–5.

Julier, C., Delepine, M., Keavney, B. et al. (1997). Genetic susceptibility for human familial essential hypertension in a region of homology with blood pressure linkage on rat chromosome 10. *Hum. Mol. Genet.*, **6**, 2077–85.

Kato, N., Sugiyama, T., Morita, H. et al. (1998). G protein beta3 subunit variant and essential hypertension in Japanese. *Hypertension*, **32**, 935–8.

Kim, H.S., Krege, J.H., Kluckman, K.D. et al. (1995). Genetic control of blood pressure and the angiotensinogen locus. *Proc. Natl Acad. Sci. U.S.A.*, **92**, 2735–9.

Kimura, S., Mullins, J.J., Bunnemann, B. et al. (1992). High blood pressure in transgenic mice carrying the rat angiotensinogen gene. *EMBO J.*, **11**, 821–7.

Kotanko, P., Binder, A., Tasker, J. et al. (1997). Essential hypertension in African Caribbeans associates with a variant of the beta$_2$-adrenoceptor. *Hypertension*, **30**, 773–6.

Kreutz, R., Hubner, N., James, M.R. et al. (1995). Dissection of a quantitative trait locus for genetic hypertension on rat chromosome 10. *Proc. Natl Acad. Sci. U.S.A.*, **92**, 8778–82.

Kreutz, R., Struk, B., Rubattu, S. et al. (1997). Role of the alpha-, beta-, and gamma-subunits of epithelial sodium channel in a model of polygenic hypertension. *Hypertension*, **29**, 131–6.

Krushkal, J., Ferrell, R,, Mockrin, S.C. et al. (1999). Genome-wide linkage analyses of systolic blood pressure using highly discordant siblings. *Circulation*, **99**, 1407–10.

Kunz, R., Kreutz, R., Beige, J., Distler, A. & Sharma, A.M. (1997). Association between the angiotensinogen 235T-variant and essential hypertension in whites: a systematic review and methodological appraisal. *Hypertension*, **30**, 1331–7.

Kurtz, T.W. (1994). Genetic models of hypertension. *Lancet*, **344**, 167–8.

Lander, E.S. & Schork, N.J. (1994). Genetic dissection of complex traits. *Science*, **265**, 2037–48.

Lang, C.C., Stein, C.M., Brown, R.M. et al. (1995). Attenuation of isoproterenol-mediated vasodilatation in blacks. *N. Engl. J. Med.*, **333**, 155–60.

Liddle, G.W., Bledsoe, T. & Coppage, W.S. (1963). A familial renal disorder stimulating primary aldosteronism but with negligible aldosterone secretion. *Trans. Assoc. Am. Phys.*, **76**, 199–213.

Lifton, R.P., Dluhy, R.G., Powers, M. et al. (1992). A chimaeric 11 beta-hydroxylase/aldosterone synthase gene causes glucocorticoid-remediable aldosteronism and human hypertension. *Nature*, **355**, 262–5.

Lockette, W., Ghosh, S., Farrow, S. et al. (1995). Alpha$_2$-adrenergic receptor gene polymorphism and hypertension in blacks. *Am. J. Hypertens.*, **8**, 390–4.

Mansfield, T.A., Simon, D.B., Farfel, Z. et al. (1997). Multilocus linkage of familial hyper-kalaemia and hypertension, pseudohypoaldosteronism type II, to chromosomes 1q31-42 and 17p11-q21. *Nat. Genet.*, **16**, 202–5.

Menard, J., Clauser, E., Bouhnik, J. & Corvol, P. (1993). Angiotensinogen: biochemistry. In: *The Renin–Angiotensin system*, ed. Robertson, J.I.S. & Nicolls, M.G., pp. 8.1–8.10. London: Mosby.

Mune, T., Rogerson, F.M., Nikkila, H., Agarwal, A.K. & White, P.C. (1995). Human hypertension caused by mutations in the kidney isozyme of 11 beta-hydroxysteroid dehydrogenase. *Nat. Genet.*, **10**, 394–9.

Munroe, P.B., Strautnieks, S.S., Farrall, M. et al. (1998). Absence of linkage of the epithelial sodium channel to hypertension in black Caribbeans. *Am. J. Hypertens.*, **11**, 942–5.

Niu, T., Yang, J., Wang, B. et al. (1999). Angiotensinogen gene polymorphisms M235T/T174M: no excess transmission to hypertensive Chinese. *Hypertension*, **33**, 698–702.

Phimster, B. (ed.) (1999). Chipping Forecast. *Nat. Genet.*, **21**, (suppl.), 1–60.

Pickering, G.W. (1965). Hyperpiesis: high blood pressure without evident cause: essential hypertension. *Br. Med. J.*, **2**, 1021–6.

Platt, R. (1963). Heredity in hypertension. *Lancet*, **1**, 899–904.

Risch, N. & Zhang, H. (1995). Extreme discordant sib pairs for mapping quantitative trait loci in humans. *Science*, **268**, 1584–9.

Rotimi, C., Morrison, L., Cooper, R. et al. (1994). Angiotensinogen gene in human hypertension. Lack of an association of the 235T allele among African Americans. *Hypertension*, **24**, 591–4.

Sham, P.C. & Curtis, D. (1995). An extended transmission/disequilibrium test (TDT) for multi-allele marker loci. *Ann. Hum. Genet.*, **59**, 323–36.

Sharma, P., Fatibene, J., Ferraro, F. et al. (2000). A genome-wide search for susceptibility loci to human essential hypertension. *Hypertension*, **35**, 1291–6.

Shimkets, R.A., Warnock, D.G., Bositis, C.M. et al. (1994). Liddle's syndrome: heritable human hypertension caused by mutations in the beta subunit of the epithelial sodium channel. *Cell*, **79**, 407–14.

Siffert, W. & Dusing, R. (1995). Sodium–proton exchange and primary hypertension. An update. *Hypertension*, **26**, 649–55.

Siffert, W., Rosskopf, D., Siffert, G. et al. (1998). Association of a human G-protein beta$_3$ subunit variant with hypertension [see comments]. *Nat. Genet.*, **18**, 45–8.

Smithies, O. (1997). Theodore Cooper memorial lecture. A mouse view of hypertension. *Hypertension*, **30**, 1318–24.

Spielman, R.S. & Ewens, W.J. (1996). The TDT and other family-based tests for linkage disequilibrium and association. *Am. J. Hum. Genet.*, **59**, 983–9.

Spielman, R.S., McGinnis, R.E. & Ewens, W.J. (1993). Transmission test for linkage disequilibrium: the insulin gene region and insulin-dependent diabetes mellitus (IDDM). *Am. J. Hum. Genet.*, **52**, 506–16.

Svetkey, L.P., McKeown, S.P. & Wilson, A.F. (1996a). Heritability of salt sensitivity in black Americans. *Hypertension*, **28**, 854–8.

Svetkey, L.P., Timmons, P.Z., Emovon, O. et al. (1996b). Association of hypertension with beta$_2$- and alpha$_2$c10-adrenergic receptor genotype. *Hypertension*, **27**, 1210–15.

Svetkey, L.P., Chen, Y.T., McKeown, S.P., Preis, L. & Wilson, A.F. (1997). Preliminary evidence of linkage of salt sensitivity in black Americans at the beta$_2$-adrenergic receptor locus. *Hypertension*, **29**, 918–22.

Tripodi, G., Valtorta, F., Torielli, L. et al. (1996). Hypertension-associated point mutations in the adducin alpha and beta subunits affect actin cytoskeleton and ion transport. *J. Clin. Invest.*, **97**, 2815–22.

Tsai, C.H., Yeh, H.I., Chou, Y. et al. (2000). G protein beta3 subunit variant and essential hypertension in Taiwan – a case-control study. *Int. J. Cardiol.*, **73**, 191–5.

Victor, R.G. & Mark, A.L. (1995). The sympathetic nervous system in human hypertension. In: *Hypertension. Pathophysiology, Diagnosis and Management*, ed. Laragh, J.H. & Brenner, B.M., pp. 863–78. New York: Raven Press.

Walker, W.G., Whelton, P.K., Saito, H., Russell, R.P. & Hermann, J. (1979). Relation between blood pressure and renin, renin substrate, angiotensin II, aldosterone and urinary sodium and potassium in 574 ambulatory subjects. *Hypertension*, **1**, 287–91.

Watt, G.C., Harrap, S.B., Foy, C.J. et al. (1992), Abnormalities of glucocorticoid metabolism and the renin–angiotensin system: a four-corners approach to the identification of genetic determinants of blood pressure. *J. Hypertens.*, **10**, 473–82.

Whelton, P.K. (1994). Epidemiology of hypertension. *Lancet*, **344**, 101–6.

White, P.C. (1996). Inherited forms of mineralocorticoid hypertension. *Hypertension*, **28**, 927–36.

Xu, X., Rogus, J.J., Terwedow, H.A. et al. (1999). An extreme-sib-pair genome scan for genes regulating blood pressure. *Am. J. Hum. Genet.*, **64**, 1694–701.

9

The endothelium in health and disease

Beverley J. Hunt[1] and Karen M. Jurd[2]

[1] Departments of Haematology and Rheumatology, Guy's and St Thomas' Trust, London.
[2] Protection and Performance Department, Centre for Human Sciences, DERA Alverstoke, Gosport

Introduction

The endothelium is far from the inert lining to blood vessels that it was originally considered to be, but a highly specialized, metabolically active organ. Resting endothelial cells form a monolayer maintaining a barrier between blood constituents and the extravascular space, but they also exert multifunctional homeostatic effects (Table 9.1). Although only one cell thick, the endothelium constitutes a dynamic interface between the blood and the rest of the body. It is also increasingly recognized that endothelial cells are heterogeneous, in that the function and phenotype of endothelial cells are specialized according to their particular site, e.g. cerebral endothelial cells lack thrombomodulin (see below), and not all endothelial cells constitutively express histocompatibility locus A (HLA) class II molecules. Discussion of the endothelium in disease is a confusing area. In many circles the term 'endothelial dysfunction' is a synonym for impaired endothelial-dependent vasodilatation. The aim of this chapter is to emphasize that the pathophysiological responses of the endothelium involve multiple effects and play a critical role in many diseases (Table 9.2).

Endothelial cell activation

The quiescent endothelium maintains a status quo, but under the stimulation of certain agents such as interleukin-1 (IL-1) and tumour necrosis factor-α (TNF-α) it undergoes a series of metabolic changes and participates in the inflammatory process; this is known as endothelial cell activation (ECA) and is a central pathophysiological event.

The term 'ECA' was coined in the late 1960s when Willms-Kretschmer et al. (1967) noted that in delayed hypersensitivity reactions venules became leaky and their endothelial cell linings became plump and protruded into the lumen. These

Table 9.1 Functions of the vascular endothelium

Maintenance of selective permeability
Integration and transduction of blood-borne signals
Regulation of inflammatory and immune reactions
Regulation of vascular tone
Maintenance of thromboresistance
Modulation of leukocyte interactions with tissues
Regulation of vascular growth

Table 9.2 Diseases where the endothelium is critically involved

Adult respiratory distress syndrome
Atherosclerosis
Diabetic vasculopathy
Haemolytic–uraemic syndrome/thrombotic thrombocytopenic purpura
Kawasaki's syndrome
Transplant rejection, both allograft and xenograft
Pulmonary hypertension
Systemic inflammatory response syndrome
Vasculitis

endothelial cells also displayed increased quantities of biosynthetic organelles (such as endoplasmic reticulum). The authors referred to these endothelial cells as being 'activated', implying that there was a functional consequence to the altered morphology. In the 1970s this view of the endothelium having a dynamic function was ignored and the endothelium was considered to be inert and passive.

In the 1980s, however, there was growing realization that when endothelial cells were exposed in vitro to cytokines which mediate the inflammatory response they exhibited new surface molecules and biological functions. To emphasize that this process did not represent sublethal injury with consequent dysfunction, Pober (1988) reintroduced the term 'ECA' with the following definition: 'a quantitative change in the level of expression of certain gene products (i.e. proteins) that, in turn, endow endothelial cells with the new capacities that cumulatively allow endothelial cells to perform new functions' (Pober, 1988).

Today the extraordinary multifunctional ability of endothelial cells to control and mediate inflammation is recognized by many in basic science and clinical science conferences focusing on the endothelium. Few scientists study all aspects of ECA, but concentrate on the area relevant to them. Meetings on endothelial cells are characterized by the diversity of approaches used to study these multi-functional cells. Due to the complexity of the subject many are working on one aspect without being aware of the other areas. To an immunologist ECA means the upregulation of MHC class II antigens, the expression of cell adhesion molecules and the production of certain cytokines. To those involved in thrombosis, ECA produces a change in phenotype from antithrombotic to prothrombotic. To the vascular biologist there is alteration in tone, due to changes in prostacyclin and nitric oxide, which also promote platelet aggregation. In fact all these changes are present in ECA; biological functions cannot be pigeon-holed and are often mutually dependent and interactive. For example, there is integration of haemostatic and immunological responses of the endothelium. Immunoregulatory cytokines such as IL-1 stimulate tissue factor (TF) expression, while thrombin, a central molecule in haemostasis, has a number of bioregulatory roles, such as being chemotactic for monocytes in addition to activating platelets and cleaving fibrinogen. Hence proinflammatory and prothrombotic responses are interlinked as part of host defence and the physical and biological behaviour of cells involved in these mechanisms can be dramatically affected by interactions between them.

Agents causing ECA include the cytokines IL-1 and TNF-α, bacterial endotoxin (lipopolysaccharide: LPS), complement, viral infections and immune complexes. Knowledge concerning ECA is largely based on in vitro stimulation by IL-1, TNF-α or LPS. Pober and Cotran (1991) have distinguished two types of endothelial cell response: the first, 'endothelial cell stimulation', or type I ECA, does not require de novo protein synthesis or gene upregulation (e.g. the release of von Willebrand factor: vWF); the second, 'endothelial cell activation', or type II ECA, does. Thus endothelial cell activation requires a period of time for the stimulating agent to cause effect (e.g. expression of TF by endothelial cells in culture occurs after 4–6 h), whereas in endothelial cell stimulation the response occurs within seconds.

Type I activation involves retraction of endothelial cells from one another, exposing the underlying subendothelium. This is accompanied by expression of P-selectin and release of vWF and secretion of platelet-activating factor (PAF). Type II activation includes progressive induction, at the level of transcription, of many genes including leukocyte adhesion molecules (E-selectin, intercellular adhesion molecule 1 (ICAM-1) and vascular cell adhesion molecule 1 (VCAM-1), cytokines (IL-1, IL-6, IL-8 and monocyte chemoattractant protein (MCP)), and tissue factor (TF) which is the main initiator of coagulation. Thrombomodulin and other functionally important molecules are lost from the surface of endothelial cells (Bach et al., 1995).

The changes in endothelial cell activation

There are five main changes associated with ECA: loss of vascular integrity; expression of leukocyte adhesion molecules; secretion of cytokines; prothrom-

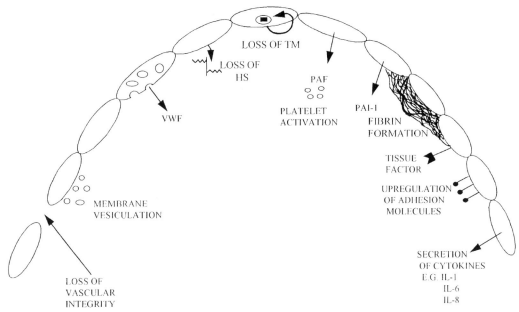

Figure 9.1   Changes associated with endothelial cell activation. TM, thrombomodulin; HS, heparan sulphate; VWF, von Willebrand factor; PAF, platelet-activating factor; PAI-1, plasminogen activator inhibitor type 1.

botic changes and upregulation of HLA molecules. They are reviewed below and summarized in Figure 9.1.

Loss of vascular integrity

In type I ECA, after stimulation with agents such as thrombin or histamine, endothelial cells retract from one another leaving gaps that allow cells and proteins to pass from the intravascular space to the underlying tissue space.

Expression of leukocyte adhesion molecules

Leukocyte–endothelial interactions involve the four sequential steps of tethering, triggering, strong adhesion and migration (Figure 9.2). Tethering of circulating leukocytes to the endothelium results in their rolling along the vessel wall. Triggering agents, mainly cytokines, activate cell adhesion molecules resulting in strong adhesion and flattening of leukocytes which then become motile and migrate into the tissues. This sequence of events can be viewed as a cascade reaction similar to the complement and coagulation cascades.

Tethering is mediated by the selectins. The selectin family comprises E-, L- and P-selectin (CD62E, CD62L and CD62P respectively) composed of a lectin domain, an epidermal growth factor (EGF)-like region and complement regulatory-like

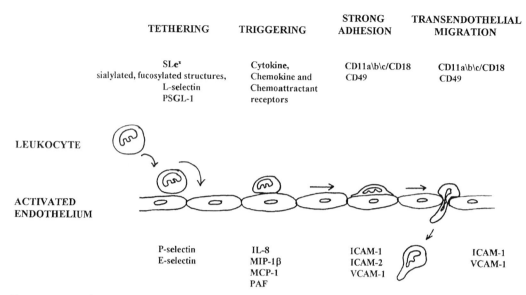

TETHERING	TRIGGERING	STRONG ADHESION	TRANSENDOTHELIAL MIGRATION
SLe^x sialylated, fucosylated structures, L-selectin PSGL-1	Cytokine, Chemokine and Chemoattractant receptors	CD11a\b\c/CD18 CD49	CD11a\b\c/CD18 CD49

LEUKOCYTE

ACTIVATED ENDOTHELIUM

| P-selectin E-selectin | IL-8 MIP-1β MCP-1 PAF | ICAM-1 ICAM-2 VCAM-1 | ICAM-1 VCAM-1 |

Figure 9.2   Leukocyte adhesion. Simplified representation of leukocyte–endothelial adhesion reactions. Tethering of leukocytes to activated endothelium is mediated by low-affinity interactions between selectins. Strong adhesion and transendothelial migration are dependent on higher-affinity reactions involving integrins and the IgG supergene family of adhesion molecules. PSGL-1, P-selectin glycosylation ligand 1; IL-8, interleukin 8; MIP-1β, monocyte inducible protein 1β; MCP-1, monocyte chemotactic protein 1; PAF, platelet-activating factor; ICAM-1, intercellular adhesion molecule 1; VCAM-1, vascular cell adhesion molecule 1. The interactions shown are simplified and are not exclusive.

modules (Bevilacqua and Nelson, 1993). L-selectin binds to mucin-like endothelial glycoproteins whilst E and P-selectins bind sulphated polysaccharides and sialylated Lewis x-related structures (Rosen and Bertozzi, 1994). E-selectin is synthesized and expressed by endothelial cells when activated by cytokines (Pober et al., 1986) and binds neutrophils, monocytes and a subpopulation of memory T cells. P-selectin is expressed by activated endothelium and platelets. It is present on the inner surface of intracellular storage bodies, known as Weibel Palade bodies in the cytoplasm of endothelial cells (Bonfani et al., 1989), and is also found in the α granules of platelets (Israels et al., 1992). Upon stimulation of endothelial cells the Weibel Palade bodies fuse with the endothelial cell surface membrane, discharging their contents and exposing P-selectin. L-selectin is constituitively expressed on most leukocytes and is shed upon their activation (Kishimoto et al., 1989). It is mainly concentrated at the microvilli of leukocytes, a site important for its adhesive function (Stein et al., 1999).

Each selectin recognizes specific carbohydrate motifs on either endothelial cells or leukocytes through their lectin domain. Endothelial cell selectins extend beyond the surrounding glycocalyx so allowing capture of circulating leukocytes that express the appropriate receptor. This loose association of leukocyte and endothelium allows exposure to triggering factors which activate leukocyte integrins.

Integrins consist of α and α subunits (Plow and Ginsberg, 1989) and can be grouped according to their β subunit. At least four leukocyte integrins mediate strong adhesion. These are the β_2-integrins, CD11a/b/c (Sanches-Madrid et al., 1983); and β_1-integrin CD49d (Maxfield et al., 1989). CD11a is present on lymphocytes and CD11b (Mac-1) on neutrophils and monocytes; CD49d is expressed by lymphocytes and monocytes. Activation of leukocytes triggers an increase in avidity caused by a conformational change in the integrin heterodimer. Once activated, the leukocyte integrins bind to counterreceptors on the endothelium–endothelial cell adhesion molecules, which are members of the immunoglobulin gene superfamily (Hogg et al., 1991). β_2-integrins bind to ICAM-1 and ICAM-2. ICAM-2 is constituitively expressed on the endothelium, but ICAM-1 is increased with ECA and inflammation (Pober and Cotran, 1991). The β_1-integrin mediates binding of lymphocytes and monocytes to VCAM-1 which is induced by proinflammatory cytokines (Osborn et al., 1989).

Important triggering factors are IL-8, produced by the endothelium itself or underlying inflammatory cells; PAF, a phospholipid that is rapidly produced by endothelium in response to thrombin, histamine or leukotrienes; monocyte inductible protein 1β (MIP-1β) bound to endothelial proteoglycans; bacterial wall components; and complement activation products. Following strong adhesion to the endothelium leukocytes migrate into the tissues. Many of the cytokines that trigger strong adhesion are also chemotactic; IL-8 induces adhesion and chemotaxis of neutrophils and MIP-1β induces adhesion and migration of T cells.

In addition to host defence, endothelial-leukocyte interactions contribute to pathological inflammatory conditions such as reperfusion injury after ischaemia, autoimmunity, graft rejection and allergic reactions. Diseases characterized by acute inflammation and neutrophil infiltration show increased expression of E- and P-selectin, whereas in chronic lymphocytic inflammation there is increased VCAM-1 expression. E-selectin, ICAM-1 and VCAM-1 are transcriptionally regulated by cytokines, LPS and other inflammatory mediators. Different combinations of cytokines can differentially modulate their induction. There are also differences in the ability to express these molecules between endothelium in large vessels and in the microvasculature.

Cytokine production

Cytokines are important mediators of inflammation. They promote innate immunity and host defence in infectious disease, but also augment the pathogenesis of noninfectious inflammatory states contributing to tissue injury. In addition to

Table 9.3 Cytokines produced by the endothelium

Cytokine	Function
IL-1	Lymphocyte activation
	Local and systemic inflammation
	Acute phase response
	Haematopoiesis
IL-6	Lymphocyte activation
	Acute phase response
	Haematopoiesis
CSFs	Leukocyte recruitment and activation
	Haematopoiesis
	EC proliferation
Chemotactic factors (MCP-1, IL-8)	Leukocyte recruitment and activation
PDGF	Smooth muscle cell proliferation

IL-1, interleukin 1; CSFs, colony-stimulating factors; EC, endothelial cell; MCP-1, monocyte chemotactic protein-1; PDGF, platelet-derived growth factor.

acting as a target for the action of cytokines the endothelium is an important source of these molecules (Table 9.3). Endothelium stimulated with IL-1, TNF-α, interferon-γ (IFN-γ) or LPS produces cytokines. Endothelial cells can synthesize IL-6 that affects the proliferation of T and B cells and regulates production of acute-phase proteins in the liver. Stimulation of the endothelium with LPS, TNF-α or IL-1 itself induces IL-1 production by endothelial cells, which amplifies the inflammatory response. The endothelium also releases chemoattractants such as IL-8 and MCP-1 (Mantovani and Dejana, 1989).

Prothrombotic changes

The antithrombotic effects of the resting endothelium can be separated into antiplatelet, anticoagulant and fibrinolytic. The prothrombotic effects of the endothelium are due to loss of antithrombotic effects and expression of pro-thrombotic molecules. These changes are reviewed below.

Antiplatelet/vasoactive effects

Key molecules: nitric oxide (NO), prostacyclin (PGI$_2$), PAF, endothelin-1 (ET-1), ecto-ADPase

Endothelial cells exhibit an antithrombotic effect by reducing platelet reactivity by synthesizing and releasing prostacyclin PGI$_2$, NO and also ecto-ADPase (for reviews, see Hamblin, 1990; Bach et al., 1994; Marcus, 1994; Davies et al., 1995).

PGI$_2$ is a potent inhibitor of platelet aggregation and a powerful vasodilator. It is transiently and rapidly secreted in response to a variety of agonists, including thrombin, histamine and adenosine diphosphate (ADP), thereby acting locally to inhibit the spread of thrombus.

NO is a potent inhibitor of platelet aggregation and works synergistically with PGI_2. The vascular relaxant and platelet-inhibitory actions of NO are mediated via stimulation of soluble guanylate cyclase, thus elevating cyclic guanosine mono-phosphate (GMP) levels in smooth muscle cells and platelets. This contrasts with the biological actions of PGI_2, many of which are mediated via elevation of cyclic adenosine monophosphate (AMP) levels. Unlike PGI_2, NO also inhibits platelet adhesion to the subendothelium.

NO is synthesized by NO synthetase. There are three main classes of NO ·synthetase: inducible NO synthase (iNOS) endothelial NO synthetase (eNOS) and neuronal NO synthase (nNOS). cNOS is expressed by endothelial cells, neuronal cells and several other cell types and is regulated by Ca^{2+} and calmodulin. NO is released from the endothelium under basal conditions, and also in response to a number of physiological stimuli such as shear stress, circulating hormones (noradrenaline (norepinephrine), vasopressin, bradykinin) and various autacoids (acetylcholine, histamine, substance P). Shear stress, in particular, appears to be a major stimulus for NO release, for NO activity is highest in largest-diameter arteries that are subject to greater variation in pulsatile flow and shear stress (see Chapter 3).

iNOS is found in endothelium, vascular smooth muscle cells, macrophages and neutrophils. It is induced after cytokine exposure and is capable of generating far greater quantities of NO than cNOS; at high concentrations NO is cytotoxic and thus plays a key role in the immune response to bacteria and other pathogens.

The endothelins (ETs) are 21-amino-acid peptides produced in a number of different tissues. Originally discovered in 1988 (Yanagisiwa et al., 1988), three ETs are now known – ET-1, ET-2 and ET-3. Endothelial cells produce ETs, mainly ET-1, in response to a number of different factors including hypoxia, hyperoxia, pressure, low shear stress, catecholamines, thrombin, low-density lipoproteins, vasopressin, angiotensin II and TGF-β (Schriffin, 1995). ET-1 is the most potent vasoconstrictor known and is produced by posttranslational processessing of preproET-1, the 212-amino-acid ET-1 precursor, to proET-1 or big ET-1 which is subsequently converted to the ET-1 peptide (Denault et al., 1995). This occurs both intracellularly and at the membrane in endothelial cells and on the surface of smooth muscle cells in the vascular wall through the action of ET-converting enzyme (ECE). ECE is found on the cell surface as an ectoenzyme and colocalized with big ET-1 in intracellular vesicles where it is recycled from the luminal membrane (Barnes et al., 1998). ECE-1α, ECE-1β and ECE-2 are differing iso-forms of ECE.

After binding to specific receptors, ET-1 promotes influx of calcium ions and release of calcium from intracellular stores, resulting in phosphorylation of myosin light chains and initiation of smooth muscle contraction. There are two ET receptor subtypes, ET_A and ET_B (Hosoda et al., 1992, Arai et al., 1993). ET-1 is secreted mainly toward underlying smooth muscle and binds ET_A and ET_B receptors to bring about contraction, proliferation and hypertrophy. Receptor binding is rapid but dissociation is very slow, accounting for the long-lasting vasoconstrictor effect. ET-1 also acts on endothelial ET_B receptors, which induces release of NO and PGI_2, so inducing vasodilatation. A critical balance exists between NO and ET-1: this may be a major determinant in the regulation of local and systemic haemodynamic function and cellular proliferation. The distribution of receptor subtypes is tissue and cell-specific. Vascular smooth muscle cells possess mainly ET_A receptors, whereas endothelial cells contain only ET_B receptors. In the coronary circulation ET_B receptors are virtually absent, thus ET-1 behaves mainly as a coronary vasoconstrictor (Russell et al., 1997).

ET-1 may play a role in the pathophysiology of a variety of cardiovascular disorders, including heart failure, coronary heart disease, primary pulmonary hypertension, arterial hypertension and atherosclerosis (Schiffrin and Touyz, 1998). In these conditions there is evidence of increased plasma ET levels, increased ET-1 mRNA in endothelial cells and smooth muscle cells or response to ET antagonists. Although ET-1 is known as a potent vasoconstictor there is accumulating evidence that ET-1 acts as a cytokine. It may play a part in inflammation by priming neutrophils and inducing neutrophil aggregation, adhesion and elastase release (Gomez-Garre et al., 1992, Lopez-Farre et al., 1993); by activating mast cells (Uchida et al., 1992); increasing cell adhesion molecule expression (McCarron et al., 1993); stimulating monocytes and macrophages to release proinflammatory cytokines (McMillen and Sumpio, 1995); stimulating IL-6 production by endothelial cells (Xin et al., 1995); and by inducing release of growth factors (Jaffe et al., 1990).

Rapid production of PAF is induced by many of the agonists that induce PGI_2 synthesis and causes platelet secretion and aggregation. Activated platelets release adenosine triphosphate (ATP) and ADP from their dense granules. Adenine nucleotides are relatively stable and a system to degrade them is provided by ectonucleotidases at the endothelial cell surface, thus endothelial cells inhibit platelet aggregation, in part, by ecto-ADPase activity. Ecto-ADPase catalyses hydrolysis of ATP and ADP to AMP and orthophosphate. Endothelial cells convert AMP to adenosine, which has an antiaggregating effect. When endothelial cells are activated in vitro, platelet aggregation occurs associated with loss of ecto-ADPase activity, which will permit accumulation of ADP, a potent stimulus to platelet thrombosis.

Anticoagulant pathways

Key molecules: antithrombin/heparan sulphate; thrombomodulin, tissue factor
pathway inhibitor (TFPI)

Aortic, venous and microvascular endothelia exert a profound anticoagulant effect by expressing heparan sulphate proteoglycans, consisting of a protein core to which heparan sulphate glycosaminglyocan chains are attached. Heparan sulphate potentiates antithrombin (AT) activity, which is a major physiological anti-coagulant. AT is an irreversible inhibitor of not only thrombin, as the name suggests, but of the majority of intrinsic coagulation proteases. Heparan sulphate, expressed on endothelial cell surfaces in vivo, acts as an endogenous catalyst for the anticoagulant actions of AT.

Heparan sulphate proteoglycans are the predominating proteoglycans of the endothelium. Cytokines stimulate synthesis of the glycosaminoglycans whilst physical injury, hypoxia and viral infection decrease its synthesis (Ihrcke et al., 1996). During inflammation heparan sulphate is released from the endothelium. Mechanisms causing this release include cleavage of the glycosaminoglycan chains by heparanases, produced by many cell types, including activated platelets, ac-tivated endothelial cells and activated T cells; through proteolysis of the protein core by proteases from activated T cells and neutrophil elastase, binding of antibodies to endothelial cells and the activation of complement.

Apart from its anticoagulant function, heparan sulphate is also important in maintaining vascular integrity and its loss from the surface may result in oedema and exudation of plasma proteins. There is also evidence that heparan sulphate can influence cellular immune responses through interactions with antigen-presenting cells and it tethers extracellular superoxide dismutase (SOD) to the vessel wall. The loss of heparan sulphate during ECA thus results in both loss of anticoagulant and anti-free radical mechanisms.

Thrombomodulin is an endothelial cell surface-expressed glycoprotein, and is a critical receptor in the protein C anticoagulant system (Esmon and Owen, 1981). This system is activated when coagulation is initiated and thrombin is generated. Thrombin bound to thrombomodulin on the surface of endothelial cells allows the activation of protein C. (Thrombin, once bound to thrombomodulin, loses its coagulant activity and is no longer able to convert fibrinogen to fibrin, or activate platelets.) Activated protein C, together with its cofactor protein S, act as anti-coagulants by inactivating factors Va and VIIIa, thus limiting further thrombin generation.

ECA results in the loss of thrombomodulin from the endothelial cell surface. This is due to internalization of thrombomodulin, decreased transcription of mRNA and subsequent downregulation of thrombomodulin synthesis (Moore et al., 1989).

TFPI is produced by the endothelium and inhibits the first steps of the extrinsic coagulation pathway by inhibiting factor Xa and the TF–VIIa complex (Rapaport, 1991). Much of circulating TFPI is bound to lipoprotein, and platelets carry about 10% of circulating TFPI which they release upon activation. It is also released into the circulation in response to heparin (Sandset et al., 1988) and other glycosaminoglycans to a lesser degree. It has been suggested that TFPI is bound to endothelial cell glycosaminoglycans, but this is not certain. The main physiological role of TFPI appears to be in the inhibition of small amounts of TF and is essential for maintaining a normal haemostatic balance. The effect of ECA on TFPI levels is uncertain, but it is increased in plasma by endotoxin, suggesting it may be upregulated at the same time as TF.

Procoagulant effects

Key molecules: vWF, TF, vesicles with prothrombinase activity

vWF is stored in Weibel Palade bodies in endothelial cells and in the α granules of platelets. It is also present free in plasma and anchored in the subendothelium (Wagner, 1990). When platelets are activated, vWF acts as the ligand for platelet adhesion by binding to a specific receptor, glycoprotein Ib. Following type 1 ECA, Weibel Palade bodies fuse with the endothelial cell membrane, releasing vWF. The inner surface of the Weibel Palade bodies is coated with P-selectin, which is thus expressed on the endothelial cell surface. In the plasma vWF is also the carrier for factor VIII, thus levels of factor VIII are reduced with levels of vWF in von Willebrand's disease. Levels of vWF have been used as a marker of disease activity in the vasculitides; but they are not ideal because vWF also behaves as an acute-phase protein.

TF is an integral membrane component that serves as the essential cofactor for coagulation factor VII/VIIa which subsequently activates factor X, but has also been shown to activate factor IX. TF is strongly expressed on all solid tissues, especially vascular adventitial cells, forming a haemostatic envelope around blood vessels. Thus if a vessel is injured, extraendothelial TF initiates coagulation (Drake et al., 1989). It is not expressed on endothelium, but expression is induced in vitro on monocytes and endothelium 2–6 h after stimulation with IL-1, TNF-α or LPS and will thus cause activation of coagulation and clot formation. It remains unclear whether endothelial TF can be upregulated in vivo: the current consensus is that it probably is not, and that monocyte TF expression is the main activator in pathological situations.

Stimulation of platelets or endothelium by complement results in deposition of C5-9 and subsequent vesiculation of their membranes. These vesicles are endowed with prothrombinase activity. This phenomenon also occurs with ECA (Berckmans et al., 2001).

Fibrinolytic effects

The fibrinolytic system is responsible for clot breakdown and thus healing. Plasmin is produced from its inactive precursor plasminogen by the action of tissue plasminogen activator (tPA) which, with its inhibitor, plasminogen activator inhibitor type I (PAI-1), is produced by the endothelium. Stimulation of endothelial cells with cytokines such as TNF-α or with LPS leads to unaltered or decreased secretion of tPA, but enhanced PAI-1 release. Thus, overall there is a reduction of fibrinolytic activators resulting in reduced fibrinolytic potential (Schleef et al., 1988).

Upregulation of expression of class I and II HLA molecules

The term 'antigen presenting cell' means that the cell is able to present antigen to resting T cells in a form they recognize as foreign and thus cause activation of T cells. T cells recognize antigens as foreign in two ways: 'direct' recognition is when they see, and are activated by, major histocompatibility complex (MHC) molecules of a different type from their own, while 'indirect' recognition occurs when a foreign antigen is processed and 'presented' to them by self MHC molecules. Thus, in transplant rejection, recipient T cells will see MHC molecules on donor cells as foreign and become activated. This is discussed in Chapter 18, as is the controversy over whether endothelial cells can act as antigen-presenting cells.

MHC loci are the major target of immune response following allograft rejection. It has also been suggested that aberrant expression of autologous MHC is involved in the pathogenesis of some autoimmune diseases. MHC expression is not a constant feature of endothelial cells; they can be upregulated by cytokines. Moreover, an increase in expression will alter the magnitude of the immune response. Thus the distribution and the MHC will determine both the target and the strength of the immune response. Under standard culture conditions human endothelial cells express class I MHC molecules (HLA-A, B and C) but not class II (HLA-DR, DP, DQ). Treatment of cultured endothelial cells with IFN-β, IFN-α, TNF-α, lymphotoxin or CD40 ligand increases the level of expression of class I molecules without inducing class II molecules. IFN-γ also increases the level of class I MHC molecule expression and, on human endothelial cells, is uniquely able to induce expression of class II MHC molecules. In general, the MHC patterns of expression in vivo are the same as exhibited by cultured endothelial cells. Human endothelial cells are uniformly positive for class I molecules. Class II MHC molecules are expressed constitutively on some endothelial cells, including most postcapillary venules, veins and some arteries. This expression is altered at sites of inflammation and rejection, e.g. on quiescent pulmonary endothelium HLA class II MHC are variably expressed; however, in chronic rejection there is enhanced and consistent expression of class II on endothelial cells (for review, see Pober et al., 1996; see Chapter 18).

The intracellular mechanisms underlying endothelial cell activation

The diverse effects of ECA share a common intracellular control mechanism which 'switch on' the facets of endothelial cell activation ECA by altering gene transcription (Baldwin, 1996). After a stimulating agent attaches to its receptor on the endothelial cell surface, the message is transmitted intracellularly to a transcription factor, nuclear factor κB (NF-κB). Most inducible transcription factors are activated by a limited number of physiological agents, but NF-κB is activated by a large variety of agents representing a threat to the organism. The genes which are upregulated during ECA (e.g. TF, PAI-1, E-selectin) contain binding sites for NF-κB in their promoter area. NF-κB is stored in an inactive form in the cytoplasm, and is activated by the removal of an inhibitory subunit, IκB. This is initiated by phosphorylation followed by proteolysis (Henkel et al., 1993). In the absence of IκB, exposed sequences on the NF-κB dimer composed of p50 and p65 (RelA) subunits are recognized by a receptor and transported into the nucleus where binding to DNA regulatory sequences initiates transcription of the genes involved in ECA. NF-κB-binding sites are found in the regulatory region of essentially all the genes studied that are induced as part of ECA (Collins et al., 1993).

Endothelial cell activation in disease

Systemic inflammatory response syndrome (SIRS)

SIRS is defined as the clinical response to a nonspecific insult resulting in two or more of the following: (1) temperature greater than 38 °C or less than 36 °C; (2) heart rate greater than 90 beats/min; (3) respiratory rate greater than 20 breaths/min or a $P\text{CO}_2$ less than 32 mmHg; or (4) white blood cell count greater than $12.0 \times 10^9/\text{l}$ or less than $4.0 \times 10^9/\text{l}$ or the presence of more than 10% immature neutrophils. Sepsis refers to the presence of SIRS in association with a confirmed infectious process. Septic shock is defined as sepsis with hypotension in spite of adequate fluid resuscitation, or hypoperfusion (manifest as lactic acidosis, oliguria or altered mental status). Epidemiological evidence suggests that these occur sequentially and that a clinical progression from SIRS to sepsis to septic shock occurs. A stepwise increase in mortality rates exists for the hierarchy of SIRS, sepsis and septic shock: 7%, 16% and 46% respectively. The likelihood of end-organ dysfunction (acute respiratory distress syndrome (ARDS), acute renal failure, disseminated intravascular coagulation (DIC)) increases directly as two, three and four criteria for SIRS are met (Rangel-Frauso et al., 1995). Overwhelming infection with Gram-negative bacteria results in the release of endotoxin, an LPS component of bacterial cell walls that stimulates production of proinflammatory cytokines. Widespread ECA in response to the sequential release of TNF-α, IL-1, IL-6 and IL-8 is thought to be the mechanism underlying SIRS and its sequelae (Van Zee et al., 1991).

Excess NO production may mediate the hypotension and myocardial depression associated with septic shock. Endotoxin and subsequent cytokine generation is capable of initiating iNOS in macrophages and vascular smooth muscle cells. Once synthesized, iNOS produces abundant amounts of NO, resulting in the vasodilatation and hypotension that characterize septic shock (Petro et al., 1991). Because it is apparent that NO is integrally involved in the pathophysiology of septic shock, L-arginine analogues have been used as specific inhibitors of iNOS. Glucocorticoids inhibit induction of iNOS after exposure to endotoxin. Methylene blue (an NO inactivator) reverses hypotension secondary to sepsis in association with normalizing plasma NO levels (Keaney et al., 1994). Although it appears that NO inhibition may be an effective therapy for the treatment of hypotension secondary to sepsis, there is no evidence that NOS inhibitors reduce mortality, and there is concern that complete, nonselective inhibition of NO synthesis may have deleterious side-effects. In animal models of sepsis, higher doses of an NOS inhibitor lead to higher mortality and glomerular thrombosis (Nava et al., 1992). Thus, NO release during sepsis may be necessary to ensure adequate local perfusion to vital organs and to prevent vascular thrombosis in small arterioles both by minimizing vascular resistance and impairing platelet activation.

Inducing septicaemia in primates results in widespread expression of E-selectin, especially in the kidney, lung, and liver – all involved at an early stage of the development of multiorgan failure. At the same time there is a rapid influx of neutrophils into the lungs and central organs which parallels the expression of E-selectin (see Dinarello et al., 1993, for review of animal models of SIRS).

The infusion of endotoxin into healthy volunteers results in early rises in TNF-α levels (at 30 min) followed by rises in IL-1 and IL-6 (Suffredini et al., 1989; van Deventer et al., 1990); and increase in coagulation activation as measured by thrombin–antithrombin complexes and prothrombin fragment 1.2, and also an increase in tPA activity soon to be offset by the release of PAI-1. Rises in plasma vWF are also observed. These changes are consistent with ECA type I and type II.

DIC is common during SIRS and is a strong predictor of death and multiple organ failure in the setting of SIRS. Nonsurvivors of septic shock have a stronger activation of coagulation and a more marked inhibition of fibrinolysis than survivors (Gando et al., 1995). Recently a polymorphism within the promoter area of the PAI-1 gene, which is known to produce a greater increase in PAI-1 levels after IL-1, has been shown to be an adverse survival factor in meningococcal septicaemia (Hermans et al., 1999; Westendorp et al., 1999). Upregulation of TF on the endothelium and monocytes may be the initiator of the activation of coagulation. Treatment with antithrombin concentrates and protein C concentrates has been used to negate the effects of activation of coagulation, but the studies have been small and poorly controlled (Taylor et al., 1987; Fourier et al., 1993). The administration of TFPI following a bacterial infusion into baboons resulted in the prolongation of survival time and attenuation of coagulopathy (Creasey et al., 1993). In addition, the inhibition of an endotoxin-induced co-agulopathy has been achieved in chimpanzees by a monoclonal antibody specific for TF (Levi et al., 1994). As yet there are no comprehensive studies of their use in humans.

Anticytokine strategies aimed at TNF-α and IL-1 have been employed in animal models of SIRS (for review, see Dinarello et al., 1993). Specific blockade of TNF by soluble forms of the TNF-α receptor or neutralizing antibodies reduce mortality and severity of disease. Similar results have been obtained with IL-1 receptor antagonists and soluble IL-1 receptors. Clinical studies have demonstrated that blockade of these cytokines may also be useful in treating human SIRS (Boermeester et al., 1995), but the outcome is not always beneficial and further studies are needed.

Ischaemia–reperfusion injury

Ischaemic–reperfusion injury contributes to the pathophysiology of a number of clinical disorders. These include stroke and myocardial infarction, organ preservation, the use of fibrinolytic agents and surgery where blood vessels are cross-clamped. The length of time a tissue can survive oxygen deprivation varies but eventually all ischaemic tissue becomes necrotic. (For recent excellent reviews of ischaemia–reperfusion, see Grace, 1994; Cohen, 1995).

There is abundant evidence to suggest that cell damage following ischaemia is biphasic, with injury being initiated during ischaemia and exacerbated during reperfusion. Ischaemic injury has been well characterized: the cell is deprived of the energy needed to maintain ionic gradients and homeostasis, and failure of enzyme systems leads to cell death. Reperfusion is obviously a prerequisite for recovery from ischaemic injury and removal of toxic metabolites. However, the return of toxic metabolites to the circulation may have serious metabolic consequences and, paradoxically, reperfusion of ischaemic tissue may induce further local tissue injury. Reperfusion injury is mediated by the interaction of free radicals, neutrophils and activated endothelial cells (see Figure 9.3 for simplified series of events).

A free radical is an unstable molecule containing one or more unpaired electrons. The hydroxyl radical is formed via the iron-catalysed Haber–Weiss reaction. Superoxide radicals (which are a byproduct of normal cellular

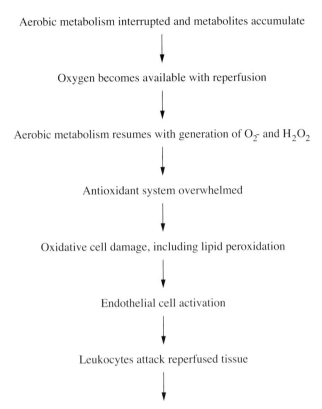

Aerobic metabolism interrupted and metabolites accumulate

↓

Oxygen becomes available with reperfusion

↓

Aerobic metabolism resumes with generation of O_2^- and H_2O_2

↓

Antioxidant system overwhelmed

↓

Oxidative cell damage, including lipid peroxidation

↓

Endothelial cell activation

↓

Leukocytes attack reperfused tissue

↓

'Postischaemia syndrome' – cytokines released into systemic circulation

Figure 9.3   Likely sequence of events in ischaemia–reperfusion injury.

metabolism and produced by xanthine oxidase in postischaemic tissue) release iron from ferritin which in turn reacts with hydrogen peroxide to produce hydroxyl radicals. It is probably responsible for most of the cellular damage that occurs from free radicals. The most damaging effect of free radicals is lipid peroxidation which produces structural and functional cell damage.

Reperfusion is associated with accumulation of neutrophils in the microvasculature; neutrophil–endothelial cell interactions are a prerequisite for the microvascular injury of ischaemia–reperfusion. Neutrophils adhere to, and migrate across, the endothelium via adhesion molecules and cause local damage by releasing free radicals, proteolytic enzymes and peroxidase.

In ischaemia–reperfusion NO release is impaired or the released NO is immediately inactivated by haemoglobin or oxygen-derived free radicals before it can exert its vasodilator effects. It has also been suggested that NO may react with superoxide to yield secondary cytotoxic species via peroxynitrite ($ONOO^-$). Some animal work has actually suggested that it may be causally involved in myocardial reoxygenation injury. ET-1 may also play a role in the pathogenesis of ischaemic injury. Raised circulating plasma ET-1 concentrations have been found in vivo in arterial injury and in the early hours after myocardial infarction, with sustained increase in patients with continuing ischaemia. Watanabe and colleagues demonstrated that administration of endothelin antibody reduced myocardial infarct size in rats (Watanabe et al., 1991). Endothelial damage and impaired NO release occur during ischaemia, resulting in inhibition of vasodilatation. Ischaemia and decreased shear stress will stimulate ET-1 release, which in turn results in vasoconstriction, continuing ischaemia and further infarction.

There are different opportunities of reducing the damage. The first is to prevent generation of free radicals and hydrogen peroxide directly. Allopurinol inhibits the production of xanthine oxidase, and has been shown to reduce infarct size in animal models and in some clinical trials. Desferrioxamine is a powerful iron-chelating agent; because iron is essential for the Haber–Weiss reaction and production of the free radical it has been used with beneficial effects during ischaemia–reperfusion injury (Ambrosia et al., 1987). A second option is to enhance the tissues' capacity to trap free radicals. A number of antioxidants and free radical scavengers have been investigated. Recombinant superoxide dismutase (SOD) is an enzyme that detoxifes O_2^-. Results of its use in clinical trials have so far been variable.

The use of monoclonal antibodies against key cytokines, IL-1 and TNF-α, reduced leg muscle injury in a rat leg model of ischaemia–reperfusion, while antibodies to adhesion molecules in animals have also shown success.

Ischaemic preconditioning is a term used to cover the phenomenon whereby resistance of a tissue to a lethal period of ischaemia is enhanced by a preceding period of sublethal ischaemia. Ischaemic preconditioning from animal experiments appears to be a biphasic phenomenon: there is an early phase of protection that lasts for about 2 h after the preconditioning stimulus, and a second window of protection that occurs 24 h later (Marber et al., 1993). Adenosine and heat shock proteins are implicated in this phenomenon.

Heat shock proteins are produced by all living organisms, in response to adverse changes in the environment. This defensive process, called the heat-shock response, occurs in response to a wide range of stimuli, including ischaemia preconditioning (Lindquist, 1986). How they work is unclear: experimental work suggests that they are associated with increased production of free radical scavengers, especially catalase and SOD (Karmazyn et al., 1990).

Adenosine is a ubiquitous product of ischaemia. The early phase of ischaemic preconditioning appears to be effected by the intervention of A_1 receptors and protein kinase C in myocytes, for if adenosine receptors are blocked then preconditioning does not have an effect. Similar effects are seen with inhibitors and agonists of the protein kinase C pathway (Cophen and Downey, 1993).

Currently there is no clearcut solution to the management of ischaemia–reperfusion injury. The future may be in the use of combination therapy with better techniques for reperfusion, and the use of antioxidants with neutrophil inhibitors.

Antiendothelial cell antibodies

There have been studies in many conditions suggesting a causative role for antiendothelial antibodies. They have been reported in patients with various types of connective tissue disorders and autoimmune state, including Behçet's disease, retinal vasculitis, Kawasaki's disease, haemolytic–uraemia syndrome, inflammatory bowel disease, multiple sclerosis, acute preeclampsia and some viral infections. In spite of the interest, no definite conclusions have been drawn about their clinical significance or their pathogenic role. All studies should be reviewed carefully, especially the methodology, for it is difficult to identify true antiendothelial cell antibodies. The endothelium is bathed in plasma containing antibodies and many antiendothelial cell assays are based on measuring binding of antibodies to endothelial cells. Thus, binding of low-titre immunoglobulins may have little pathological significance. In addition the assays are often performed in vitro on human umbilical vein endothelial cells following three or more passages in vitro. This can alter the endothelial cell surface phenotype or the response to standard stimuli. Finally, there is enormous endothelial cell heterogeneity, depending on their site, so antiendothelial cell antibodies could be specific for certain antigens present only on a few types of endothelium.

Antiendothelial cell antibodies have been described in active systemic lupus erythematosus (SLE). In culture they bind to the endothelium, deposit complement, cause platelets to adhere, can upregulate TF and disrupt the endothelial cell monolayer. The addition of peripheral blood mononuclear cells has been shown to induce endothelial cell cytotoxicity in combination with antiendothelial cell antibodies (Meroni et al., 1995).

Immune complexes

Normally the mononuclear phagocytic system is an efficient scavenger of immune complexes. However, under certain circumstances, immune complexes apparently escape the system and are deposited on tissues, causing inflammation. The association of serum sickness with systemic necrotizing vasculitis is widely recognized. Animal models have formed the basis of our current understanding (for review, see Cochrane and Koffler, 1973).

If antigen is injected into the skin of sensitized animals then this is followed by a vasculitis mediated by the formation of immune complexes (the Arthus reaction). These immune complexes are removed within 24–48 h by neutrophils. Activated neutrophils release proteases that digest proteins and they also generate free radicals. These cause endothelial cell detachment and lysis, with vessel wall damage and occlusion (Kniker and Cochrane, 1965).

SLE is considered a prototype disease mediated by immune complexes. Serum complement levels are reduced in active lupus and improve with treatment (Schur and Sandson, 1968). Complement deposition has been identified in inflamed tissues (Tann and Kunkel, 1966). Anti-double-stranded DNA antibodies are considered to be a marker of lupus activity, and DNA and anti-DNA antibodies are found in renal tissue and skin (Fournie, 1988), although there are some patients with very high serum levels and apparently inactive disease and vice versa.

Immune complex-mediated vasculitis occurs with hepatitis B infection. Cases of polyarteritis nodosa associated with chronic carriage of hepatitis B were first described in 1970 (Gocke et al., 1970). Circulating immune complexes from patients with vasculitis in association with chronic carriage of hepatitis B contain viral antigen, and vasculitis is accompanied by low complement levels, cryo-globulins and deposits of immunoglobulin and complement in affected vessel walls (Shusterman and London, 1984). In vitro studies suggest this would cause activation of local endothelial cells.

vWF levels are also elevated in the systemic vasculitides and there is some evidence to show that plasma levels reflect disease activity; many authors feel the levels reflect the extent of ECA but it must be remembered that levels are also increased as part of the acute-phase response (Nusinow et al., 1984). (For further details, see Chapter 16)

Summary

ECA appears to be an effect mechanism in the inflammatory response and thus a component of the pathophysiological response to injury. ECA may play an important role in the pathogenesis of many diseases. However it must be remembered that many of the mechanisms described here have only been observed in vitro or in animal models: there is considerable scope for future research.

In future there may be more fundamental approaches to switching off ECA, at the level of NF-κB. Intriguingly, glucocorticosteroids stimulate the production of IκB, thus locking up NF-κB, while the glucocorticoid receptor complex binds to NF-κB, preventing it from binding to DNA and thus preventing increased gene activity (Marx, 1995). The design of a pharmaceutical agent behaving in the same way but without the side-effects of glucocorticoids would have obvious benefits. Aspirin, a widely used antiinflammatory drug and platelet inhibitor, inhibits activation of NF-κB by preventing proteolytic degradation of IκB (Kopp and Ghosh, 1994). Inhibition of NF-κB activation by antioxidants and specific protease inhibitors may also prove useful. Other approaches at switching off NF-κB are being actively explored. There is clearly great potential for interference with the mechanism of NF-κB activation and hence prevention of ECA, which may aid in the treatment of many conditions.

Endothelial responses to hypoxic stress

Physiologically there are wide variations in oxygen tension within the body, which are transduced by the endothelial cell through regulated gene expression into homeostatic signals to the surrounding tissues. Normally, the P_{O_2} of arterial blood is approximately 150 mmHg, while oxygen tensions in the tissues have been measured at 40 mmHg, and lower in conditions of hypoxaemia. Endothelial cells sense and respond to oxygen tensions falling below 70 mmHg. In contrast to the homeostatic effect that occurs with 'normal' oxygenation, prolonged or severe hypoxia represents a major stress and the genetic response can cause permanent detrimental effects (Graven et al., 1993).

Changes in the environmental oxygen tension result in a differential expression of specific genes within the endothelial cell. These produce a specific set of proteins which are responsible for erythropoiesis, glycolysis and angiogenesis. Changes in oxygen tension appears to signal through a novel oxygen sensor that alters the levels and DNA-binding activity of transcription factors such as activating protein-1 (AP-1), nuclear kappa NF-κB and hypoxia-inducible transcription factor-1 (HIF). Thus, this results in the transcription induction of genes encoding vasoconstrictors, smooth muscle mitogens and genes encoding matrix or re-modelling molecules. The vasoconstrictors and smooth muscle mitogens include PDGF-β, ET-1, vascular endothelial growth factor (VEGF) and thrombospondin-1 (TSP-1). The remodelling molecules include collagenase IV and thrombospon-din-TSP-1. There is also reciprocal transcription inhibition of vasodilator and/or antimitogenic effects through eNOS.

The oxygen sensor

The nature of this has not been fully elucidated. It has been hypothesized that it consists of a haem-binding protein that binds O_2-like molecules and attains a relaxed form in the bound state or a 'tense' configuration in the unbound state (Faller, 1999). Certainly, inhibitors of haem biosynthesis blunt the hypoxic response in endothelial cells. Furthermore, transition metals that can substitute for iron in the haem structure, but which are incapable of binding oxygen (cobalt and nickel) render the sensing molecule unresponsive to oxygen tension. Further research is required.

Second messenger systems

Several transcription factors have been found to be activated by hypoxia, including hypoxia-inducible transcription factor (HIF), AP-1 and NF-κB. The induction of cyclooxygenase-2 (COX-2) gene by hypoxia is mediated via the NF-κB p65 transcription factor in human vascular endothelial cells (Schmedtje et al., 1997), but the role of NF-κB in mediating other hypoxia-responsive genes remains unclear. A number of endothelial cell vasoactive genes that are transcriptionally activated by hypoxia, including PDGF-B, ET-1, TSP-1 and VEGF, are also known to be inducible by phorbol esters through an AP-1 binding site.

Genes upregulated by hypoxia in the endothelium

See Figure 9.4 for a summary of gene regulation in hypoxia.

PDGF-β is a mitogenic peptide that causes proliferation of vascular smooth muscle cells and is also a paracrine vasoconstrictor. Hypoxia increases PDGF-β mRNA 8–12-fold within 24–48 h (Kourembanas et al., 1990). ET-1 is the most powerful vasoconstrictor agent released by endothelial cells. Production increases rapidly in in vitro hypoxia and persists for at least 48 h. TSP-1 is a 450 kDa matrix-associated glycoprotein. It is involved in platelet aggregation, cell adhesion, smooth muscle and fibroblast proliferation and migration. Hypoxia increases transcription. In vitro hypoxia increases transcription sixfold. Like PDGF-β and ET-1, eNOS and VEGF, the effect of low oxygen tension is reversible.

Vascular endothelial growth factor

This is a dimeric glycoprotein which is a potent mitogen for endothelial cells, mediating endothelial cell growth and tissue neovascularization (Goldberg and Schneider, 1994; Minchenko et al., 1994), which plays an important role in response to ischaemic injury, wound healing and tumour pathogenesis. The receptors for both ET-1 and VEGF (Flt-1 and Flk-1) are upregulated in vascular tissue in parallel with their respective ligands by low oxygen tension. The VEGF gene is regulated at both the transcriptional and posttranscriptional level. Hypoxia increases the rate of transcription threefold and the stability of VEGF mRNA is enhanced by hypoxia, and by hypoglycaemia, both of which are a consequence of ischaemia (Stein et al., 1995).

Endothelial nitric oxide synthase (eNOS) and NO

eNOS produces NO, a potent inorganic vasodilator from arginine, and promotes relaxation of neighbouring smooth muscle cells. ENOS is constituitively expressed but activation of the calcium–calmodulin pathway is required for maximal activation. Exposure of endothelial cells to low oxygen tensions (20–40 mmHg) results in a dramatic fall in transcription of eNOS and thus a subsequent fall in eNOS

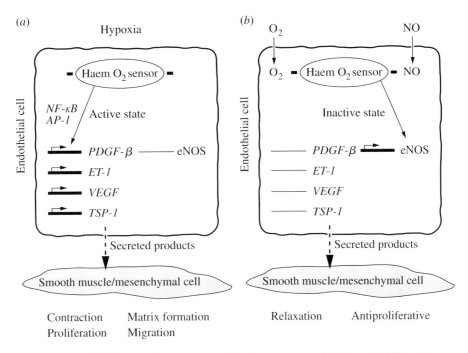

Figure 9.4   Schemative model of vasoactive gene regulation by oxygen and nitric oxide (NO). (*a*)
Under hypoxic conditions, the haem-containing oxygen sensor is activated (unbound,
tense conformation), leading to activation of genes whose products can act upon
underlying vascular smooth muscle and stromal cells to cause constriction, proliferation,
migration and matrix deposition and the suppression of genes whose products counteract
these effects. (*b*) Conversely, in the presence of ligands for the haem-containing oxygen
sensor, such as oxygen or NO, the sensor attains an inactive state (bound, relaxed
conformation), resulting in the production of vasoconstrictor or mitogenic factors. NF-κB,
nuclear factor κB; AP-1, activating protein-1; PDGF-β, platelet-derived growth factor-β;
eNOS, endothelial nitric oxide synthase; ET-1, endothelin-1; VEGF, vascular endothelial
growth factor; TSP-1, thrombospondin-1; from Douglas V. Faller, 'Endothelial cell responses
to hypoxic stress', *Clinical and Experimental Pharmacology Physiology* (1999) 26, 74–84.
Figure no 1, reproduced with permission.

protein levels (Phelan and Faller, 1996). NO itself regulates the genes encoding
vasoactive factors, i.e. NO and oxygen transduce similar genes, and thus their
absence leads to the same pattern of gene expression. Thus NO can feed back and
modulate signals induced by hypoxia and vice versa. For example, NO, which can
act directly on smooth muscle cells as a vasodilator, can also facilitate vasodilatation indirectly by reversing the production of vasoconstrictors induced by hypoxia
(Faller, 1999).

In vivo effects of chronic hypoxia

Short-term exposure of endothelial cells to low oxygen tensions results in predominantly vasoconstrictor effects. However, chronic hypoxia can lead to remodelling of the vasculature, for it generates factors that induce smooth muscle proliferation and remodelling. This will have the effect of causing irreversible remodelling of the vasculature and surrounding tissues with smooth muscle proliferation and fibrosis (Voelkel and Tudor, 1995).

PDGF-β and ET-1 may mediate much of the tissue remodelling as both are strong chemoattractants and mitogens for fibroblast and smooth muscle cells. A major inhibitor of these effects, as well as endothelial cell migration, mitogenesis and proliferation, is NO, the production of which is inhibited by hypoxia. Over time the mitogenic effects of PFGF-β, VEGF, ET-1 and TSP-1 will result in structural remodelling and smooth muscle hypertrophy that is seen in chronic pulmonary artery hypertension, whether due to hypoxia in the newborn or primary or secondary pulmonary hypertension, seen in adults.

Endothelial cell heterogeneity

Endothelial cells not only have to perform multiple homeostatic functions but also integrate different extracellular signals and cellular responses in different regions of the vascular tree. One can imagine that the predominant functions of an endothelial cell in the liver might be different from those in the brain.

Let us consider the diversity of the haemostatic function of endothelial cells. Firstly, the level of mRNA can vary from one vascular bed to another, as does vWF (Bahnak et al., 1989). Histochemical studies of the thrombomodulin receptor have revealed high levels within the endothelium of the lungs and heart and yet barely detectable levels within the brain (Ishii et al., 1986). Similarly, there are variations in expression of tPA, PAI-1 and urokinase plasminogen activator. Experimentation with knockout mice has confirmed that some aspects of the endothelium are regulated in a tissue-specific manner (Aird et al., 1995). For example, mice that are homozygous for a point mutation in thrombomodulin that deletes its anticoagulant function have fibrin deposits in lungs, heart and spleen, illustrating these organs' endothelial dependence on thrombomodulin as an anticoagulant. Under hypoxic conditions there is a 10-fold increase in fibrin deposition in the lungs, suggesting that the environment interacts with the genotype to alter phenotypic expression (Weiler-Guettler et al., 1998).

The mechanisms responsible for generating a tissue-specific phenotype for the endothelium are slowly being unravelled. Firstly, it is recognized that an array of signals, including growth factors, cytokines, mechanical forces, extracellular matrix and neighbouring cells, will exert their effect on local endothelium. For example, the degree of shear stress is different, levels of shear will vary during the phases of the cardiac cycle and exercise and are higher in arteries than veins and is accentuated at sites just distal to bifurcations in vessels. Shear appears to play a particularly important role because it stimulates the release of vasoactive proteins and changes gene expression and thus cell phenotype (Davies, 1995). This is illustrated by the increased presence of atherosclerotic lesions at branch points of the arterial tree where there is flow reversal and low shear stresses. These endothelial cells demonstrate increased lipoprotein uptake, upregulation of leukocyte adhesion molecules and secretion of growth and chemotactic factors causing monocyte/macrophage and smooth muscle cell proliferation (Ku et al., 1985, Mondy et al., 1997).

A second mechanism that contributes to the formation of tissue-specific phenotypes is signalling pathways specific to cell subtypes. For example, in the heart, only some of the microvascular endothelial cells in the myocardium express the gene for vWF. This is dictated by the presence of different receptors for platelet-derived growth factor (PDGF) AB heterodimers; some have the appropriate receptors and can transduce the signal and produce vWF, while others cannot (Edelberg et al., 1998). The PDGF is produced by underlying myocytes. Thus, the range of responses of the endothelial cell is shaped by the extracellular milieu and the ability to transduce the local signals.

A final mechanism is found at the level of transcription. It seems that some endothelial cell genes are regulated by different pathways in different regions of the vascular tree. Returning to vWF again, studies in transgenic mice have shown that a short region of the vWF promoter directed expression of vWF exclusively in the brain. However, a promoter that contained additional DNA elements up- and downstream directed expression in the heart and skeletal muscles (Aird et al., 1997). Further studies showed that this level of transcription control was due to microenvironmental factors and led to these genes being expressed by brain or lung tissues.

In conclusion, there appears to be cross-talk between local environment and endothelium that operates at varying levels from molecular to cellular.

REFERENCES

Aird, W.C., Jahroudi, N., Weiler-Guettler, H. et al. (1995). Human von Willebrand factor gene sequences target expression to a subpopulation of endothelial cells in transgenic mice. *Proc. Natl Acad. Sci. U.S.A.*, **92**, 4567–71.

Aird, W.C., Edelberg, J.M., Weiler-Guettler, H. et al. (1997). Vascular bed-specific expression of an endothelial cell gene is programmed by the tissue microenvironment. *J. Cell Biol.*, **138**, 117–24.

Ambrosia, G., Zweier, J., Jacobus, W.E. et al. (1987). Improvement of postischaemic myocardial function and metabolism induced by administration of desferroxamine at the time of reflow: the role of iron in the pathogenesis of reperfusion injury. *Circulation*, **76**, 906–15.

Arai, H., Nakao, K., Takaya, K. et al. (1993). The human endothelin-B receptor gene: structural organisation and chromosomal assignment. *J. Biol. Chem.*, **268**, 3463–70.

Bach, F.H., Robson, S.C., Ferran, C. et al. (1994). Endothelial cell activation and thromboregulation during xenograft rejection. *Immunol. Rev.*, **141**, 5–30.

Bach, F.H., Robson, S.C., Winkler, H. et al. (1995). Barriers to xenotransplantation. *Nat. Med.*, **1**, 869–73.

Bahnak, B.R., Wu, Q.Y., Coulonbel, L. et al. (1989). Expression of von Willebrand factor in porcine vessels: heterogeneity at the level of von Willebrand factor mRNA. *J. Cell Physiol.*, **138**, 305–10.

Baldwin, A.S. (1996). The NF-κB and IκB proteins: New discoveries and insights. *Ann. Rev. Immunol.*, **14**, 649–81.

Barnes, K., Brown, C. & Turner, A.J. (1998). Endothelin-converting enzyme: ultrastructural localisation and its recycling from the cell surface. *Hypertension*, **31**, 3–9.

Berckmans, R.J., Nieuwland, R., Boing, A.N. et al. (2001). Cell-derived microparticles circulate in healthy humans and support low grade thrombin generation. *Thromb. Haemost.*, **85**, 639–46.

Bevilacqua, M.P. & Nelson, R.M. (1993). Selectins. *J. Clin. Invest.*, **91**, 379–87.

Boermeester, M.A., van Leewen, P.A.M., Coyle, S.M. et al. (1995). IL-1 blockade attenuates mediator release and dysregulation of the haemostatic mechanism during human sepsis. *Arch. Surg.*, **130**, 739–48.

Bonfani, R., Furie, B.C., Furie, B. & Wagner, D.D. (1989). PADGEM (GMP-140) is a component of Weibel-Palade bodies of human endothelial cells. *Blood*, **73**, 1109–12.

Cochrane, C.G. & Koffler, D. (1973). Immune complex disease in experimental animals and men. *Adv. Immunol.*, **16**, 185.

Cohen, R.A. (1995). The role of nitric oxide and other endothelium derived vasoactive substances in vascular disease. *Prog. Cardiovasc. Dis.*, **XXXVIII**, 105–28.

Collins, T., Palmer, H.J., Whitley, M.Z., Neish, A.S. & Williams, A.J. (1993). A common theme in endothelial activation – insights from the structural analysis of the genes for E-selectin and VCAM-1. *Trends Cardiovasc. Med.*, **3**, 92–7.

Cophen, M.V. & Downey, J.M. (1993). Ischaemic preconditioning: can the protection be bottled? *Lancet*, **342**, 6.

Creasey, A.A., Chang, A.C.K., Feigen, L. et al. (1993). Tissue factor pathway inhibitor reduces mortality from *E. Coli* septic shock. *J. Clin. Invest.*, **91**, 2850–60.

Davies, P. (1995). Flow-mediated endothelial mechanotransduction. *Physiol. Rev.*, **75**, 519–60.

Davies, M.G., Fulton, G.J. & Hagen, P.O. (1995). Clinical biology of nitric oxide. *Br. J. Surg.*, **82**, 1598–1610.

Denault, J.-B., Claing, A., D'Orleans-Juste, P. et al. (1995). Processing of proendothelin-1 by human furin convertase. *FEBS Lett.*, **362**, 276–80.

Dinarello, C.A., Gelfand, J.A. & Wolff, S.M. (1993). Anticytokine strategies in the treatment of the systemic inflammatory response syndrome. *J.A.M.A.*, **269**, 1829–35.

Drake, T.A., Morissey, J.H. & Edgington, T.S. (1989). Selective cellular expression of tissue factor in human tissues. Implications for disorders of haemostasis and thrombosis. *Am. J. Pathol.*, **134**, 1087–97.

Edelberg, J.M., Aird, W.C., Wu, W. et al. (1998). PDGF mediates cardiac microvascular communication. *J. Clin. Invest.*, **102**, 837–43.

Esmon, C.T. & Owen, W.G. (1981). Identification of an endothelial cell cofactor for the thrombin-catalysed activation of protein C. *Proc. Natl Acad. Sci.*, **78**, 2249–54.

Faller, D.V. (1999). Endothelial cell responses to hypoxic stress. *Clin. Exp. Pharmacol. Physiol.*, **26**, 74–84.

Fourier, F., Chopin, F.C., Huart, J.J. et al. (1993). Double-blind placebo controlled trial of antithrombin III concentrates in septic shock with disseminated intravascular coagulation. *Chest*, **104**, 882–8.

Fournie, G.J. (1988). Circulating DNA and lupus nephritis. *Kidney Int.*, **33**, 487–97.

Gando, S., Nakanishi, Y. & Tedo, I. (1995). Cytokines and plasminogen activator inhibitor-1 in post-trauma disseminated intravascular coagulation: relationship to multiple organ dysfunction syndrome. *Crit. Care Med.*, **23**, 1835–42.

Gocke, D.J., Hsu, K., Morgan, C. et al. (1970). Association between polyarteritis and Australian antigen. *Lancet*, **2**, 1149–53.

Goldberg, M.A. & Schneider, T.J. (1994). Similarities between the oxygen-sensing mechanisms regulating the expression of vascular endothelial growth factor and erythropoietin. *J. Biol. Chem.*, **269**, 4355–9.

Gomez-Garre, D., Guerra, M., Gonzalez, E. et al. (1992). Aggregation of human polymorphonuclear leucocytes by endothelin: role of platelet activating factor. *Eur. J. Pharmacol.*, **224**, 167–72.

Gonzalez-Amaro, R., Diaz-Gonzalez, F. & Sanchez-Madrid, F. (1998). Adhesion molecules in inflammatory diseases. *Drugs*, **56**, 977–88.

Grace, P.A. (1994). Ischaemia–reperfusion injury. *Br. J. Surg.*, **81**, 637–47.

Graven, K.K., Zimmerman, L.H., Dickson, E.W., Weinhouse, G.L. & Farber, H.W. (1993). Endothelial cell hypoxia associated proteins are cell and stress specific. *J. Cell. Physiol.*, **157**, 544–54.

Hamblin, T.J. (1990). Endothelins. *Br. Med. J.*, **301**, 568.

Henkel, T., Machleidt, T., Alkalay, I. et al. (1993). Rapid proteolysis of IκB is necessary for activation of transcription factor NF-κB. *Nature*, **365**, 182.

Hermans, P.W., Hibberd, M.L., Booy, R. et al. (1999). 4G/5G promoter polymorphisms in the plasminogen-activator-inhibitor-1 gene and outcome of meningococcal disease. *Lancet*, **354**, 556–60.

Hogg, N., Bates, P.A. & Harvey, J. (1991). Structure and function of intercellular adhesion molecule-1. Integrins and ICAM-1. In: *Immune Responses*, vol. 50, ed. Hogg, N., pp. 98–115. Basel: Karger.

Hosoda, K., Nakao, K., Tamura, H. et al. (1992). Organisation, structure, chromosomal assignment, and expression of the gene encoding the human endothelin-A receptor. *J. Biol. Chem.*, **267**, 18797–804.

Ihrcke, N.S., Wrenshall, L.E., Lindman, B.J. & Platt, J.L. (1996). Role of heparan sulphate in immune system–blood vessel interactions. *Immunol. Today*, **14**, 500–5.

Ishii, H., Salem, H.H., Bell, C.E. et al. (1986). Thrombomodulin, an endothelial anticoagulant protein, is absent from the human brain. *Blood*, **67**, 362–7.

Israels S.J., Gerrard, J.M., Jacques, Y.V. et al. (1992). Platelet dense granule membranes contain both granulophisin and P-selectin (GMP-140). *Blood*, **80**, 143–50.

Jaffer, F.E., Knauss, T.C., Poptic, E. et al. (1990). Endothelin stimulates PDGF secretion in cultured human mesangial cells. *Kidney Int.*, **38**, 1193–8.

Karmazyn, M., Mailer, K. & Curie, R.W. (1990). Acquisition and decay of heat-shock enhanced postischaemic ventricular recovery. *Am. J. Physiol.*, **259**, 424–31.

Keaney, J.F., Puyana, J.-C., Francis, S. et al. (1994). Methylene blue reverses endotoxin-induced hypotension. *Circ. Res.*, **74**, 1121–5.

Kishimoto, T.K., Jutila, M.A., Berg, E.L. & Butcher, E.C. (1989). Neutrophil Mac-1 and MEL-14 adhesion proteins inversely regulated by chemotactic factors. *Science*, **245**, 1238–41.

Kniker, W. & Cochrane, C.G. (1965). Pathogenic factors in vascular lesions of experimental serum sickness. *J. Exp. Med.*, **122**, 83–98.

Kopp, E. & Ghosh, S. (1944). Inhibition of NF-κB by sodium salicylate and aspirin. *Science*, **265**, 956–9.

Kourembanas, S., Hannan, R.L. & Faller, D.V. (1990). Oxygen tension regulates the expression of the platelet-derived growth factor-B chain gene in human endothelial cells. *J. Clin. Invest.*, **86**, 670–4.

Ku, D.N., Giddens, D.P., Zarins, C.K. & Glagov, S. (1985). Pulsatile flow and atherosclerosis in the human carotid bifurcation: positive correlation between plaque location and low oscillating shear stress. *Arteriosclerosis*, **5**, 293–302.

Levi, M., ten Cate, H., Bauer, K. et al. (1994). Inhibition of endotoxin-induced activation of coagulation and fibrinolysis by pentoxifylline or by monoclonal anti-tissue factor antibody in chimpanzees. *J. Clin. Invest.*, **93**, 114–20.

Lindquist, S. (1986). The heat-shock response. *Annu. Rev. Biochem.*, **55**, 1151–91.

Lopez-Farre, A., Riesco, A., Espinosa, G. et al. (1993). Effect of endothelin on neutrophil adhesion to endothelial cells and perfused heart. *Circulation*, **88**, 1166–71.

Mantovani, A. & Dejana, E. (1989). Cytokines as communication signals between leucocytes and endothelial cells. *Immunol. Today*, **10**, 370–5.

Marber, M.S., Latchman, D.S., Walker, J.M. & Yellon, D.M. (1993). Cardiac stress protein elevation 24 hours after brief ischaemia or heat stress is associated with resistance to myocardial infarction. *Circulation*, **88**, 1264–72.

Marcus, A.J. (1994). Thrombosis and inflammation as multicellular processes: significance of cell–cell interaction. *Semin. Hematol.*, **31**, 261–9.

Marx, J. (1995). How the glucocorticoids suppress immunity. *Science*, **270**, 232–3.

Maxfield, S.R., Moulder, K., Koning, F. et al. (1989). Murine T-cells express a cell-surface receptor for multiple extracellular-matrix proteins – identification and characterisation with monoclonal antibodies. *J. Exp. Med.*, **169**, 2173–90.

McCarron, R.M., Wang, L., Stanimirovic, D.B. et al. (1993). Endothelin induction of adhesion molecule expression on human brain microvascular endothelial cells. *Neurosci Lett.*, **156**, 31–4.

McMillen, M.A. & Sumpio, B.E. (1995). Endothelins: polyfunctional cytokines. *J. Am. Coll. Surg.*, **180**, 621–37.

Meroni, P., Khamashta, M.A., Younou, P. & Shoenfield, Y. (1995). Mosaic of anti-endothelial cell antibodies. Review of the first international workshop on antiendothelial cell antibodies, clinical and pathological significance. *Lupus*, **4**, 95–9.

Minchenko, A., Bauer, T., Salceda, S. & Caro, J. (1994). Hypoxic stimulation of vascular endothelial growth factor expression in vitro and in vivo. *Lab. Invest.*, **71**, 374–9.

Mondy, J.S., Linder, V., Miyashiro, J.K. et al. (1997). Platelet derived growth factor ligand and receptor expression in response to altered blood flow in vitro. *Circ. Res.*, **81**, 320–7.

Moore, K.L., Esmon, C.T. & Esmon, C.L. (1989). TNF leads to the internalization and degradation of thrombomodulin from the surface of bovine endothelial cells in culture. *Blood*, **73**, 159–65.

Nava, E., Palmer, R.M.J. & Moncada, S. (1992). The role of nitric oxide in endotoxic shock. *J. Cardiovasc. Pharmacol.*, **20**, 5132–4.

Nusinow, S.R., Federeci, A.D., Zimmerman, T.S. & Curd, J.G. (1984). Increased von Willebrand factor antigen in the plasma of patients with vasculitis. *Arthritis Rheum.*, **27**, 1405–10.

Osborn, L., Hession, C., Tizzard, R. et al. (1989). Direct expression of vascular cell adhesion molecule 1, a cytokine-induced endothelial protein that binds to lymphocytes. *Cell*, **59**, 1203–11.

Petro, A., Bennet, D. & Vallance, P. (1991). Effect of nitric oxide synthase inhibitors on hypotension in patients with septic shock. *Lancet*, **338**, 1557–8.

Phelan, M.W. & Faller, D.V. (1996). Hypoxia decreases constitutive nitric oxide synthase transcript and protein in cultured endothelial cells. *J. Cell. Physiol.*, **167**, 469–76.

Plow, E.F. & Ginsberg, M.H. (1989). Cellular adhesion: GPIIb/IIIa as a prototypic adhesion receptor. *Prog. Haemostas. Thromb.*, **9**, 117–56.

Pober, J.S. (1988). Cytokine-mediated activation of vascular endothelium. *Am. J. Pathol.*, **133**, 426–33.

Pober, J.S. & Cotran, R.S. (1991). The role of endothelial cells in inflammation. *Transplantation*, **50**, 536–44.

Pober, J.S., Gimbrone, M.J., Lapierre, L.A. et al. (1986). Overlapping patterns of activation of human endothelial cells by interleukin 1, tumor necrosis factor, and immune interferon. *J. Immunol.*, **137**, 1893–6.

Pober, J.S. & Orosz, C.G., Rose, M.L. & Savage, C.O. (1996). Can graft endothelial cells initiate a host antigraft immune response? *Transplantation*, **61**, 343–9.

Rangel-Frauso, M.S., Pittet, D., Costigan, M. et al. (1995). The natural history of the systemic inflammatory response syndrome. *J.A.M.A.*, **273**, 117–23.

Rapaport, S.I. (1991). The extrinsic pathway inhibitor: a regulator of tissue factor-dependent blood coagulation. *Thromb. Haemost.*, **66**, 6–15.

Rosen, S.D. & Bertozzi, C.R. (1994). The selectins and their ligands. *Curr. Opin. Cell Biol.*, **6**, 663–73.

Russell, F.D., Skepper, J.N. & Davenport, A.P. (1997). Detection of endothelin receptors in human coronary artery vascular smooth muscle cells but not endothelial cells by using electron microscope autoradiography. *J. Cardiovasc. Pharmacol.*, **29**, 820–6.

Sanches-Madrid, F., Nagy, J.A., Robbins, E., Simon, P. & Springer, T.A. (1983). A human leukocyte differentiation antigen family with distinct α subunits and common β subunit. *J. Exp. Med.*, **158**, 1785–803.

Sandset, P.M., Abildgaard, U. & Larsen, M.L. (1988). Heparin induces release of extrinsic pathway inhibitor (EPI). *Br. J. Haematol.*, **72**, 391–6.

Schiffrin, E.L. (1995). Endothelin: potential role in hypertension and vascular hypertrophy. Brief review. *Hypertension*, **25**, 1135–43.

Schiffrin, E.L. & Touyz, R.M. (1998). Vascular biology of endothelin. *J. Cardiovasc. Pharmacol.*, **32**, S2–13.

Schleef, R.R., Bevilacqua, M.P., Sawdey, M. et al. (1988). Cytokine activation of vascular endothelium: effects on tissue type plasminogen activator and type one plasminogen activator inhibitor. *J. Biol. Chem.*, **263**, 5797–803.

Schmedtje, Jr, J.F., Ji, Y.-S., Liu, W.L., Dubois, R.N. & Runge, M.S. (1997). Hypoxia induces cyclooxygenase-2 via the NF-κB p65 transcription factor in human vascular endothelial cells. *J. Biol. Chem.*, **272**, 601–8.

Schur, P.H. & Sandson, J. (1968). Immunological factors and clinical activity in systemic lupus erythematosus. *N. Engl. J. Med.*, **278**, 533–8.

Shusterman, M. & London, W.T. (1984). Hepatitis B and immune complex disease. *N. Engl. J. Med.*, **310**, 43–5.

Stein, I., Neeman, M., Shweiki, D., Itin, A. & Keshet, E. (1995). Stabilisation of vascular endothelial growth factor mRNA by hypoxia and hypoglycaemia and coregulation with other ischaemia-induced genes. *Mol. Cell Biol.*, **15**, 5363–8.

Stein, J.V., Cheng, G., Stockton, B.M. et al. (1999). L-selectin-mediated leukocyte adhesion in vivo: microvillous distribution determines tethering efficiency, but not rolling velocity. *J. Exp. Med.*, **189**, 37–49.

Suffredini, A.F., Harpel, P.C. & Parillo, J.E. (1989). Promotion and subsequent inhibition of plasminogen activation after administration of intravenous endotoxin to normal subjects. *N. Engl. J. Med.*, **320**, 1165–72.

Tann, E.M. & Kunkel, H.G. (1966). An immunofluorescent study of skin lesions in systemic lupus erythematosus. *Arthritis Rheum.*, **9**, 37–46.

Taylor, F.B., Chang, A., Esmon, C.T. et al. (1987). Protein C prevents the coagulopathic and lethal effects of *E. Coli* infusion in the baboon. *J. Clin. Invest.*, **79**, 918–25.

van Deventer, S.J.H., Buller, H.R. & ten Cate, J.W. (1990). Experimental endotoxaemia in humans: analysis of cytokine release and coagulation, fibrinolytic and complement pathways. *Blood*, **76**, 2520–6.

Van Zee, K.J., DeForge, L.E., Fischer, E. et al. (1991). IL-8 in septic shock, endotoxaemia and after IL-8 administration. *J. Immunol.*, **146**, 3478–82.

Voelkel, N.F. & Tudor, R.M. (1995). Cellular and molecular mechanisms in the pathogenesis of severe pulmonary hypertension. *Eur. Respir. J.*, **8**, 2129–38.

Wagner, D.D. (1990). Cell biology of von Willebrand factor. *Annu. Rev. Cell Biol.*, **6**, 217–46.

Watanabe, T., Suzuki, N., Shimamoto, N. et al. (1991). Contribution of endogenous endothelin to the extension of myocardial infarct size in rats. *Circ. Res.*, **69**, 370–7.

Weiler-Guettler, H., Christie, P.D., Beeler, D.L. et al. (1998). A targeted point mutation in thrombomodulin generates viable mice with a prethrombotic state. *J. Clin. Invest.*, **101**, 1983–91.

Westendorp, R.G., Hottenga, J.J. & Slagboom, P.E. (1999). Variation in plasminogen-activator-inhibtor-1 gene and risk of meningococcal septic shock. *Lancet*, **354**, 561–3.

Willms-Kretschmer, K., Flax, M.H. & Cotran, R.S. (1967). The fine structure of the vascular response in hapten-specific delayed hypersensitivity and contact dermatitis. *Lab. Invest.*, **17**, 334–49.

Xin, X., Cai, Y., Matsumoto, K. et al. (1995). Endothelium induced interleukin-6 production by rat aortic endothelial cells. *Endocrinology*, **136**, 132–7.

Yanagisawa, M., Kurihara, H., Kimura, S. et al. (1988). A novel potent vasoconstrictor peptide produced by vascular endothelial cells. *Nature*, **332**, 411–15.

10

Nitric oxide

Norman Chan and Patrick Vallance

Rayne Institute, University College London, London

Introduction

Since the discovery of endothelial-derived nitric oxide (NO) as a potent vasodilator, NO has been implicated in a variety of biological roles. This chapter aims to
provide a general overview of the role of NO in normal physiology of the
vasculature as well as pathophysiology in disease states.

From EDRF to nitric oxide

In 1980, Furchgott and Zawadzki demonstrated that the presence of vascular
endothelial cells is essential for acetylcholine (ACh) to induce relaxation of
isolated rabbit aorta. If the vascular endothelium is injured or mechanically
removed, the blood vessel fails to relax to ACh but still responds to glyceryl
trinitrate (GTN). This endothelial-dependent relaxation of vascular smooth
muscle to ACh is mediated by a humoral factor, initially named endothelium-
derived relaxing factor (EDRF; Furchgott and Zawadzki, 1980). The exact biochemical identity of EDRF was the focus of intense research and in 1986 Furchgott
and Ignarro independently suggested that NO might account for the biological
properties of EDRF (Furchgott, 1988; Ignarro et al., 1988). This was confirmed a
year later (Ignarro et al., 1987; Palmer et al., 1987).

The L-arginine–nitric oxide pathway

Endothelium-derived NO is synthesized from one of the guanidine-nitrogen
atoms of the amino acid L-arginine by the endothelial isoform of NO synthase,
yielding L-citrulline as a byproduct (Palmer et al., 1988; Schmidt et al., 1988). NO
is labile and has a short half–life (10–60 s; Knowles and Moncada, 1992). It is
rapidly oxidized to nitrite and then nitrate by oxygenated haemoglobin, molecular
oxygen and superoxide anions before being excreted into the urine (Wennmalm et

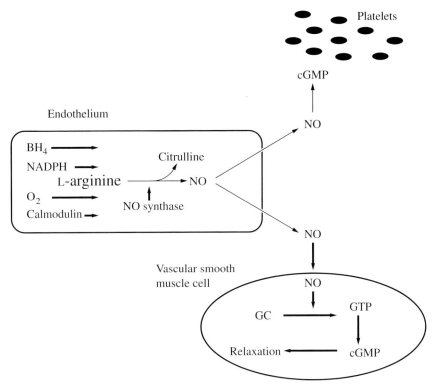

Figure 10.1   The L-arginine–nitric oxide (NO) pathway. BH_4, tetrahydrobiopterin; NADPH, nicotinamide-adenine dinucleotide phosphate; cGMP, cyclic guanosine 3,5-monophosphate; GC, guanylate cyclase; GTP, guanosine triphosphate.

al., 1992; Moncada and Higgs, 1993). The biosynthesis of NO from L-arginine requires several cofactors, including nicotinamide-adenine dinucleotide phosphate (NADPH), flavin mononucleotide, flavin adenine dinucleotide, tetrahydrobiopterin (BH_4), calmodulin and oxygen (Bredt and Snyder, 1990; Lewis et al., 1993; Moncada and Higgs, 1995). Endothelium-derived NO then diffuses across the endothelial cell membrane and enters the vascular smooth muscle cells (VSMC) where it activates guanylate cyclase (GC) leading to an increase in intracellular cyclic guanosine-3',5-monophosphate (cGMP) levels (Figure 10.1; Gruetter et al., 1981; Ignarro et al., 1984; Luscher and Vanhoutte, 1989; Moncada and Higgs, 1993). As a secondary messenger, cGMP mediates many of the biological effects of NO including the control of vascular tone and blood pressure, platelet activation and neurotransmission. In addition, NO has other molecular targets which include haem proteins, DNA and thiols. These effects may mediate changes in functions of certain enzymes or channels. NO may also interact with some enzymes of the respiratory chain including complex I and II, and aconitase (Radi et al., 1994), and exert an effect on tissue mitochondrial respiration through

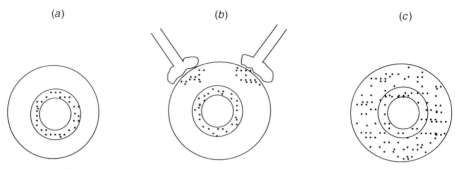

Figure 10.2 (*a*) In most, if not all, vessels nitric oxide (NO) is synthesized within the endothelium. (*b*) In certain vessels (e.g. cerebral vessels) NO is also synthesized by nerves in the adventitia (nitrogenic nerves). (*c*) After exposure to endotoxin or cytokines, inducible nitric oxide synthase (iNOS) is expressed throughout the vessel wall and produces large amounts of NO.

these mechanisms. Interaction of NO with superoxide anion can attenuate physio-logical responses mediated by NO (Gryglewski et al., 1986) and can produce irreversible inhibitory effects on mitochondrial function as a result of peroxynit-rite (ONOO⁻) formation (Castro et al., 1994; Wolin, 1996).

Nitric oxide synthase isoforms: expression and regulation

Three isoforms of nitric oxide synthase (NOS) have been identified, the en-dothelial isoform (eNOS), neuronal isoform (nNOS) and macrophage or in-ducible isoform (iNOS; Forstermann et al., 1994). All three NOS isoforms play distinct roles in the regulation of vascular tone. eNOS and nNOS are constituents of healthy cells (Figure. 10.2). The genes encoding eNOS and nNOS are located on chromosome 7 and 12 respectively. The levels of eNOS and nNOS expression and activity are tightly regulated and may be induced under different physiological conditions (e.g. shear stress or nerve injury). Inducible NOS is encoded by a gene located on chromosome 17 (Xu et al., 1994). Under normal physiological condi-tions, iNOS is not expressed in vascular cells and its expression is seen mainly in conditions of acute infection or inflammation. To classify iNOS as 'nonconstitu-tive' is not strictly correct since it is also expressed constitutively in certain epithelial cells (Guo et al., 1995). Similarly, it is clear that the 'constitutive' isoforms are transcriptionally regulated and may be induced.

Regulation by calcium and calmodulin

eNOS isoform is activated by elevation of intracellular calcium and the subsequent binding of calcium/calmodulin. This process can be induced by several substances, including ACh, bradykinin, substance P, thrombin and adenosine 5'-triphosphate, all of which may lead to an increase in intracellular free calcium in endothelial cells (Furchgott and Vanhoutte, 1987; Moncada, 1992). In contrast, iNOS is irreversibly bound to calcium/calmodulin and its activation is largely independent of calcium.

Caveolae

The simplistic calcium/calmodulin-dependent, eNOS-mediated signalling mechanism has been refined following the discovery that eNOS is located in specialized cell surface signal-transducing domains termed plasmalemmal caveolae (Feron et al., 1996; Shaul et al., 1996). Caveolae are cholesterol-rich and have a rigid structure. They produce a microenvironment for eNOS and other transporter localization such as cationic amino acid transporter 1 (CAT1). The colocalization of these transporters forms a caveolar complex which facilitates the uptake of arginine in the formation of NO (McDonald et al., 1997). Caveolin, the principal transmembrane protein in caveolae, may interact with eNOS, resulting in enzyme inhibition, a reversible process modulated by calcium/calmodulin (Michel et al., 1997).

Acylation

The targeting of eNOS to caveolae involves acylation by saturated fatty acids myristate (myristoylation) and palmitate (palmitoylation). Myristoylation of eNOS is irreversible whereas eNOS palmitoylation is reversible and the enzymes involved in these processes remain unidentified. Agonists such as bradykinin promote eNOS depalmitoylation, thus stimulating NO production by the endothelium (Robinson and Michel, 1995). Upon formation of eNOS–caveolin heteromeric complex, it may undergo cycles of dissociation and reassociation modulated by calcium-mobilizing agonists such as calcium ionophore A23187 and muscarinic agonists such as carbachol (Feron et al., 1998). Alteration of this cycle directly affects the NO-dependent signalling in the vascular wall. While mechanisms for eNOS targeting of caveolae are fairly well established, it remains unclear whether nNOS and iNOS targeting also occurs.

Phosphorylation

Endothelial NO production is also regulated by phosphorylation of eNOS with various protein kinases, including protein kinase A, protein kinase B (Akt), protein kinase C and calmodulin kinase. This process is independent of intracellular calcium concentrations. Several amino acid residues (for example, serine, threonine and tyrosine) are involved in the phosphorylation of eNOS (Michel et al., 1993; Garcia-Cardena et al., 1996; Fleming et al., 1998). The effect of phosphorylation on eNOS activity depends on the specific residue phosphorylated and

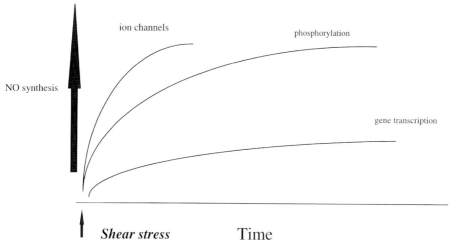

Figure 10.3   Mechanisms of different time course through which shear stress induces nitric oxide (NO) generation.

the binding domain. While the Akt-mediated serine phosphorylation of eNOS increases enzyme activity (Dimmeler et al., 1999), phosphorylation of serine (741) in the calcium/calmodulin domain of nNOS prevents the binding of calmodulin and decreases enzyme activity (Zoche et al., 1997).

Regulation by shear stress

Haemodynamic shear stress exerted by the viscous drag of flowing blood is an important physiological stimulus in the regulation of NO release from the endothelial cells (Davies, 1995). The mechanism of shear stress-induced NO release is complex, involving an extremely rapid initiation via ion channel activation and subsequent upstream events related to signalling pathway activation, such as phosphorylation and eNOS transcription (Figure 10.3). These complex events allow rapid and short-lasting as well as slow-onset and sustained vasodilatation which is important in maintaining vascular tone. A more detailed analysis of flow-mediated events is provided in Chapter 3, but a short summary will now be given.

Ultraquick: ion channels

Numerous in vitro studies provided strong evidence that ion channels, including certain calcium, potassium and chloride ion channels, are involved in the mechanotransduction by the vascular endothelium seconds after exposure to haemodynamic shear stress (Resnick et al., 2000). Application of shear stress to bovine aortic endothelial cells by fluid perfusion led to an immediate marked increase in intracellular free calcium within 1 min followed by a rapid decline (Ando et al., 1988). Notably, the increase in intracellular calcium occurs only in response to pulsatile flow and not to steady flow (Helmlinger et al., 1995) and is independent of flow rate (Ando et al., 1993). The detection of potassium-selective current with whole cell patch-clamp recordings of arterial endothelial cells suggests activation of a distinct potassium channel in response to shear stress. This stress-activated current desensitizes slowly and recovers rapidly and fully on flow cessation (Olesen et al., 1988). Recently, a flow-activated chloride-selective membrane current in vascular endothelial cell was demonstrated which is distinct from the potassium current (Barakat et al., 1999). The balance between anionic and cationic current determines the net membrane potential and the subsequent change in calcium that alters NO output.

Quick: phosphorylation

Mechanical activation of eNOS as induced by shear stress also occurs via phosphorylation and the effect is independent of intracellular calcium concentrations (Kuchan & Frangos, 1994; Ayajiki et al., 1996; Corson et al., 1996; Fleming et al., 1998). It has been shown that, in response to shear stress, the serine/threonine protein kinase B (Akt) directly phosphorylates eNOS and activates eNOS (Dimmeler et al., 1999; Fulton et al., 1999; Fisslthaler et al., 2000) with a maximal increase up to sixfold after 1 h of exposure to shear stress (Dimmeler et al., 1999). The stimulation of Akt phosphorylation by shear stress appears to be mediated by phosphoinositide 3-OH kinase (Dimmeler et al., 1999).

Slow: increased transcription

Shear stress also stimulates eNOS gene transcription to maintain long-term NO production (Resnick et al., 2000). Application of shear stress for 3 h resulted in an induction of eNOS mRNA in a dose-dependent manner in both bovine and human aortic endothelial cells. This increase in eNOS mRNA is prevented by incubation with a potassium channel antagonist (Uematsu et al., 1995). Furthermore, exposure of endothelium to laminar shear stress induces the expression of transforming growth factor β_1 also modulated by potassium channel currents (Ohno et al., 1995).

These in vitro experimental data demonstrated the complexity of short, medium and long-term regulation of NO release in response to shear stress.

Agonist activation of eNOS

In addition to shear stress, activation of eNOS can be induced by hormones (such as catecholamines, vasopressin, oestrogen), autacids (such as bradykinin and histamine) and platelet-derived mediators (such as serotonin and adenine diphosphate). Specific receptors for these stimuli mediate eNOS activation through coupling with G proteins (e.g. serotonin receptors; Boulanger and Vanhoutte, 1997). Inhibition of eNOS activities may also be induced by the association of eNOS with caveolin-1 and caveolin-3 in endothelial cells and myocytes respectively (Garcia-Cardena et al., 1997). This negative effect on eNOS activities may be a result of interference with calcium/calmodulin binding and electron transfer (Ghosh et al., 1998). Thus the balance between activation and inhibition mechanisms mediated by various receptors and caveolin regulates eNOS activity.

Genetic variation in NOS isoforms

The genetic sequence and chromosomal location for each of the NOS isoforms in human have been identified (Wang and Marsden, 1995). There is significant genetic sequence variation for eNOS between individuals (Nadaud et al., 1994; Wang et al., 1996; Markus et al., 1998; Miyamoto et al., 1998; Hingorani et al., 1999). Recently, it has been shown that one eNOS gene polymorphism involves a point mutation (G $\rightarrow$ T subsitution) in exon 7 of the gene which predicts an amino acid substitution, glutamic acid $\rightarrow$ aspartic acid at residue 298 of the mature protein (Yoshimura et al., 1998; Hingorani et al., 1999). The Asp/Asp protein is more susceptible to proteolytic degradation. In some studies, this mutation has been associated with essential hypertension (Miyamoto et al., 1998), coronary artery disease (Cai et al., 1999; Hingorani et al., 1999; Liao et al., 1999) and acute myocardial infarction (Hibi et al., 1998; Shimasaki et al., 1998) but further studies are needed. Additional genetic polymorphism involving mutations in the 5'-flanking region of the eNOS gene (T-786 $\rightarrow$ C) has been demonstrated and appears more prevalent in Japanese patients with coronary spasm. This mutation results in a significant reduction in eNOS gene promotor activity leading to reduced eNOS expression, at least in vitro (Nakayama et al., 1999). Polymorphism of the variable number of tandem repeats (VNTR) in intron 4 of the eNOS gene was found to contribute to variation in fasting plasma levels of NO in healthy human subjects and with a variety of cardiovascular diseases (Wang et al., 1997). However, its functional significance is uncertain since in itself it should not affect eNOS expression or activity.

Biological effects of NO on the vasculature

Endothelium-derived NO is a very potent vasodilator in the vasculature and the balance between NO and various endothelium-derived vasoconstrictors (such as endothelin) and the effects of the sympathetic nervous system maintains the blood vessel tone. In addition, NO has antiatherogenic properties including suppression of platelet aggregation, leukocyte migration and cellular adhesion to the endothelium (Radomski et al., 1987, 1990; Bath et al., 1991; Kubes et al., 1991; Bode-Boger et al., 1994) and inhibition of VSMC mitogenesis, proliferation (Garg and Hassid, 1989; Nakaki et al., 1990; Scott-Burden and Vanhoutte, 1993) and migration (Sarkar et al., 1996). Furthermore, NO inhibits the activation and expression of certain adhesion molecules (De Caterina et al., 1995; Biffl et al., 1996; Khan et al., 1996; Takahashi et al., 1996), production of superoxide anion (Clancy et al., 1992) and oxidation of low-density lipoprotein (LDL) (Hogg et al., 1993). Loss of endothelium-derived NO would be expected to promote a vascular phenotype more prone to atherogenesis, a concept supported by studies in experimental animals (Carvalho et al., 1987; Chataigneau et al., 1999).

Nitric oxide release from the vascular endothelium

There is a continuous basal release of NO from the vascular endothelium to maintain the resting vascular tone. A number of chemical and physical stimuli may activate eNOS which leads to increased NO production contributing to the control and regulation of the vascular tone (Busse et al., 1993).

Basal nitric oxide release

The synthesis of NO in vascular endothelial cells in culture and in fresh vascular tissue can be inhibited by N^G-monomethyl-L-arginine (L-NMMA), an analogue of L-arginine in which one of the guanidino nitrogen atoms is methylated (Palmer et al., 1988). This inhibitory effect of L-NMMA is readily reversed by L-arginine and the inactive stereoisomer (D-NMMA) has no effect on the L-arginine – NO pathway (Vallance et al., 1989a). This NOS-inhibitor has been used to examine the role of NO in various vascular beds in vitro and in vivo in both human and animal models.

In rings of rabbit aorta, L-NMMA causes significant endothelium-dependent contraction (Rees et al., 1989a). Intravenous infusion of L-NMMA induced a dose-related increase in blood pressure which is reversed by intravenous administration of L-arginine in guinea pigs (Aisaka et al., 1989), rats (Whittle et al., 1989) and rabbits (Rees et al., 1989a). These in vitro and in vivo data suggest a pivotal role of basal NO synthesis in maintaining vascular tone.

In the human forearm vasculature, infusion of L-NMMA via the brachial artery causes substantial dose-dependent vasoconstriction, indicating that continuous generation of NO is crucial in maintaining peripheral vasodilatation (Figure 10.4; Vallance et al., 1989a). Basal NO production also occurs in every other vascular bed studied, including cerebral (White et al., 1997), pulmonary (Stamler et al., 1994), renal (Haynes et al., 1993) and coronary arteries (Lefroy et al., 1993).

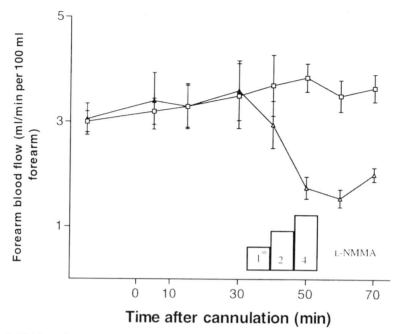

Figure 10.4   Inhibition of endogenous nitric oxide NO by L-N^G-monomethyl-L-arginine (L-NMMA) produced a dose-dependent reduction in forearm blood flow.

In the venous system, however, inhibitors of NOS do not lead to an increase in basal tone in a variety of venous preparations from animals (Ekelund and Mellander, 1990; Martin et al., 1992). Identical findings have also been shown in humans (Vallance et al., 1989b; Yang et al., 1991), suggesting that basal NO production does not have a major role in the maintenance of the resting tone in most veins.

Agonist-stimulated NO release

Many chemical substances, such as ACh, bradykinin, serotonin and substance P, are able to induce endothelium-dependent vasodilatation in experimental settings. In rings of rabbit aorta, endothelium-dependent relaxation induced by ACh, calcium ionophore A23187 or substance P is inhibited by L-NMMA (Rees et al., 1989a). This provides in vitro evidence that vasorelaxation induced by endothelium-dependent agonists is NO-mediated. This was also supported by in vivo animal studies. L-NMMA has been shown to inhibit the hypotensive effect of ACh but not that of GTN in rabbits (Rees et al., 1989b) and rats (Whittle et al., 1989). However, the blockade is far from complete and there is now growing evidence for additional mechanisms underlying endothelium-dependent response, particularly in resistance vessels.

Table 10.1 Phenotypes of nitric oxide synthase knockout mice

Mutant mice	Phenotype
eNOS −/−	Elevation of systemic blood pressure
	Increased pulmonary vasoconstrictor response to hypoxia
	Diminished vasodilatory responses to muscarinic agonists
nNOS −/−	Resistance to ischaemic and inflammatory injury to the brain
	Gastroparesis
	Pyloric stenosis
	Bladder–urethral sphincter dysfunction
	Impaired NANC neurotransmission of gastrointestinal and bronchial smooth muscles
iNOS −/−	Increased susceptibility to bacterial infection
	Resistance to sepsis-induced hypotension

eNOS, endothelial nitric oxide synthase; nNOS, neuronal nitric oxide synthase; iNOS, inducible nitric oxide synthase; NANC, nonadrenergic noncholinergic.

Similarly, in humans, L-NMMA inhibits agonist-stimulated relaxation in both resistance (Vallance et al., 1989a; Lefroy et al., 1993; Cockcroft et al., 1994; Quyyumi et al., 1995) and conduit vessels in vivo (Thom et al., 1987; Schoeffter et al., 1988; Yasue et al., 1990; Yang et al., 1991; Collins et al., 1993; Jovanovic et al., 1994). However, the degree of inhibition to agonist varies depending on the specific vascular bed, suggesting that mechanisms (e.g. prostaglandins and endothelium-derived hyperpolarizing factors) other than that mediated by NO may also be involved.

Vascular phenotype of NOS knockouts

Endothelium-derived NO from any of the NOS isoforms can be involved in vasodilatory responses. Pharmacological blockade of NO production with L-NMMA affects all isoforms of NOS and is unable to distinguish their individual physiological roles (Griffith and Gross, 1996). However, with the use of genetically modified animals lacking one or other isoform of NOS (knockouts), it is possible to distinguish the roles of NO from various NOS isoforms in regulating intravascular pressure and flow under different physiological conditions. The phenotypes of various NOS knockouts are summarized in Table 10.1.

eNOS

eNOS knockout mice are hypertensive (Huang et al., 1995; Shesely et al., 1996; Godecke et al., 1998) and lack vasodilatory responses to ACh in several major vessels. These include the aorta (Huang et al., 1995; Gregg et al., 1998; Chataigneau et al., 1999; Kojda et al., 1999; Lake-Bruse et al., 1999), carotid (Faraci et al., 1998; Chataigneau et al., 1999), coronary (Godecke et al., 1998; Chataigneau et al., 1999) and pulmonary arteries (Steudel et al., 1997). These observations provide direct evidence that endothelium-dependent vasorelaxation is mediated by eNOS-derived NO. Interestingly, small-resistance vessels from these animals show a preserved response to ACh, suggesting that ACh has complex and NO-independent actions. Flow-mediated dilatation is also preserved in the eNOS knockouts and it appears that prostaglandins compensate for the loss of NO.

The importance of eNOS-derived NO in the modulation of vascular tone is further demonstrated by studies of heterozygous eNOS-deficient mice (eNOS +/ −). In eNOS +/− mice, there is increased pulmonary vasoconstrictor responses to hypoxia (Fagan et al., 1999). Additionally, low-dose ACh produced relaxation whereas high doses of ACh produced paradoxical vasoconstriction in this genotype (Faraci et al., 1998). Thus even partial loss of eNOS expression is sufficient to alter vascular tone–a phenomenon known as 'gene-dosing' effect.

nNOS

In the central nervous system, nNOS-derived NO is involved (in addition to eNOS) in the regulation of blood pressure by reducing vascular sympathetic tone, and regulates local cerebral blood flow by a direct paracrine action on adjacent VSMCs. Mice with nNOS gene deletion are resistant to ischaemic and inflammatory injury. Occlusion of the middle cerebral artery after 1–3 days resulted in a reduced infarct volume and neurological deficit in nNOS knockout mice compared to controls (Huang et al., 1994). This protective role of nNOS knockout was also found in response to malonate-induced neurotoxicity and in N-methyl-D-aspartate-treated isolated cortical neurons (Schulz et al., 1996).

iNOS

Mice lacking iNOS, iNOS −/−, have increased susceptibility to bacterial infection but are more resistant to sepsis-induced hypotension (Laubach et al., 1995; MacMicking et al., 1995; Wei et al., 1995).

Limitations of knockout studies

Although study of genetically altered mice is a powerful tool in examining the impact of specific genes on complex physiological system, there are potential drawbacks. Following deletion of the target gene, compensatory mechanisms may result which could influence vascular responses to pharmacological agents. For instance, in eNOS knockout mice, synthesis of nNOS may be upregulated to compensate for the lack of eNOS in mediating cerebral artery responses to ACh (Meng et al., 1998). It has also been shown that in eNOS $-/-$ mice, response to exogenous NO donors is increased as a result of increased guanylate cyclase sensitivity to NO compared to the wild-type mice (eNOS $+/+$) (Hussain et al., 1999; Brandes et al., 2000). Furthermore, near-normal flow-induced dilatation in gracilis muscle arterioles of eNOS $-/-$ mice was maintained due to enhanced release of endothelial dilator prostaglandins (Sun et al., 1999). In nNOS-deficient mice, carbon dioxide inhalation augments cerebral blood flow to the same extent as in wild-type mice. However, inhibition of other NOS isoforms failed to decrease cerebral blood flow, indicating that cerebral circulation response is compensated by mechanisms not involving the L-arginine – NO pathway (Irikura et al., 1995). Hence, compensatory mechanisms may cause considerable difficulties when comparing endothelium-dependent and endothelium-independent mechanisms in genetically modified mouse models.

Assessing NO response using acetylcholine

Vascular response to agonists varies depending on the blood vessel type as well as the specific vascular bed studied. For instance, ACh causes relaxation of human conduit (Thom et al., 1987; Schoeffter et al., 1988; Yasue et al., 1990; Yang et al., 1991; Collins et al., 1993; Jovanovic et al., 1994) and resistance vessels but has only minimal effect on hand veins (Vallance et al., 1989b; Collier and Vallance, 1990) and saphenous veins (Thom et al., 1987; Lawrie et al., 1990; Yang et al., 1991). A biphasic response to ACh has been observed in superficial hand veins (Collier and Vallance, 1990) and the coronary artery (Angus et al., 1991) in humans with vasodilatation at low doses of ACh and vasoconstriction at high doses. Furthermore, in eNOS knockout mice, ACh-induced vasorelaxation of femoral and mesenteric vessels occurs. This is thought to be due to the release of endothelial-derived hyperpolarizing factor (EDHF; Waldron et al., 1999), an unidentified diffusable substance distinct from NO which contributes to endothelium-dependent relaxation by opening potassium channels in the VSMCs (Beny and Brunet, 1988; Kauser et al., 1989).

Clearly, the mechanism of ACh-induced vascular response is complex and may involve several components. These include endothelium-dependent relaxation (Bruning et al., 1994), endothelium-independent contraction as a result of a direct effect on muscarinic receptors on VSMCs (Penny et al., 1995), vasorelaxation through inhibition of noradrenaline (norepinephrine) release as a result of its action on presynaptic muscarinic receptors (Vanhoutte, 1974), and vasorelaxation through the release of prostaglandins and/or EDHF (Chen and Cheung, 1992; Bauersachs et al., 1996; Garland and Plane, 1996; Hutcheson et al., 1999). The relative contribution of each mechanism depends on the vascular bed, size of the vessel (Shimokawa et al., 1996) and pathophysiological condition studied (Rosolowsky et al., 1990; Najibi et al., 1994). For this reason, caution should be exercised when interpreting changes in ACh responses as being indicative of changes in the L-arginine – NO pathway.

Biochemical detection of NO in vivo

Given the difficulty in interpreting NO-mediated vascular responses induced by ACh and other agonists, direct quantification of NO might help to resolve the issue. However, there are considerable difficulties in the direct biochemical measurement of NO. Electrochemical methods such as a porphyrinic microsensor have been used to detect free NO (Malinski et al., 1993; Vallance et al., 1995). These methods are, however, unsuitable for quantitative measurement of NO due to the instability of NO in vivo (Baylis and Vallance, 1998). Measurement of plasma and urinary nitrate, the stable endproduct of NO metabolism, has limited value as it does not distinguish exogenous nitrate (present in diet) from endogenous nitrate. Furthermore, plasma nitrate concentration does not differentiate the finer differences in NO production since the rate of NO production, excretion and its volume of distribution are all factors that can influence the plasma concentration.

Production of NO can also be quantified by measuring ^{15}N nitrate excretion in urine after intravenous administration of the isotope L-[^{15}N]$_2$-guanidino arginine (Hibbs et al., 1992; Forte et al., 1997; Macallan et al., 1997). This method has the advantage of ensuring that the measured urinary ^{15}N nitrate is endogenous. However, it does not distinguish the cellular origin of NO production. Even accurate direct measurement of total body nitrate production does not reflect biologically active NO, nor does it provide information regarding the target tissue response to the available NO. Given these various drawbacks in the measurement and interpretation of NO production and activities, measurement of NO metabolites should be interpreted with caution and ideally in conjunction with functional outcomes (vascular responses).

Loss of NO and predisposition to atherogenesis

Since NO has a number of antiatherogenic effects, it would be logical to assume that loss of NO or a reduction in its activities promotes atherogenesis. Indeed, a reduction in NO activity (manifested as impaired endothelial-dependent vasodilatation) occurs very early in experimental and human hypercholesterolaemia, even before any structural changes in the vascular wall. The impaired endothelial-dependent vasodilatation can be reversed with L-arginine (Cooke et al., 1991; Drexler et al., 1991). The antiatherogenic role of NO is further supported by studies of long-term NOS inhibition. Aortic rings from rabbits fed with cholesterol-rich diet had impaired endothelial-dependent vasorelaxation in response to ACh. Furthermore, blockade of NO with nitro-L-arginine methylester (L-NAME) caused structural changes with development of greater lesion surface area in the aorta of hypercholesterolaemic rabbits (Naruse et al., 1994).

Endothelial dysfunction in disease states

Hypercholesterolaemia and atherosclerosis

Impaired endothelium-dependent vasorelaxation to ACh occurs in models of atherosclerosis and hypercholesterolaemic animals (Bossaller et al., 1987; Shimokawa and Vanhoutte, 1989). In these studies, relaxation to endothelium-independent NO donors such as GTN and sodium nitroprusside (SNP) was unaffected, indicating impairment of the L-arginine – NO pathway rather than a reduced VSMC response to NO. Similar findings were also confirmed in human coronary and peripheral circulation in vivo (Ludmer et al., 1986; Werns et al., 1989; Creager et al., 1990; Zeiher et al., 1991). In patients with early coronary artery disease (CAD), abnormal responses to ACh were found even in angiographically normal segments of coronary artery (Werns et al., 1989). Similarly, in patients with established CAD, the degree of endothelium dysfunction in the conduit vessels as assessed by flow-mediated dilatation is also impaired. This impairment correlates with the extent of the CAD (Neunteufl et al., 1997). Furthermore, in hypercholesterolaemic subjects, impaired endothelium-dependent vasodilatation occurs in both coronary and peripheral vessels before the development of clinical atherosclerosis (Drexler et al., 1991; Chowienczyk et al., 1992). Restoration of this impaired endothelium-dependent vasodilatation in the forearm resistance vessels of hypercholesterolaemic subjects can be achieved after 24 weeks of lipid-lowering therapy (John et al., 1998).

Hypertension

A large body of evidence from animal studies (Konishi and Su, 1983; Luscher and Vanhoutte, 1986; Carvalho et al., 1987) and in vivo human studies indicates that ACh-induced relaxation is impaired in individuals with hypertension (Panza et al., 1993a, b; Taddei et al., 1993; Cardillo et al., 1998). However, at least one study has found no difference in endothelium-dependent vasodilator response to ACh or carbachol between patients with essential hypertension and matched normotensive controls (Cockcroft et al., 1994). This may reflect differences in methodology and in population subgroup in this heterogeneous condition.

Additionally, basal NO release is reduced in essential hypertension (Calver et al., 1992b; Forte et al., 1997). Current data would be most consistent with hypertension causing a decrease in NO-mediated dilatation rather than the loss of NO being causative in essential hypertension (Vallance, 1999). This notion is supported by the observation that impaired endothelium-dependent vasodilatation in essential hypertension can be restored with antihypertensive therapy (Hirooka et al., 1992; Panza et al., 1993c; Calver et al., 1994); and that endothelium-dependent vasodilatation is impaired following acute elevation of blood pressure in normotensive subjects (Millgard and Lind, 1998).

Impairment of NO-mediated dilatation occurs not only in essential hypertension but also in secondary hypertension due to primary hyperaldosteronism, renovascular hypertension (Taddei et al., 1993), cortisol-induced hypertension (Kelly et al., 1998) and preeclampsia (Delacretaz et al., 1995).

Diabetes mellitus

Endothelial function can be affected in diabetes mellitus in several ways. There may be reduced basal and/or stimulated NO release, decreased bioavailability of NO or reduced VSMC responsiveness. The vasodilating effect of insulin in skeletal muscle has been shown to be mediated via an increase in NO release (Steinberg et al., 1994). Hence in the presence of insulin deficiency in type 1 diabetes mellitus, there may be reduced NO release. Even if NO release is normal, its bioavailability may be reduced since advanced glycation endproducts as a result of chronic hyperglycaemia may quench NO in vitro (Bucala et al., 1991). Alternatively, there may be a defective response to NO since hyperglycaemia interferes with NO-induced GC activation (Weisbrod et al., 1993). There is considerable controversy regarding the extent of endothelial dysfunction in type 1 diabetes mellitus (Chan et al., 2000), as endothelial function studies in both animal and human models of type 1 diabetes mellitus have produced conflicting results. For example, agonist-stimulated endothelium-dependent vasodilatation has been found to be either impaired (Johnstone et al., 1993; O'Driscoll et al., 1997) or unchanged (Calver et al., 1992a; Huvers et al., 1999; Smits et al., 1993; Meeking et al., 2000). Endothelial function is modulated by several factors associated with diabetes such as degree of acute hyperglycaemia (Schaffler et al., 1998; Williams et al., 1998), chronicity of hyperglycaemia (disease duration), accumulation of advanced glycosylated end-product (Bucala et al., 1991), insulin levels (Scherrer et al., 1994), diabetic complications such as autonomic neuropathy (Makimattila et al., 1997) and microalbuminuria (Elliot et al., 1993). Variation in these factors between subjects in different studies may in part explain the conflicting results. At present, there is no clear consensus about the level at which the disease might alter NO signalling. Several aetiological factors may account for endothelial dysfunction in diabetic vasculopathies. These include excess oxygen free radicals, abnormalities in the aldose reductase and polyol pathway, activation of protein kinase C and accumulation of advanced glycation endproducts. The contribution of each of the above factors in diabetic vasculopathy has been reviewed recently (Chan et al., 2000) and is beyond the scope of this chapter, but Chapter 15 provides a detailed account of the diabetic vasculopathies.

Links between risk factors and atherogenesis

In addition to various disease states, endothelium-dependent vasodilatation is impaired in old age (Celermajer et al., 1994; Lyons et al., 1997), young healthy subjects with a family history of premature CHD (Clarkson et al., 1997) and cigarette smoking (Celermajer et al., 1993). The age-related endothelial dysfunction may partially explain the increased cardiovascular risk in the elderly. In asymptomatic young smokers, impairment of endothelium-dependent vasodilatation is reversible with smoking cessation (Celermajer et al., 1993). It may be that tobacco has a direct toxic effect on the vascular endothelium (Davis et al., 1985; Nagy et al., 1997). Additionally, depletion of the cofactor BH_4 for eNOS in chronic smokers may contribute to decreased NO synthesis (Heitzer et al., 2000). This is supported by the finding that BH_4 supplementation restores endothelial function in chronic smokers (Ueda et al., 2000). Thus, various effects on the L-arginine – NO pathway exerted by hypertension, diabetes, hyperlipidaemia, ageing, cigarette smoking and family history of CHD may form a link between risk factors and atherogenesis.

Chronic heart failure

Chronic heart failure (CHF) is characterized by a reduced vasodilator response to exercise and increased vasoconstriction. In addition to various compensatory neurohumoral mechanisms and markedly increased vasoconstrictor production, the endothelium plays an important role in abnormal dilator response (Kiowski et al., 1998). In patients with CHF, there is a reduced endothelium-dependent vasodilator response to ACh (Katz et al., 1993; Nakamura et al., 1994a; Carville et al., 1998) and serotonin (Maguire et al., 1998) in peripheral resistance vessels. Interestingly, the endothelium-independent vasodilator response to NO donor is also attenuated (Katz et al., 1993; Maguire et al., 1998) and the degree of impairment relates to the severity of CHF (Carville et al., 1998). Furthermore, vasoconstriction response is also diminished (Carville et al., 1998; Yoshida et al., 1998) or lost (Maguire et al., 1998), suggesting that mechanisms other than the L-arginine – NO pathway may contribute to abnormal basal vascular tone in this condition. Treatment of CHF with angiotensin-converting enzyme (ACE) inhibitor has been shown to improve endothelium-dependent vasodilatation induced by

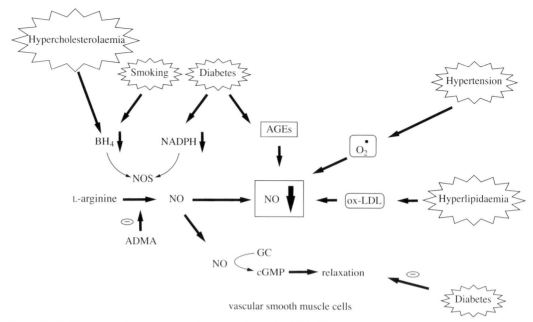

Figure 10.5 Summary of complex mechanisms through which disease states decrease nitric oxide (NO) bioactivities. For abbreviations, see text.

cholinergic stimuli (Nakamura et al., 1994b; Drexler et al., 1995), an effect which may contribute to the improved cardiovascular mortality associated with this form of treatment. Recently, the addition of spironolactone to conventional therapy for CHF has been shown to reduce mortality substantially (Pitt et al., 1999). It has subsequently been shown in a randomized placebo-controlled study in patients with moderate to severe CHF, spironolactone increased vasodilator response to ACh with an associated increase in vasoconstriction to L-NMMA, suggestive of enhanced basal NO-mediated dilatation (Farquharson and Struthers, 2000). Whether these beneficial effects on endothelial NO account for the favourable outcome remains to be determined.

How might diseases alter the L-arginine – NO pathway?

The involvement of the L-arginine – NO pathway in disease states is complex and it can be altered in several ways (Figure. 10.5).

Decreased NO production

Cofactor deficiency

In diabetes, chronic hyperglycaemia increases aldose reductase activity, leading to an increase in glucose metabolism through the polypol pathway (Asahina et al., 1995). Aldose reductase is the rate-limiting enzyme in the conversion of glucose to

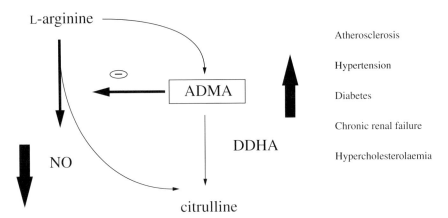

Figure 10.6 Asymmetric dimethylarginine (ADMA) is synthesized from L-arginine by protein methylase I and subsequently metabolized by dimethylarginine dimethylaminochydrolase (DDHA) yielding citrulline. ADMA acts as an endogenous inhibitor of nitric oxide NO synthesis and its synthesis is increased in certain disease states.

sorbitol. This process is dependent on NADPH, resulting in increased utilization (Asahina et al., 1995). Since NADPH is also an essential cofactor for NOS, its depletion as a result of chronic hyperglycaemia could lead to a reduction in NO synthesis. Furthermore, insulin resistance was associated with deficiency of BH$_4$, resulting in impaired vascular relaxation (Shinozaki et al., 1999). In hypercholesterolaemia, impaired endothelial-dependent vasodilatation can be restored with BH$_4$ supplementation (Stroes et al., 1997) suggesting that BH$_4$ deficiency plays an important role in impaired vascular function in this condition.

Role of endogenous inhibitors of NOS

Overproduction of endogenous inhibitors of NOS in certain disease states may contribute to reduced NO synthesis. Asymmetric and symmetric dimethylarginine (ADMA and SDMA) have been identified in the human plasma. ADMA has similar properties to L-NMMA (Vallance et al., 1992a). It is synthesized by the human endothelial cells from arginine and is metabolized to citrulline (MacAllister et al., 1996) before excretion into the urine (Figure 10.6; Vallance et al., 1992a). The enzyme responsible for ADMA metabolism in the human vascular endothelial cells is dimethylarginine dimethylaminohydrolase, of which two isoforms (DDAH I and II) have been identified, sequenced and cloned (MacAllister et al., 1996; Kimoto et al., 1997; Leiper et al., 1999). Circulating ADMA is increased in certain disease states. This includes animal models of hypertension (Matsuoka et al., 1997), diabetes (Masuda et al., 1999), hypercholesterolaemia (Yu et al., 1994; Bode-Boger et al., 1996a) and atherosclerosis (Boger et al., 1997). In humans, elevated ADMA concentrations were found in chronic renal failure (Vallance et al., 1992b), childhood hypertension (Goonasekera et al., 1997), preeclampsia (Fickling et al., 1993), thrombotic microangiopathy (Herlitz et al., 1997), hyper-cholesterolaemia (Boger et al., 1998) and atherosclerosis (Miyazaki et al., 1999). The mechanism whereby various disease states are associated with increased ADMA levels remains unclear but may involve alteration in DDHA activity, which may be important in atherogenesis.

Decreased NO bioavailability

Role of oxidative stress

Even with adequate production, NO may not reach its biological targets (VSMCs and platelet) to exert its effect due to the lack of its bioavailability. For example, in hyperlipidaemia, excess LDL synthesis increases the formation of oxidized LDL superoxide anions. The resultant increase of oxidative stress enhances NO destruction (Chin et al., 1992), thereby reducing its biological effects. In atherosclerotic rabbit aorta, despite a threefold increase in total NO synthesis compared to normal rabbits, there is markedly impaired endothelium-dependent vasodilatation (Minor et al., 1990). This impaired vascular response was partially restored following treatment with superoxide dismutase (Mugge et al., 1991), suggesting that superoxide-induced NO inactivation plays a major role. In humans, hyper-triglyceridaemia with or without diabetes may have greater potential than cholesterol to increase superoxide production by leukocytes (Hiramatsu, 1988; Pronai et al., 1991). Other atherogenic factors such as free fatty acids and low levels of high-density lipoproteins also increase oxidative stress (Sattar et al., 1998), contributing to reduced NO bioavailability. In addition to the associated atherogenic phenotype and oxidative stress, hyperglycaemia per se increases free radical production through increased arachidonic acid metabolism (Tesfamariam and Cohen, 1992). In human aortic endothelial cells, although prolonged exposure to high glucose concentration causes increased eNOS expression, it also leads to a concomitant increase in superoxide anion production, resulting in NO inactivation (Cosentino et al., 1997).

Advanced glycation endproducts

Inactivation or quenching of NO also occurs in diabetes as a result of accumulation of advanced glycation endproducts (AGEs), the product of nonenzymatic glycation and cross-linking of collagen protein in sustained hyperglycaemia. In experimentally induced diabetic rats, there is in vitro and in vivo evidence that reactive intermediates resulting from glycation quench NO rapidly (< 5 s, Bucala et al., 1991). Additionally, impairment of endothelium-dependent vasodilatation in diabetic rats can be partially restored by aminoguanidine, an inhibitor of AGE formation (Bucala et al., 1991).

Decreased VSMC sensitivity

The VSMC sensitivity may be decreased even with adequate NO supply. In human in vivo vascular studies, nitrovasodilators or NO donors (such as GTN or sodium nitroprusside) have frequently been used as controls for agonist-stimulated endothelium-dependent vasodilatation. These agents act directly upon VSMC and the resultant vasodilatation is endothelium-independent. There is evidence to suggest that VSMC sensitivity to NO is reduced in diabetes since hyperglycaemia interferes with NO-induced GC activation in vitro (Weisbrod et al., 1993). Consistent with this finding, impaired vascular response to NO donors in vivo have been demonstrated in patients with type 1 diabetes (Calver et al., 1992a; Zenere et al., 1995; Clarkson et al., 1996).

Endotoxaemia, septic shock and inflammation: overproduction of NO

Bacterial endotoxin and certain proinflammatory cytokines can lead to profound vasodilatation and decreased vasopressor responsiveness – the main clinical features of septic shock. These cardiovascular effects result from excessive NO production due to induction of iNOS (Suffredini et al., 1989; Fleming et al., 1990; Wang et al., 1994b; Wong and Biliar, 1995; Rees et al., 1998). Under normal physiological conditions, iNOS is not expressed in the vasculature. Exposure to bacterial lipopolysaccharide (LPS) in sepsis stimulates the iNOS expression. The subsequent transcriptional induction and activation of iNOS are mediated by release of proinflammatory cytokines such as tumour necrosis factor-α (TNF-α), interleukin-1β (IL-1β) and interleukin-6 (IL-6; for review, see Bhagat and Vallance, 1999). In experimental animals, administration of TNF-α in doses similar to those produced endogenously during endotoxaemia rapidly results in a fall in arterial pressure (Mitaka et al., 1994; Lodato et al., 1995) and longer exposure to TNF-α and IL-1β in vitro leads to vasopressor hyporesponsiveness (Myers et al., 1994).

Several animal studies provide evidence for iNOS involvement in the pathogenesis of sepsis. Administration of bacterial LPS causes an increase in nitrite concentration, which is attenuated by a selective iNOS inhibitor in mice (Tunctan et al., 1998). Moreover, selective inhibition of iNOS markedly increased vascular catecholamine reactivity in experimental mice with sepsis but not in control mice (Hollenberg et al., 1999). A major limitation in these inhibitor studies is the lack of isoform specificity. More direct evidence comes from iNOS knockout studies. In wild-type mice, treatment of carotid arteries with LPS leads to impaired constrictor responses which were improved with selective iNOS inhibitors. In contrast, LPS treatment caused no impairment of vasoconstrictor responses in carotid arteries from iNOS-deficient mice (Gunnett et al., 1998).

In human sepsis the evidence for iNOS involvement has been less consistent. Some studies have suggested an increased iNOS activity, for example, in urinary leukocytes from patients with urinary tract infection (Wheeler et al., 1997), in alveolar macrophages from patients with acute respiratory distress syndrome (ARDS) following sepsis (Kobayashi et al., 1998) and in peripheral blood mononuclear cells and macrophages isolated from putrescent muscle areas in patients with cellulitis (Annane et al., 2000). However, other studies demonstrated the involvement of eNOS rather than iNOS in sepsis. In an in vitro study using human umbilical vein endothelial cells cultured with IL-1β and TNF-α, the resultant increase in NO production was shown to originate from eNOS as a result of activation of guanosine triphosphate cyclohydrolase (GTPCH-I), the rate-limiting enzyme responsible for the synthesis of BH_4 (Rosenkranz Weiss et al., 1994). Similar findings have recently been demonstrated in vivo (Bhagat et al., 1999). Whilst it is clear that overproduction of NO contributes to vasodilatation in human sepsis (Petros et al., 1991, 1994), the molecular mechanisms and isoform of NOS activated are unclear. It is also not known whether inhibition of NO generation is beneficial.

Future therapeutic possibilities

The extensive involvement of NO in various disease states makes the L-arginine – NO pathway a target for therapeutic modulation. Depending on the underlying disease process, beneficial effects may be achieved with either strategy to increase NO production or to increase NOS inhibition.

Potential therapies to increase NO production

L-arginine

Supplementation of the NO substrate L-arginine has beneficial effects in certain conditions in both animals and humans. Dietary L-arginine for 10 weeks has been shown to prevent intimal thickening in the coronary arteries (Wang et al., 1994a) and attenuates platelet reactivity in hypercholesterolaemic rabbits (Tsao et al., 1994). Furthermore, oral L-arginine administration reduces neointimal formation following balloon catheter-induced injury in both hypercholesterolaemic (Greenlees et al., 1997) and normocholesterolaemic rabbit models (McNamara et al., 1993). In humans, dietary L-arginine supplementation reduces the increased platelet reactivity in hypercholesterolaemic subjects (Wolf et al., 1997). Additionally, intravenous L-arginine infusion reduces peripheral vascular resistance (Bode-Boger et al., 1994), decreases both systolic and diastolic blood pressure (Hishikawa et al., 1992), improves endothelium-dependent coronary vasodilatation in response to intracoronary ACh in hypercholesterolaemic subjects (Drexler et al., 1991) and improves blood flow in critical lower-limb ischaemia (Kobayashi et al., 1998).

The arginine paradox

The beneficial effects of exogenous L-arginine to the vasculature in various disease states with increase of plasma nitrate and cGMP levels during L-arginine administration suggest that adequate L-arginine supply is essential for NOS activity. However, it is perplexing that the extracellular arginine administration drives NO production even when intracellular arginine levels are available in excess (Arnal et al., 1995), a phenomenon known as the 'arginine paradox'. This was first demonstrated in hypercholesterolaemic rabbits (Girerd et al., 1995) and has also been observed in patients with pulmonary hypertension (Mehta et al., 1995). Several explanations have been proposed to account for this paradox. Firstly, it is possible that the endogenous inhibitor of NOS, ADMA (Vallance et al., 1992a), might antagonize the normal intracellular concentrations of L-arginine and additional arginine supplementation could overcome NOS substrate deficiency. Secondly, since eNOS is preferentially localized to caveolae (Feron et al., 1996; Garcia-Cardena et al., 1996; Shaul et al., 1996), local concentration of L-arginine in this microenvironment may differ considerably from that within the endothelial cell. It remains unclear how specific localization of eNOS by caveolae might affect local substrate availability but may involve the colocalization of certain arginine transporters such as CAT1 (McDonald et al., 1997). The formation of such a caveolar complex seems to facilitate arginine delivery to eNOS.

Evidence has also emerged that the vasodilatory effects of L-arginine are not all mediated directly by NO. L-arginine may inhibit peripheral sympathetic tone leading to vasodilatation via its metabolite, agmatine (Wu and Morris, 1998), which stimulates central α_2-adrenoceptors (Li et al., 1994). Additionally, arginine also stimulates the release of several other hormones such as glucagon, prolactin and growth hormone (MacAllister et al., 1995a; Petrinelli et al., 1995). It is possible that these hormonal changes induced by L-arginine could contribute to the vasodilatatory effects (Steinberg et al., 1994; Giugliano et al., 1997; Boger, 1999). The complex mechanisms whereby L-arginine improves cardiovascular function merit further investigation.

Nitrovasodilators/NO donors

This group of drugs includes amyl, nitrite, GTN, SNP and molsidomine. They are all prodrugs and exert their pharmacological effects after metabolism into NO, hence termed 'NO donor'. Nitrovasodilators have conventionally been used for the treatment of cardiac failure and angina based on their venodilatory properties. Nitrosoglutathione, a compound in the class of nitrosothiols, has been studied extensively in humans. It has profound antiplatelet effects and more balanced arterial and venous vasodilatory effects in contrast to organic nitrates (de Belder et al., 1994; MacAllister et al., 1995b; Ramsey et al., 1995). Nitrosoglutathione has been shown to inhibit platelet activation in the coronary artery following angioplasty (Langford et al., 1994) as well as in coronary bypass grafts (Salas et al., 1998). Hence, these nitrosothiols are potential pharmacological agents in the treatment of NO-deficient conditions and it is possible that novel NO donors could be developed that differ significantly from existing drugs.

Inhalation of NO

Administration of NO as inhalation therapy has been shown to improve several conditions affecting the pulmonary vasculature including persistent pulmonary hypertension of the newborn (Kinsella et al., 1992), pulmonary hypertension secondary to chronic hypoxia (Pepke-Zaba et al., 1991; Frostell et al., 1993) and ARDS (Rossaint et al., 1993; Johannigman et al., 1997). In ARDS, selective delivery of NO to the pulmonary vasculature reduces the pulmonary arterial pressure and increases arterial oxygenation by improving the matching of ventilation with perfusion. As the NO is rapidly inactivated by haemoglobin, inhalation of NO gas does not cause systemic vasodilatation. However, whether this form of NO therapy will improve survival outcome in patients with ARDS remains to be determined by randomized controlled clinical trials. It does have potential adverse effects, such as pulmonary oedema and methaemoglobinaemia, which are largely due to its metabolic intermediates (e.g. $ONOO^-$). There is as yet no clear guidelines regarding the effective dose of inhaled NO for the above pulmonary conditions.

Antioxidants

Since oxidative stress has been strongly implicated for endothelial dysfunction, numerous studies have examined the role of antioxidants in vascular function and in the prevention of cardiovascular disease. Intrabrachial administration of ascorbic acid (vitamin C) improves endothelium-dependent vasodilatation in type 2 diabetes, smokers, patients with hypercholesterolaemia and heart failure (Heitzer et al., 1996; Ting et al., 1996, 1997; Hornig et al., 1998). Similarly, oral administration of ascorbic acid in patients with CHD also improves flow-mediated vasodilatation. This beneficial effect has been shown to occur rapidly after 2 h (Levine et al., 1996) and can be sustained for 30 days (Gokce et al., 1999). Furthermore, intravenous infusion of ascorbic acid improved endothelium-dependent vasodilatation in epicardial arteries in hypertensive patients without CHD (Solzbach et al., 1997). In patients with CHD, intracoronary coinfusion of vitamin C with L-arginine caused markedly increased vasodilatation (Tousoulis et al., 1999). Despite these observations, not all experiments have shown beneficial effects and further studies are required.

Several epidemiological studies have shown that increased dietary antioxidant vitamin E was associated with a lower risk of CHD in men (Rimm et al., 1993), premenopausal and postmenopausal women (Stampfer et al., 1993; Kushi et al., 1996). However, there was no association between vitamin C intake and CHD risk (Rimm et al., 1993; Kushi et al., 1996). The role of oxidative stress in preeclampsia has been the subject of much recent interest and is discussed in detail in Chapter 19. Clearly, large-scale randomized controlled-trials are required to determine whether improved endothelial function by antioxidants can be translated into reduction in cardiovascular end-points.

Gene transfer

The direct transfer of NOS isoform genes to the vessel wall alters vasomotor function and may have a role in the treatment of cardiovascular diseases (for review, see Kibbe et al., 1999). This approach has been shown to be effective in a variety of animal models of vascular disease. Vascular gene therapy delivered to specific tissues enhances NO production at the site of interest in a sustained manner. In 1995, NOS gene transfer was first reported when eNOS cDNA, complexed with the haemagglutinating virus of Japan, was delivered to rat carotid arteries intraluminally following balloon injury (von der Leyden et al., 1995). This resulted in a marked reduction in neointima formation at 14 days. Shortly after, similar results were confirmed by other research groups not only in the carotid artery but also in iliac, coronary arteries (Chen et al., 1998; Janssens et al., 1998; Shears et al., 1998; Varenne et al., 1998) and vein grafts (Matsumoto et al., 1998). Gene therapy has also been extended from local to systemic delivery. Delivery of a single injection of naked eNOS cDNA into the systemic circulation through the tail vein of spontaneously hypertensive rats resulted in increased production and excretion of cGMP and nitrite/nitrate, and was associated with a significant reduction in systolic blood pressure lasting up to 12 weeks (Lin et al., 1997).

Potential therapies to decrease NO production
NOS inhibitors

Inhibition of iNOS has been shown to improve NO-mediated haemodynamic changes in experimental models of septic shock (Wolfe and Dasta, 1995). Intravenous administration of the arginine analogue, L-NMMA, reverses the decrease in peripheral vascular resistance and fall in arterial blood pressure in endotoxaemic dogs (Kilbourn et al., 1990). The same effects with L-NMMA were also confirmed in humans in a randomized, double blind, placebo-controlled trial (Petros et al., 1991, 1994). A major pitfall in this therapeutic strategy is that none of the currently available NOS inhibitors is specific for the iNOS and this may therefore lead to potential hazardous effects (Peterson et al., 1992). Indeed, both pulmonary hypertension and reduced cardiac output have been reported following NOS inhibition (Petros et al., 1994; Robertson et al., 1994; Avontuur et al., 1998). Furthermore, it remains unclear what degree of iNOS inhibition and duration is required in septic shock. It has been shown in rats that a low dose of L-NMMA is ineffective in reversing endotoxin-induced hypotension while a higher dose accelerated the fall in systemic blood pressure and caused death (Nava et al., 1991). Future drug development in this area should focus on NOS specificity as well as degree of iNOS inhibition in order to produce an optimal pharmacological effect. Ultimately, large-scale randomized controlled trials will be needed to examine its effect on mortality in septic shock.

REFERENCES

Aisaka, K., Gross, S.S., Griffith, O.W. & Levi, R. (1989). N^G-methylarginine, an inhibitor of endothelium-derived nitric oxide synthesis, is a potent pressor agent in the guinea pig: does nitric oxide regulate blood pressure in vivo? *Biochem. Biophys. Res. Commun.*, **160**, 881–6.

Ando, J., Kawamura, T. & Kamiya, A. (1988). Cytoplasmic calcium response to fluid shear stress in cultured vascular endothelial cells. *In Vitro Cell Dev. Biol.*, **24**, 871–7.

Ando, J., Ohtsuka, A., Korenaga, R., Kawamura, T. & Kamiya, A. (1993). Wall shear stress rather than shear rate regulates cytoplasmic calcium responses to flow in vascular endothelial cells. *Biochem. Biophys. Res. Commun.*, **190**, 716–23.

Angus, J.A., Cocks, T.M., McPherson, G.A. & Broughton, A. (1991). The acetylcholine paradox: a constrictor of human small coronary arteries even in the presence of endothelium. *Clin. Exp. Pharmacol. Physiol.*, **18**, 33–6.

Annane, D., Sanquer, S., Sebille, V. et al. (2000). Compartmentalised inducible nitric-oxide synthase activity in septic shock. *Lancet*, **355**, 1143–8.

Arnal, J.-F., Munzel, T., Venema, R.C. et al. (1995). Interactions between L-arginine and L-glutamine change endothelial NO production. An effect independent of NO synthase substrate availability. *J. Clin. Invest.*, **95**, 2565–72.

Asahina, T., Kashiwagi, A., Nishio, Y. et al. (1995). Impaired activation of glucose oxidation and NADPH supply in human endothelial cells exposed to H_2O_2 in high-glucose medium. *Diabetes*, **44**, 520–6.

Avontuur, J.A., Biewenga, M., Buijk, S.L., Kanhai, K.J. & Bruining, H.A. (1998). Pulmonary hypertension and reduced cardiac output during inhibition of nitric oxide synthesis in human septic shock. *Shock*, **9**, 451–4.

Ayajiki, K., Kindermann, M., Hecker, M., Fleming, I. & Busse, R. (1996). Intracellular pH and tyrosine phosphorylation but not calcium determine shear stress-induced nitric oxide production in native endothelial cells. *Circ Res*, **78**, 750–8.

Barakat, A.I., Leaver, E.V., Pappone, P.A. & Davies, P.F. (1999). A flow-activated chloride-selective membrane current in vascular endothelial cells. *Circ Res.*, **85**, 820–8.

Bath, P.M., Hassall, D.G., Gladwin, A.M., Palmer, R.M. & Martin, J.F. (1991). Nitric oxide and prostacyclin. Divergence of inhibitory effects on monocyte chemotaxis and adhesion to endothelium in vitro. *Arterioscler Thromb*, **11**, 254–60.

Bauersachs, J., Popp, R., Hecker M. et al. (1996). Nitric oxide attenuates the release of endothelium-derived hyperpolarizing factor. *Circulation*, **94**, 3341–7.

Baylis, C. & Vallance, P. (1998). Measurement of nitric oxide and nitrate levels in plasma and urine – what does this measure tell us about the activity of the endogenous nitric oxide system? *Curr. Opin. Nephrol. Hypertens.*, **7**, 59–62.

Bhagat, K. & Vallance, P. (1999). Effects of cytokines on nitric oxide pathways in human vasculature. *Curr. Opin. Nephrol. Hypertens.*, **8**, 89–96.

Bhagat, K., Hingorani, A.D., Palacios, M., Charles, I.G. & Vallance, P. (1999). Cytokine-induced venodilatation in humans in vivo: eNOS masquerading as iNOS. *Cardiovasc Res.*, **41**, 754–64.

Beny, J.L. & Brunet, P.C. (1988). Electrophysiological and mechanical effects of substance P and acetylcholine on rabbit aorta. *J. Physiol*, **398**, 277–89.

Biffl, W.L., Moore, E.E., Moore, F.A. & Barnett, C. (1996). Nitric oxide reduces endothelial expression of intracellular adhesion molecule (ICAM)-1. *J. Surg. Res.*, **63**, 328–32.

Bode-Boger, S.M., Boger, R.H., Creutzig, A. et al. (1994). L-arginine infusion decreases peripheral arterial resistance and inhibits platelet aggregation in healthy subjects. *Clin. Sci.*, **87**, 303–10.

Bode-Boger, S.M., Boger, R.H., Kienke, J., Junker, W. & Frolich, J.C. (1996a). Elevated L-arginine/dimethylarginine ratio contributes to enhanced systemic NO production by dietary L-arginine in hypercholesterolemic rabbits. *Biochem. Biophys. Res. Commun.*, **219**, 598–603.

Bode-Boger, S.M., Boger, R.H., Alfke, H. et al. (1996b). L-arginine induces nitric oxide-dependent vasodilation in patients with critical limb ischaemia. A randomized, controlled study. *Circulation*, **93**, 85–90.

Boger, R.H. (1999). Nitric oxide and the mediation of the haemodynamic effects of growth hormone in humans. *J. Endocrinol. Invest.*, **22** (5 Suppl), 75–81.

Boger, R.H., Bode-Boger, S.M., Brandes, R.P. et al. (1997). Dietary L-arginine reduces the progression of atherosclerosis in cholesterol-fed rabbits; comparison with lovastatin. *Circulation*, **96**, 1282–90.

Boger, R.H., Bode-Boger, S.M., Szuba A et al. (1998). Asymmetric dimethylarginine (ADMA): a novel risk factor for endothelial dysfunction. Its role in hypercholesterolemia. *Circulation*, **98**, 1842–7.

Bossaller, C., Habib, G.B., Yamamoto, H. et al. (1987). Impaired muscarinic endothelium-dependent relaxation and cyclic guanosine 3',5'-monophosphate formation in the atherosclerotic human coronary artery and rabbit aorta. *J. Clin. Invest.*, **79**, 170–4.

Boulanger, C.M. & Vanhoutte, P.M. (1997). G proteins and endothelium-dependent relaxations. *J. Vasc. Res.*, **34**, 175–85.

Brandes, R.P., Kim, D.-Y., Schmitz-Winnenthal, F.-H. et al. (2000). Increased nitrovasodilator sensitivity in endothelial nitric oxide synthase knockout mice. Role of soluble guanylyl cyclase. *Hypertension*, **35**, 231.

Bredt, D.S. & Snyder, S.H. (1990). Isolation of nitric oxide synthase, a calmodulin-requiring enzyme. *Proc. Natl Acad. Sci. U.S.A.*, **87**, 682–5.

Bruning, T.A., Hendriks, M.G., Chang, P.C., Kuypers, E.A. & van Zwieten, P.A. (1994). In vivo characterization of vasodilating muscarinic-receptor subtypes in humans. *Circ. Res.*, **74**, 912–19.

Bucala, R., Tracey, K.L. & Cerami, A. (1991). Advanced glycosylation products quench nitric oxide and mediate defective endothelium-dependent vasodilation in experimental diabetes. *J. Clin. Invest.*, **87**, 432–8.

Busse, R., Mulsch, A., Fleming, I. & Hecker, M. (1993). Mechanisms of nitric oxide release from the vascular endothelium. *Circulation*, **87**(Suppl. V), V18–25.

Cai, H., Wilcken, D.E. & Wang, X.L. (1999). The Glu-298 → Asp (894G → T) mutation at exon 7 of the endothelial nitric oxide synthase gene and coronary artery disease. *J. Mol. Med.*, **77**, 511–14.

Calver, A., Collier, J. & Vallance, P. (1992a). Inhibition and stimulation of nitric oxide synthesis in the human forearm arterial bed of patients with insulin-dependent diabetes. *J. Clin. Invest.*, **90**, 2548–54.

Calver, A., Collier, J., Moncada, S. & Vallance, P. (1992b). Effect of local, intra-arterial N^G-monomethyl-L-arginine in patients with hypertension: the nitric oxide dilator mechanism appears abnormal. *J. Hypertens.*, **10**, 1025–31.

Calver, A., Collier, J. & Vallance, P. (1994). Forearm blood flow responses to a nitric oxide synthase inhibitor in patients with treated essential hypertension. *Cardiovasc. Res.*, **28**, 1720–5.

Cardillo, C., Kilcoyne, C.M., Quyyumi, A.A., Cannon, R.O. 3rd & Panza, J.A. (1998). Selective defect in nitric oxide synthesis may explain the impaired endothelium-dependent vasodilation in patients with essential hypertension. *Circulation*, **97**, 851–6.

Carvalho, M.H.C., Scivoletto, R., Fortes, Z.B., Nigro, D. & Cordellini, S. (1987). Reactivity of aorta and mesenteric microvessels to drugs in spontaneously hypertensive rats: role of the endothelium. *J. Hypertens.*, **5**, 377–82.

Carville, C., Adnot, S., Sediame, S. et al. (1998). Relation between impairment in nitric oxide pathway and clinical status in patients with congestive heart failure. *J. Cardiovasc. Pharmacol.*, **32**, 562–70.

Castro, L., Rodriguez, M. & Radi, R. (1994). Aconitase is readily inactivated by peroxynitrite, but not by its precursor, nitric oxide. *J. Biol. Chem.*, **269**, 29409–15.

Celermajer, D.S., Sorensen, K.E., Georgakopoulos, D. et al. (1993). Cigarette smoking is associated with dose-related and potentially reversible impairment of endothelium-dependent dilation in healthy young adults. *Circulation*, **88**, 2149–55.

Celermajer, D.S., Sorensen, K.E., Spiegelhalter, D.J. et al. (1994). Aging is associated with endothelial dysfunction in healthy man years before the age-related decline in women. *J. Am. Coll. Cardiol.*, **24**, 471–6.

Chan, N.N., Vallance, P. & Colhoun, H.M. (2000). Nitric oxide and vascular responses in type 1 diabetes. *Diabetologia*, **43**, 137–47.

Chataigneau, T., Feletou, M., Huang, P.L. et al. (1999). Acetylcholine-induced relaxation in blood vessels from endothelial nitric oxide synthase knockout mice. *Br. J. Pharmacol.*, **126**, 219–26.

Chen, G. & Cheung, D.W. (1992). Characterization of acetylcholine-induced membrane hyperpolarization in endothelial cells. *Circ. Res.*, **70**, 257–63.

Chen, L., Daum, G., Forough, R. et al. (1998). Overexpression of human endothelial nitric oxide synthase in balloon-injured carotid artery. *Circ. Res.*, **82**, 862–70.

Chin, J.A., Azhar, S. & Hoffman, B.B. (1992). Inactivation of endothelial derived relaxing factor by oxidized lipoprotein. *J. Clin. Invest.*, **89**, 10–12.

Chowienczyk, P.J., Watts, G.F., Cockcroft, J.R. & Ritter, J.M. (1992). Impairment of endothelium-dependent vasodilatation of forearm resistance vessels in hypercholesterolaemia. *Lancet*, **340**, 1430–2.

Clancy, R.M., Leszczynska-Piziak, J. & Abramson, S.B. (1992). Nitric oxide, an endothelial cell relaxation factor, inhibits neutrophil superoxide anion production via a direct action on the NADPH oxidase. *J. Clin. Invest.*, **90**, 1116–21.

Clarkson, P., Celermajer, D.S., Donald, A.E. et al. (1996). Impaired vascular reactivity in insulin-dependent diabetes mellitus is related to disease duration and low density lipoprotein cholesterol levels. *J. Am. Coll. Cardiol.*, **28**, 573–9.

Clarkson, P., Celermajer, D.S., Powe, A.J. et al. (1997). Endothelium-dependent dilatation is impaired in young healthy subjects with a family history of premature coronary disease. *Circulation*, **96**, 3378–83.

Cockcroft, J.R., Chowienczyk, P.J., Benjamin, N. & Ritter, J.M. (1994). Preserved endothelium-dependent vasodilatation in patients with essential hypertension. *N. Engl. J. Med.*, **330**, 1036–40.

Collier, J. & Vallance, P. (1990). Biphasic response to acetylcholine in human hand veins in vivo: the role of the endothelium. *Clin. Sci.*, **78**, 101–4.

Collins, P., Burman, J., Chung, H.I. & Fox, K. (1993). Haemoglobin inhibits endothelium-dependent relaxation to acetylcholine in human coronary arteries in vivo. *Circulation*, **87**, 80–5.

Cooke, J.P., Andon, N.A., Girerd, W.J., Hirsch, A.T. & Creager, M.A. (1991). Arginine restores cholinergic relaxation of hypercholesterolemic rabbit thoracic aorta. *Circulation*, **83**, 1057–62.

Corson, M.A., James, N.L., Latta, S.E. et al. (1996). Phosphorylation of endothelial nitric oxide synthase in response to fluid shear stress. *Circ. Res.*, **79**, 984–91.

Cosentino, F., Hishikawa, K., Katusic, Z.S. & Luscher, T.F. (1997). High glucose increases nitric oxide synthase expression and superoxide anion generation in human aortic endothelial cells. *Circulation*, **96**, 25–8.

Creager, M.A., Cooke, J.P., Mendelsohn, M.E. et al. (1990). Impaired vasodilation of forearm resistance vessels in hypercholesterolaemic humans. *J. Clin. Invest.*, **86**, 228–34.

Davies, P.F. (1995). Flow mediated mechanotransduction. *Physiol. Rev.*, **75**, 519–56.

Davis, J.W., Shelton, L., Eigenberg, D.A., Hignite, C.E. & Watanabe, I.S. (1985). Effects of tobacco and non-tobacco cigarette smoking on endothelium and platelets. *Clin. Pharmacol. Ther.*, **37**, 529–33.

de Belder, A.J., MacAllister, R., Radomski, M.W. Moncada, S. & Vallance, P.J. (1994). Effects of *S*-nitroso-glutathione in the human forearm circulation: evidence for selective inhibition of platelet activation. *Cardiovasc. Res.*, **28**, 691–4.

De Caterina, R., Libby, P., Peng, H.B. et al. (1995). Nitric oxide decreases cytokine-induced endothelial activation. Nitric oxide selectively reduces endothelial expression of adhesion molecules and proinflammatory cytokines. *J. Clin. Invest.*, **96**, 60–8.

Delacretaz, E., de Quay, N., Waeber, B. et al. (1995). Differential nitric oxide synthase activity in human platelets during normal pregnancy and pre-eclampsia. *Clin. Sci.*, **88**, 607–10.

Dimmeler, S., Fleming, I., Fisslthaler, B. et al. (1999). Activation of nitric oxide synthase in endothelial cells by Akt-dependent phosphorylation. *Nature*, **399**, 601–5.

Drexler, H., Zeiher, A.M., Meinzer, K. & Just, H. (1991). Correction of endothelial dysfunction in coronary microcirculation of hypercholesterolemic patients by L-arginine. *Lancet*, **338**, 1450–6.

Drexler, H., Kurz, S., Jeserich, M., Munzel, T. & Hornig, B. (1995). Effect of chronic angiotensin-converting enzyme inhibition on endothelial function in patients with chronic heart failure. *Am. J. Cardiol.*, **76**, 13E–18E.

Ekelund, U. & Mellander, S. (1990). Role of endothelium derived nitric oxide in the regulation of tonus in large-bore arterial resistance essels, arterioles and veins in cat skeletal muscle. *Acta Physiol. Scand.*, **140**, 301–9.

Elliot, T.G., Cockcroft, J.R., Groop, P.-H., Viberti, G.C. & Ritter, J.M. (1993). Inhibition of nitric oxide synthesis in forearm vasculature of insulin-dependent diabetic patients: blunted vasoconstriction in patients with microalbuminuria. *Clin. Sci.*, **85**, 687–93.

Fagan, K.A., Fouty, B.W., Tyler, R.C. et al. (1999). The pulmonary circulation of homozygous or heterozygous eNOS-null mice is hypertensive to mild hypoxia. *J. Clin. Invest.*, **103**, 291–9.

Faraci, F.M., Sigmund, C.D., Shesely, E.G., Maeda, N. & Heistad, D.D. (1998). Responses of carotid artery in mice deficient in expression of the gene for endothelial NO synthase. *Am. J. Physiol.*, **274**, H564–70.

Farquharson, C.A. & Struthers, A.D. (2000). Spironolactone increases nitric oxide bioavailability, improves endothelial vasodilator dysfunction, and suppresses vascular angiotensin I/ angiotensin II conversion in patients with chronic failure. *Circulation*, **101**, 594–7.

Feron, O., Belhassen, L., Kobzik, L. et al. (1996). Endothelial nitric oxide synthase targeting to caveolae: specific interactions with caveolin isoforms in cardiac myocytes and endothelial cells. *J. Biol. Chem.*, **271**, 22810–14.

Feron, O., Saldana, F., Michel, J.B. & Michel, T. (1998). The endothelial nitric-oxide synthase-caveolin regulatory cycle. *J. Biol. Chem.*, **273**, 3125–8.

Fickling, S.A., Williams, D., Vallance, P., Nussey, S.S. & Whitley, G.S. (1993). Plasma concentrations of endogenous inhibitor of nitric oxide synthsis in normal pregnancy and pre-eclampsia. *Lancet*, **342**, 242–3.

Fisslthaler, B., Dimmeler, S., Hermann, C., Busse, R. & Fleming, I. (2000). Phosphorylation and activation of the endothelial nitric oxide synthase by fluid shear stress. *Acta Physiol. Scand.*, **168**, 81–8.

Fleming, I., Gray, G.A., Julou-Schaeffer, G., Parratt, J.R. & Stoclet, J.C. (1990). Incubation with endotoxin activates the L-arginine pathway in vascular tissue. *Biochem. Biophys. Res. Commun.*, **171**, 562–8.

Fleming, I., Bauersachs, J., Fisslthaler, B. & Busse, R. (1998). Calcium-independent activation of the endothelial nitric oxide synthase in response to tyrosine phosphatase inhibitors and fluid shear stress. *Circ. Res.*, **82**, 686–95.

Forstermann, U., Closs, E.I., Pollock, J.S. et al. (1994). Nitric oxide synthase isoenzymes. Characterization, purification, molecular cloning, and functions. *Hypertension*, **23**, 1121–31.

Forte, P., Copland, M., Smith, L.M. et al. (1997). Basal nitric oxide synthesis in essential hypertension. *Lancet*, **349**, 837–42.

Frostell, C.G., Blomqvist, H., Hedenstierna, G., Lundberg, J. & Zapol, W.M. (1993). Inhaled nitric oxide selectively reverses human hypoxic pulmonary vasoconstriction without causing systemic vasodilation. *Anesthesiology*, **78**, 427–35.

Fulton, D., Gratton, J.P., McCabe, T.J. et al. (1999). Regulation of endothelium-derived nitric oxide production by the protein kinase Akt. *Nature*, **399**, 597–601.

Furchgott, R.F. (1988). Studies on relaxation of rabbit aorta by sodium nitrite: the basis for the proposal that the acid-activatable inhibitory factor from retractor penis is inorganic nitrite and the endothelium-derived relaxing factor in nitric oxide. In: *Vasodilatation: Vascular Smooth Muscle, Peptides, Autonomic Nerves and Endothelium*, ed. Vanhoutte, P.M., pp. 401–14. New York: Raven.

Furchgott, R.F. & Vanhoutte, P.M. (1987). Endothelium-derived relaxing and contracting factors. *FASEB J.*, **3**, 2007–18.

Furchgott, R.F. & Zawadzki, J.V. (1980). The obligatory role of endothelial cells in the relaxion of arterial smooth muscle by acetylcholine. *Nature*, **288**, 373–6.

Garcia-Cardena, G., Fan, R., Stern, D.F., Liu, J. & Sessa, W.C. (1996). Endothelial nitric oxide synthase is regulated by tyrosine phosphorylation and interacts with caveolin-1. *J. Biol. Chem.*, **271**, 27237–40.

Garcia-Cardena, G., Martasek, P., Masters, B.S.S. et al. (1997). Dissecting the interaction between nitric oxide synthase (NOS) and caveolin: functional significance of the NOS caveolin binding domain in vivo. *J. Biol. Chem.*, **272**, 25437–40.

Garg, U.C. & Hassid, A. (1989). Nitric oxide-generating vasodilators and 8-bromo-cyclic gaunosine monophosphate inhibit mitogenesis and proliferation of cultured rat vascular smooth muscle cells. *J. Clin. Invest.*, **83**, 1774–7.

Garland, C.J. & Plane, F. (1996). Relative importance of the endothelium-derived hyperpolarizing factor for the relaxation of vascular smooth muscle in different arterial beds. In: *Endothelium-Derived Hyperpolarizing Factor*, ed. Vanhoutte, P.M., pp. 173–9. Amsterdam: Harwood Academic.

Ghosh, S., Gachhui, R., Crooks, C., Wu, C., Lisanti, M. & Stuehr, D.J. (1998). Interaction between caveolin-1 and the reductase domain of endothelial nitric oxide synthase. Consequences for catalysis. *J. Biol. Chem.*, **273**, 22267–71.

Girerd, X.J., Hirsch, A.T., Cooke, J.P., Dzau, V.J. & Creager, M.A. (1995). L-arginine augments endothelium-dependent vasodilatation in cholesterol-fed rabbits. *Circ. Res.*, **67**, 1301–8.

Giugliano, D., Marfella, R., Verrazzo, G. et al. (1997). The vascular effects of L-arginine in humans. The role of endogenous insulin. *J. Clin. Invest.*, **99**, 433–8.

Godecke, A., Decking, U.K.M., Ding, Z. et al. (1998). Coronary hemodynamics in endothelial NO synthase knockout mice. *Circ. Res.*, **82**, 186–94.

Gokce, N., Keaney, J.F. Jr, Frei, B. et al. (1999). Long-trem ascorbic acid administration reverses endothelial vasomotor dysfunction in patients with coronary artery diasese. *Circulation*, **99**, 3234–40.

Goonasekera, C.D.A., Rees, D.D., Woolard, P. et al. (1997). Nitric oxide synthase inhibitors and hypertension in children and adolescents. *J. Hypertens.*, **15**, 901–9.

Greenlees, C., Wadsworth, R.M., Martorana, P.A. & Wainwright, C.L. (1997). The effects of

L-arginine on neointimal formation and vascular function following balloon injury in inheritable hyperlipidaemic rabbits. *Cardiovasc. Res.*, **35**, 351–9.

Gregg, A.R., Schauer, A., Shi, O. et al. (1998). Limb reduction defects in endothelial nitric oxide synthase-deficient mice. *Am. J. Physiol.*, **275**, H2319–24.

Griffith, O. & Gross, S.S. (1996). Inhibitors of nitric oxide synthases. In: *Methods in Nitric Oxide Research*, ed. Feelisch, M. & Stamler, J.S., pp. 187–208. New York: John Wiley.

Gruetter, C.A., Gruetter, D.Y., Lyon, J.E., Kadowitz, P.J. & Ignarro, J. (1981). Relationship between cyclic guanosine 3':5'-monophosphate formation and relaxation of coronary arterial smooth muscle by glyceryl trinitrate, nitroprusside, nitrite and nitric oxide: effects of methylene blue and methemoglobin. *J. Pharmacol. Exp. Ther.*, **219**, 181–6.

Gryglewski, R.J., Palmer, R.M.J. & Moncada, S. (1986). Superoxide ion is involved in the breakdown of endothelium-derived vascular relaxing factor. *Nature*, **320**, 454–6.

Gunnett, C.A., Chu, Y., Heistad, D.D., Loihl, A. & Faraci, F.M. (1998). Vascular effects of LPS in mice deficient in expression of the gene for inducible nitric oxide synthase. *Am. J. Physiol.*, **275**, H416–21.

Guo, F.H., De Raeve, H.R., Rice T.W. et al. (1995). Continuous nitric oxide synthesis by inducible nitric oxide synthase in normal human airway epithelium in vivo. *Proc. Natl Acad. Sci. U.S.A.*, **92**, 7809–13.

Haynes, W., Noon, J., Walker, B. & Webb, D. (1993). Inhibition of nitric oxide synthesis increases blood pressure in healthy humans. *J. Hypertens.*, **11**, 1375–80.

Heitzer, T., Just, H. & Munzel, T. (1996). Antioxidant vitamin C improves endothelial dysfunction in chronic smoker. *Circulation*, **94**, 6–9.

Heitzer, T., Brockhoff, P., Mayer, B. et al. (2000). Tetrahydrobiopterin improves endothelium-dependent vasodilation in chronic smokers. *Circ. Res.*, **86**, e36.

Helmlinger, G., Berk, B.C. & Nerem, R.M. (1995). Calcium responses of endothelial cell monolayers subjected to pulsatile and steady laminar flow differ. *Am. J. Physiol.*, **269**, C367–75.

Herlitz, H., Petersson, A., Sigstrom, L., Wennmalm, A. & Westberg, G. (1997). The arginine-nitric oxide pathway in thrombotic microandiopathy. *Scand. J. Urol. Nephrol.*, **31**, 477–9.

Hibbs, J.B. Jr, Westenfelder, C., Tainer, R. et al. (1992). Evidence for cytokine-inducible nitric oxide synthesis from L-arginine in patients receiving interleukin-2 therapy. *J. Clin. Invest.*, **89**, 867–77.

Hibi, K., Ishigami, T., Tamura, K. et al. (1998). Endothelial nitric oxide synthase gene polymorphism and acute myocardial infarction. *Hypertension*, **32**, 521–6.

Hingorani, A.D., Liang, C.F., Fatibene, J. et al. (1999). A common variant of the endothelial nitric oxide synthase (Glu298 → Asp) is a major risk factor for coronary artery disease in the UK. *Circulation*, **100**, 1515–20.

Hiramatsu, K. (1988). Increased superoxide production by mononuclear cells of patients with hypertriglyceridaemia and diabetes. *Diabetes*, **37**, 832–7.

Hirooka, Y., Imaizumi, T., Masaki, H. et al. (1992). Captopril improves impaired endothelium-dependent vasodilation in hypertensive patients. *Hypertension*, **20**, 175–80.

Hishikawa, K., Nakaki, T., Suzuki, H., Kato, R. & Saruta, T. (1992). L-arginine as an antihypertensive agent. *J. Cardiovasc. Pharmacol.*, **20** (Suppl. 12), S196–7.

Hogg, N., Kalyanaraman, B., Joseph, J., Struck, A. & Parthasarathy, S. (1993). Inhibition of low-density lipoprotein oxidation by nitric oxide. Potential role in atherogenesis. *FEBS Lett.*, **334**, 170–4.

Hollenberg, S.M., Easington, C.R., Osman, J., Broussard, M. & Parrillo, J.E. (1999). Effects of nitric oxide synthase inhibition on microvascular reactivity in septic mice. *Shock*, **12**, 262–7.

Hornig, B., Arakawa, N., Kohler, C. & Drexler, H. (1998). Vitamin C improves endothelial function of conduit arteries in patients with chronic heart failure. *Circulation*, **97**, 363–8.

Huang, Z., Huang, P.L., Panahian, N. et al. (1994). Effects of cerebral ischaemia in mice deficient in neuronal nitric oxide synthase. *Science*, **265**, 1883–5.

Huang, P.L., Huang, Z., Mashimo, H. et al. (1995). Hypertension in mice lacking the gene for endothelial nitric oxide synthase. *Nature*, **377**, 239–42.

Hussain, M.B., Hobbs, A.J. & MacAllister, R.J. (1999). Autoregulation of nitric oxide-soluble guanylate cyclase-cyclic GMP signalling in mouse thoracic aorta. *Br. J. Pharmacol.*, **128**, 1082–8.

Hutcheson, I.R., Chaytor, A.T., Howard Evans, W. & Griffith, T.M. (1999). Nitric oxide-independent relaxations to acetylcholine and A23187 involve different routes of heterocellular communication: role of gap junctions and phospholipase A$_2$. *Circ. Res.*, **84**, 53–63.

Huvers, F.C., De Leeuw, P.W., Houben, A.J.H.M. et al. (1999). Endothelium-dependent vasodilatation, plasma markers of endothelial function, and adrenergic vasoconstrictor responses in type 1 diabetes under near-normoglycemic conditions. *Diabetes*, **47**, 1300–7.

Ignarro, L.J., Burke, T.M., Wood, K.S., Wolin, M.S. & Kadowitz, P.J. (1984). Association between cyclic GMP accumulation and acetylcholine-elicited relaxation of bovine intrapulmonary artery. *J. Pharmacol. Exp. Ther.*, **288**, 682–90.

Ignarro, L.J., Buga, G.M., Wood, K.S., Byrns, R.E. & Chaudhuri, G. (1987). Endothelium-derived relaxing factor produced and released from artery and vein is nitric oxide. *Proc. Natl Acad. Sci. U.S.A.*, **84**, 9265–9.

Ignarro, L.J., Byrns, R.E. & Wood, K.S. (1988). Biochemical and pharmacological properties of endothelium-derived relaxing factor and its similarity to nitric oxide redical. In *Vasodilatation: Vascular Smooth Muscle, Peptides, Autonomic Nerves and Endothelium*, ed. Vanhoutte, P.M., pp. 401–14. New York: Raven.

Irikura, K., Huang, P.L., Ma, J. et al. (1995). Cerebrovascular alterations in mice lacking neuronal nitric oxide synthase gene expression. *Proc. Natl Acad. Sci. U.S.A.*, **92**, 6823–7.

Janssens, S., Flaherty, D., Nong, Z. et al. (1998). Human endothelial nitric oxide gene transfer inhibits vascular smooth muscle cell proliferation and neointima formation after balloon injury in rats. *Circulation*, **97**, 1274–81.

Johannigman, J.A., Davis, K. Jr, Campbell, R.S. et al. (1997). Inhaled nitric oxide in acute respiratory distress syndrome. *J. Trauma*, **43**, 904–9.

John, S., Schlaich, M., Langenfeld, M. et al. (1998). Increased bioavailability of nitric oxide after lipid-lowering therapy in hypercholesterolemic patients. *Circulation*, **98**, 211–16.

Johnstone, M.T., Creager, S.J., Scales, K.M. et al. (1993). Impaired endothelium-dependent vasodilation in patients with insulin-dependent diabetes mellitus. *Circulation*, **88**, 2510–16.

Jovanovic, A., Grbovic, L. & Tulic, I. (1994). Predominant role for nitric oxide in the relaxation induced by acetylcholine in human uterine artery. *Hum. Reprod.*, **9**, 387–93.

Katz, S.D., Schwartz, M., Yuen, J. & LeJemtel, T.H. (1993). Impaired acetylcholine-mediated vasodilation in patients with congestive heart failure. Role of endothelium-derived vasodilating and vasoconstricting factors. *Circulation*, **88**, 55–61.

Kauser, K., Stekiel, W.J., Rubanyi, G.M. & Harder, D.R. (1989). Mechanism of action of EDRF on pressurized arteries. Effect on K^+ conductance. *Circ. Res.*, **65**, 199–204.

Kelly, J.J., Tam, S.H., Williamson, P.M., Lawson, J. & Whitworth, J.A. (1998). The nitric oxide system and cortisol-induced hypertension in humans. *Clin. Exp. Pharmacol. Physiol.*, **25**, 945–6.

Khan, B.V., Harrison, D.G., Olbrych, M.T., Alexander, R.W. & Medford, R.M. (1996). Nitric oxide regulates vascular cell adhesion molecule 1 gene expression and redox-sensitive transcriptional events in human vascular endothelial cells. *Proc. Natl Acad. Sci. U.S.A.*, **93**, 9114–19.

Kibbe, M., Billiar, T. & Tzeng, E. (1999). Nitric oxide synthase gene transfer to the vessel wall. *Curr. Opin. Nephrol. Hypertens.*, **8**, 75–81.

Kilbourn, R.G., Jubran, A., Gross, S.S. et al. (1990). Reversal of endotoxin-mediated shock by N^G-methyl-L-arginine, an inhibitor of nitric oxide synthesis. *Biochem. Biophys. Res. Commun.*, **172**, 1132–8.

Kimoto, M., Sasakawa, T., Tsuji, H. et al. (1997). Cloning and sequencing of cDNA encoding N^G,N^G dimethylarginine dimethylaminohydrolase from rat kidney. *Biochem. Biophys. Acta.*, **1337**, 6–10.

Kinsella, J.P., Neish, S.R., Shaffer, E. & Abman, S.H. (1992). Low-dose inhaled nitric oxide in persistent pulmonary hypertension of the newborn. *Lancet*, **340**, 436–40.

Kiowski, W., Sutsch, G., Schalcher, C., Brunner, H.P. & Oechslin, E. (1998). Endothelial control of vascular tone in chronic heart failure. *J. Cardiovasc. Pharmacol.*, **32** (suppl. 3), S67–73.

Knowles, R.G. & Moncada, S. (1992). Nitric oxide as a signal in blood vessels. *Trends Biochem. Sci.*, **17**, 399–402.

Kobayashi, A., Hashimoto, S., Kooguchi, K. et al. (1998). Expression of inducible nitric oxide synthase and inflammatory cytokines in alveolar macrophages of ARDS following sepsis. *Chest*, **113**, 1632–9.

Kojda, G., Laursen, J.B., Ramasamy, S. et al. (1999). Protein expression, vascular reactivity and soluable guanylate cyclase activity in mice lacking the endothelial cell nitric oxide synthase: contribution of NOS isoforms to blood pressure and heart rate control. *Cardiovasc. Res.*, **42**, 206–13.

Konishi, M. & Su, C. (1983). Role of endothelium in dilator responses of spontaneously hypertensive rat arteries. *Hypertension*, **5**, 881–6.

Kubes, P., Suzuki, M. & Ganger, D.N. (1991). Nitric oxide: an endogenous modulator of leukocyte adhesion. *Proc. Natl Acad. Sci. U.S.A.*, **88**, 4651–5.

Kuchan, M.J. & Frangos, J.A. (1994). Role of calcium and calmodulin in flow-induced nitric oxide production in endothelial cells. *Am. J. Physiol.*, **266**, C628–36.

Kushi, L.H., Folsom, A.R., Prineas, R.J. et al. (1996). Dietary antioxidant vitamins and death from coronary heart disease in postmenopausal women. *N. Engl. J. Med.*, **334**, 1156–62.

Lake-Bruse, K.D., Faraci, F.M., Shesely, E.G. et al. (1999). Gene transfer of endothelial nitric oxide synthase (eNOS) in eNOS-deficient mice. *Am. J. Physiol.*, **277**, H770–6.

Langford, E.J., Brown, A.S., Wainwright, R.J. et al. (1994). Inhibition of platelet activity by S-nitrosoglutathione during coronary angioplasty. *Lancet*, **344**, 1458–60.

Laubach, V.E., Shesely, E.G., Smithies, O. & Sherman, P.A. (1995). Mice lacking inducible nitric oxide synthase are not resistant to lipopolysaccharide-induced death. *Proc. Natl Acad. Sci. U.S.A.*, **92**, 10688–92.

Lawrie, G.M., Weilbacher, D.E. & Henry, P.D. (1990). Endothelium-dependent relaxation in human saphenous vein grafts. Effects of preparation and clinicopathologic correlations. *J. Thorac. Cardiovasc. Surg.*, **100**, 612–20.

Lefroy, D.C., Crake, T., Uren, N.G., Davies, G.J. & Maseri, A. (1993). Effect of inhibition of nitric oxide synthesis on epicardial coronary artery caliber and coronary blood flow in humans. *Circulation*, **88**, 43–54.

Leiper, J.M. & Vallance, P. (1999). Biological significance of endogenous methylarginines that inhibit nitric oxide synthases. *Cardiovasc. Res.*, **43**, 542–8.

Leiper, J.M., Santa Maria, J., Chubb, A. et al. (1999). Identification of two human dimethylarginine dimethylaminohydrolases with distinct tissue distributions and homology with microbial arginine deiminases. *Biochem. J.*, **343**, 209–14.

Levine, G.N., Frei, B., Koulouris, S.N. et al. (1996). Ascorbic acid reverses endothelial vasomotor dysfunction in patients with coronary artery disease. *Circulation*, **93**, 1107–13.

Lewis, D.A., Rud, K.S. & Miller, V.M. (1993). Cofactors of constitutive nitric oxide synthase and endothelium-derived relaxations in canine femoral veins. *J. Cardiovasc. Pharmacol.*, **22**, 443–8.

Li, G., Regunathan, S., Barrow, C.J. et al. (1994). Agmatine: an endogenous clonidine-displacing substance in the brain. *Science*, **263**, 966–9.

Liao, Y.L., Saku, K., Ou, J. et al. (1999). A missense mutation of the nitric oxide synthase (eNOS) gene (Glu298Asp) in five patients with coronary artery disease – case reports. *Angiology*, **50**, 671–6.

Lin, K.F., Chao, L. & Chao, J. (1997). Prolonged reduction of high blood pressure with human nitric oxide synthase gene delivery. *Hypertension*, **30**, 307–13.

Lodato, R.F., Feig, B., Akimaru, K., Soma, G. & Klostergaard, J. (1995). Hemodynamic evaluation of recombinant human tumour necrosis factor (TNF)-alpha, TNF-SAM2 and liposomal TNF-SAM2 in an anaesthetized dog model. *J. Immunother. Emphasis Tumor Immunol.*, **17**, 19–29.

Ludmer, P., Selwyn, A., Shook, T.L. et al. (1986). Paradoxical vasoconstriction induced by acetylcholine in atherosclerotic coronary arteries. *N. Engl. J. Med.*, **315**, 1046–51.

Luscher, T.F. & Vanhoutte, P.M. (1986). Endothelium-dependent contractions to acetylcholine in the aorta of the spontaneously hypertensive rat. *Hypertension*, **8**, 344–8.

Luscher, T.F. & Vanhoutte, P.M. (1989). *The Endothelium: Modulator of Cardiovascular Function*. Boca Raton: CRC Press.

Lyons, D., Roy, S., Patel, M., Benjamin, N. & Swift, C.G. (1997). Impaired nitric oxide-mediated vasodilatation and total body nitric oxide production in healthy old age. *Clin. Sci.*, **93**, 519–25.

Macallan, D.C., Smith, L.M., Ferber, J. et al. (1997). Measurement of NO synthesis in human by L-[15N2]arginine: application to the response to vaccination. *Am. J. Physiol.*, **272**, R1888–96.

MacAllister, R.J., Calver, A.L., Collier, J. et al. (1995a). Vascular and hormonal responses to arginine: provision of substrate for nitric oxide or non-specific effects? *Clin. Sci. (Colch.)*, **89**,

183–90.

MacAllister, R.J., Calver, A.L., Riezebos, J., Collier. J. & Vallance, P. (1995b). Relative potency and arteriovenous selectivity of nitrovasodilators on human blood vessels: an insight into the targeting of nitric oxide delivery. *J. Pharmacol. Exp. Ther.*, **273**, 154–60.

MacAllister, R., Parry, H., Kimoto, M. et al. (1996). Regulation of nitric oxide synthesis by dimethylarginine dimethylaminohydrolase. *Br. J. Pharmacol.*, **119**, 1533–40.

MacMicking, J.D., Nathan, C., Hom, G. et al. (1995). Altered responses to bacterial infection and endotoxic shock in mice lacking inducible nitric oxide synthase. *Cell*, **81**, 641–50.

Maguire, S.M., Nugent, A.G., McGurk, C., Johnston, G.D. & Nicholls, D.P. (1998). Abnormal vascular responses in human chronic cardiac failure is both endothelium dependent and endothelium independent. *Heart*, **80**, 141–5.

Makimattila, S., Mantysaari, M., Groop, P.-H. et al. (1997). Hyperreactivity to nitrovasodilators in forearm vasculature is related to autonomic dysfunction in insulin-dependent diabetes mellitus. *Circulation*, **95**, 618–25.

Malinski, T., Radomski, M.W., Taha, Z. & Moncada, S. (1993). Direct electrochemical measurement of nitric oxide released from human platelets. *Biochem. Biophys. Res. Commun.*, **194**, 960–5.

Markus, H.S., Ruigrok, Y., Ali, N. & Powell, J.F. (1998). Endothelial nitric oxide synthase exon 7 polymorphism, ischaemic cerebrovascular disease, and carotid atheroma. *Stroke*, **29**, 1908–11.

Martin, G.R., Bolofo, M.L. & Giles, H. (1992). Inhibition of endothelium-dependent vasorelaxation by arginine analogues: a pharmacological analysis of agonist and tissue dependence. *Br. J. Pharmacol.*, **105**, 643–52.

Masuda, H., Goto, M., Tamaoki, S. & Azuma, H. (1999). Accelerated intimal hyperplasia and increased endogenous inhibitors for NO synthesis in rabbits with alloxan-induced hyperglycaemia. *Br. J. Pharmacol.*, **126**, 211–18.

Matsumoto, T., Komori, K., Yonemitsu, Y. et al. (1998). Hemagglutinating virus of Japan-liposome-mediated gene transfer of endothelial nitric oxide synthase inhibits intimal hyperplasia of canine vein grafts under conditions of poor runoff. *J. Vasc. Surg.*, **27**, 135–44.

Matsuoka, H., Itoh, S., Kimoto, M. et al. (1997). Asymmetrical dimethylarginine, an endogenous nitric oxide synthase inhibitor, in experimental hypertension. *Hypertension*, **29**, 242–7.

McDonald, K.K., Zharikov, S., Block, E.R. & Kilberg, M.S. (1997). A caveolar complex between the cationic aminoacid transport 1 and endothelial nitric-oxide synthase may explain the 'arginine paradox'. *J. Biol. Chem.*, **272**, 31213–16.

McNamara, D.B., Bedi, B., Aurora, H. et al. (1993). L-arginine inhibits balloon catheter-induced intimal hyperplasia. *Biochem. Biophys. Res. Commun.*, **193**, 291–6.

Meeking, D.R., Allard, S., Munday, J. et al. (2000). Comparison of vasodilator effects of substance P in human forearm vessels of normoalbuminuric type 1 diabetic and non-diabetic subjects. *Diab. Med.*, **17**, 243–6.

Mehta, S., Stewart, D.J., Langleben, D. & Levy, R.D. (1995). Short-term pulmonary vasodilatation with L-arginine in pulmonary hypertension. *Circulation*, **92**, 1539–45.

Meng, W., Ayata, C., Waeber, C., Haung, P.L. & Moskowitz, M.A. (1998). Neuronal NOS-cGMP-dependent ACh-induced relaxation in pial arterioles of endothelial NOS knockout mice. *Am. J. Physiol.*, **274**, H411–15.

Michel, T., Li, G.K. & Busconi, L. (1993). Phosphorylation and subcellular translocation of endothelial nitric oxide synthase. *Proc. Natl Acad. Sci. U.S.A.*, **90**, 6252–6.

Michel, J.B., Feron, O., Sacks, D. & Michel, T. (1997). Reciprocal regulation of endothelial nitric-oxide synthase by calcium-calmodulin and caveolin. *J. Biol. Chem.*, **272**, 15583–6.

Millgard, J. & Lind, L. (1998). Acute hypertension impairs endothelium-dependent vasodilatation. *Clin. Sci.*, **94**, 601–7.

Minor, R.L., Myers, P.R., Guerra, R.J., Bates, J.N. & Harrison, D.G. (1990). Diet-induced atherosclerosis increases the release of nitrogen oxides from rabbit aorta. *J. Clin. Invest.*, **86**, 2109–16.

Mitaka, C., Hirata, Y., Ichikawa, K. et al. (1994). Effects of TNF-alpha on hemodynamic changes and circulating endothelium-derived vasoactive factors in dogs. *Am. J. Physiol.*, **267**, H1530–6.

Miyamoto, Y., Saito, Y., Kajiyama, N. et al. (1998). Endothelial nitric oxide synthase gene is positively associated with essential hypertension. *Hypertension*, **32**, 3–8.

Miyazaki, H., Matsuoka, H., Cooke, J.P. et al. (1999). Endogenous nitric oxide synthase inhibitor – a novel marker of atherosclerosis. *Circulation*, **99**, 1141–6.

Moncada, S. (1992). The L-arginine:nitric oxide pathway. *Acta Physiol. Scand.*, **145**, 201–27.

Moncada, S. & Higgs, E.A. (1993). The L-arginine-nitric oxide pathway. *N. Engl. J. Med.*, **329**, 2002–12.

Moncada, S. & Higgs, E.A. (1995). Molecular mechanisms and therapeutic strategies related to nitric oxide. *FASEB J.*, **9**, 1319–30.

Mugge, A., Elwell, J.H., Peterson, T.E, et al. (1991). Chronic treatment with polyethyleneglycolated superoxide dismutase partially restores endothelium-dependent vascular relaxations in cholesterol-fed rabbits. *Circ. Res.*, **69**, 1293–300.

Myers, P.R., Parker, J.L., Tanner, M.A. & Adams, H.R. (1994). Effects of cytokines tumour necrosis factor alpha and interleukin 1 beta on endotoxin-mediated inhibition of endothelium-derived relaxing factor bioactivity and nitric oxide production in vascular endothelium. *Shock*, **1**, 73–8.

Nadaud, S., Bonnardeaux, A., Lathrop, M. & Soubrier, F. (1994). Gene structure, polymorphism and mapping of the human endothelial nitric oxide synthase gene. *Biochem. Biophys. Res. Commun.*, **198**, 1027–33.

Nagy, J., Demaster, E.G., Wittmann, I., Shultz, P. & Raij, L. (1997). Induction of endothelial cell injury by cigarette smoke. *Endothelium*, **5**, 251–63.

Najibi, S., Cowan, C.L., Palacino, J.J. & Cohen, R.A. (1994). Enhanced role of potassium channels in relaxations to acetylcholine in hypercholesterolemic rabbit carotid artery. *Am. J. Physiol.*, **266**, H2061–7.

Nakaki, T., Nakayama, M. & Kato, R. (1990). Inhibition by nitric oxide and nitric oxide-producing vasodilators of DNA synthesis in vascular smooth muscle cells. *Eur. J. Pharmacol.*, **189**, 347–53.

Nakamura, M., Ishikawa, M., Funakoshi, T. et al. (1994a). Attenuated endothelium-dependent peripheral vasodilation and clinical characteristics in patients with chronic heart failure. *Am.*

Heart J., **128**, 1164–9.

Nakamura, M., Funakoshi, T., Arakawa, N. et al. (1994b). Effect of angiotensin-converting enzyme inhibitors on endothelium-dependent peripheral vasodilation in patients with chronic heart failure. *J. Am. Coll. Cardiol.*, **24**, 1321–7.

Nakayama, M., Yasue, H., Yoshimura, M. et al. (1999). T-786 → C mutation in the 5'-flanking region of the endothelial nitric oxide synthase gene is associated with coronary spasm. *Circulation*, **99**, 2864–70.

Naruse, K., Shimizu, K., Muramatsu, M. et al. (1994). Long-term inhibition of NO synthesis promotes atherosclerosis in the hyperchoolesrterolemic rabbit thoracic aorta. *Arterioscler. Thromb.*, **14**, 746–52.

Nava, E., Palmer, R.M.J. & Moncada, S. (1991). Inhibition of nitric oxide synthesis in septic shock: how much is beneficial? *Lancet*, **338**, 1555–7.

Neunteufl, T., Katzenschlager, R., Hassan, A. et al. (1997). Systemic endothelial dysfunction is related to the extent and severity of coronary artery disease. *Atherosclerosis*, **129**, 111–18.

O'Driscoll, G., Green, D., Rankin, J., Stanton, K. & Taylor, R. (1997). Improvement in endothelial function by angiotensin converting enzyme inhibition in insulin-dependent diabetes mellitus. *J. Clin. Invest.*, **100**, 678–84.

Ohno, M., Cooke, J.P., Dzau, V.J. & Gibbons, G.H. (1995). Fluid shear stress induces endothelial transforming growth factor beta-1 transcription and production. Modulation by potassium channel blockade. *J. Clin. Invest.*, **95**, 1363–9.

Olesen, S.P., Clapham, D.E. & Davies, P.F. (1988). Haemodynamic shear stress activates a K^+ current in vascular endothelial cells. *Nature*, **331**, 168–70.

Palmer, R.M.J., Ferrige, A.G. & Moncada, S. (1987). Nitric oxide release accounts for the biological activity of endothelial-derived relaxing factor. *Nature*, **327**, 524–6.

Palmer, R.M.J., Ashton, D.S. & Moncada, S. (1988). Vascular endothelial cells synthesize nitric oxide from L-arginine. *Nature*, **333**, 664–6.

Panza, J.A., Casino, P.R., Kilcoyne, C.M. & Quyyumi, A.A. (1993a). Role of endothelium-derived nitric oxide in the abnormal endothelium-dependent vascular relaxation of patients with essential hypertension. *Circulation*, **87**, 1468–74.

Panza, J.A., Casino, P.R., Badar, D.M. & Quyyumi, A.A. (1993b). Effect of increased availability of endothelium-derived nitric oxide precursor on endothelium-dependent vascular relaxation in normal subjects and in patients with essential hypertension. *Circulation*, **87**, 1475–81.

Panza, J.A., Quyyumi, A.A., Callahan, T.S. & Epstein, S.E. (1993c). Effect of antihypertensive treatment on endothelium-dependent vascular relaxation in patients with essential hypertension. *J. Am. Coll. Cardiol.*, **21**, 1145–51.

Penny, W.F., Rockman, H., Long. J. et al. (1995). Heterogenicity of vasomotor response to acetylcholine along the human coronary artery. *J. Am. Coll. Cardiol.*, **25**, 1046–55.

Pepke-Zaba, J., Higenbottam, T.W., Dinh-Xuan, A.T., Stone, D. & Wallwork, J. (1991). Inhaled nitric oxide as a cause of selective pulmonary vasodilatation in pulmonary hypertension. *Lancet*, **338**, 1173–4.

Peterson, D.A., Peterson, D.C., Archer, S. & Weir, E.K. (1992). The non specificity of specific nitric oxide synthase inhibitors. *Biochem. Biophys. Res. Commun.*, **187**, 797–801.

Petrinelli, R., Ebel, M., Catapano, G. et al. (1995). Pressor, renal and endocrine effects of

L-arginine in essential hypertensives. *Eur. J. Clin. Pharmacol.*, **48**, 195–201.

Petros, A., Bennett, D. & Vallance, P. (1991). Effects of nitric oxide synthase inhibitors on hypotension in patients with septic shock. *Lancet*, **338**, 1557–8.

Petros, A., Lamb, G., Leone, A. et al. (1994). Effects of a nitric oxide synthase inhibitor in humans with septic shock. *Cardiovasc Res*, **28**, 34–9.

Pitt, B., Zannad, F., Remme, W.J. et al. (1999). The effect of spironolactone on morbidity and mortality in patients with severe heart failure. Randomized aldactone evaluation study investigators. *N. Engl. J. Med.*, **341**, 709–17.

Pronai, L., Hiramatsu, K., Saiusa, Y. & Nakazawa, H. (1991). Low superoxide scavenging activity associated with enhanced superoxide generation by monocytes from male hypertriglycaemics with and without diabetes. *Atherosclerosis*, **90**, 39–47.

Quyyumi, A.A., Dakak, N., Andrews, N.P. et al. (1995). Contribution of nitric oxide to metabolic coronary vasodilation in the human heart. *Circulation*, **92**, 320–6.

Radi, R., Rodriguez, M., Castro, L. & Telleri, R. (1994). Inhibition of mitochondrial electron transport by peroxynitrite. *Arch. Biochem. Biophys.*, **308**, 89–95.

Radomski, M.W., Palmer, R.M. & Moncada, S. (1987). Endogenous nitric oxide inhibits human platelet adhesion to vascular endothelium. *Lancet*, **2**, 1057–8.

Radomski, M.W., Palmer, R.M. & Moncada, S. (1990). Characterization of the L-arginine:nitric oxide pathway in human platelets. *Br. J. Pharmacol.*, **101**, 325–8.

Ramsey, B., Radomski, M., de Belder, A., Martin, J.F. & Lopez-Jaramillo, P. (1995). Systemic effects of *S*-nitro-glutathione in the human following intravenous infusion. *Br. J. Clin. Pharmacol.*, **40**, 101–2.

Rees, D.D., Palmer, R.M., Hodson, H.F. & Moncada, S. (1989a). A specific inhibitor of nitric oxide formation from L-arginine attenuates endothelium-dependent relaxation. *Br. J. Pharmacol.*, **96**, 418–24.

Rees, D.D., Palmer, R.M. & Moncada, S. (1989b). Role of endothelium-derived nitric oxide in the regulation of blood pressure. *Proc. Natl Acad. Sci. U.S.A.*, **86**, 3375–8.

Rees, D.D., Monkhouse, J.E., Cambridge, D. & Moncada, S. (1998). Nitric oxide and the haemodynamic profile of endotoxin shock conscious mouse. *Br. J. Pharmacol.*, **124**, 540–6.

Resnick, N., Yahav, H., Schubert, S., Wolfovitz, E. & Shay, A. (2000). Signalling pathways in vascular endothelium activated by shear stress: relevance to atherosclerosis. *Curr. Opin. Lipidol.*, **11**, 167–77.

Rimm, E.B., Stampfer, M.J., Ascherio, A. et al. (1993). Vitamin E consumption and the risk of coronary heart disease in men. *N. Engl. J. Med.*, **328**, 1450–6.

Robertson, F.M., Offner, P.J., Ciceri, D.P., Becher, W.K. & Pruitt, B.A. Jr. (1994). Detrimental hemodynamic effects of nitric oxide synthase inhibition in septic shock. *Arch. Surg.*, **129**, 149–55.

Robinson, L.J. & Michel, T. (1995). Mutagenesis of palmitoylation sites in endothelial nitric oxide synthase identifies a novel motif for dual acylation and subcellular targeting. *Proc. Natl Acad. Sci. U.S.A.*, **92**, 11776–80.

Rosenkranz Weiss, P., Sessa, W.C., Milstien, S. et al. (1994). Regulation of nitric oxide synthesis by proinflammatory cytokines in human umbilical vein endothelial cells. Elevations in tetrahydrobiopterin levels enhance endothelial nitric oxide synthase specific activity. *J. Clin.*

Invest., **93**, 2236–43.

Rosolowsky, M., Falck, J.R., Willerson, J.T. & Campbell, W.B. (1990). Synthesis of lipoxygenase and epoxygenase products of arachidonic acid by normal and stenosed canine coronary arteries. *Circ. Res.*, **66**, 608–21.

Rossaint, R., Falke, K.J., Lopez, F. et al. (1993). Inhaled nitric oxide for the adult respiratory distress syndrome. *N. Engl. J. Med.*, **328**, 399–405.

Salas, E., Langford, E.J., Marrinan, M.T. et al. (1998). S-nitrosoglutathione inhibits platelet activation and deposition in coronary artery saphenous vein grafts in vitro and in vivo. *Heart*, **80**, 146–50.

Sarkar, R., Meinberg, E.G., Stanley, J.C., Gordon, D. & Webb, R.C. (1996). Nitric oxide reversibly inhibits the migration of cultured vascular smooth muscle cells. *Circ. Res.*, **78**, 225–30.

Sattar, N., Petrie, J.R. & Jaap, A.J. (1998). The atherogenic lipoprotein phenotype and vascular endothelial dysfunction. *Atherosclerosis*, **138**, 229–35.

Schaffler, A., Arndt, H., Scholmerich, J. & Palitzsch, K. (1998). Acute hyperglycaemia causes severe disturbances of mesenteric microcirculation in an in vivo rat model. *Eur. J. Clin. Invest.*, **28**, 886–93.

Scherrer, U., Randin, D., Vollenweider, P., Vollenweider, L. & Nicod, P. (1994). Nitric oxide release accounts for insulin's vascular effects in humans. *J. Clin. Invest.*, **94**, 2511–15.

Schmidt, H.H.H.W., Nau, H., Wittfoht, W. et al. (1988). Arginine is a physiological precursor of endothelium-derived nitric oxide. *Eur. J. Pharmacol.*, **154**, 213–16.

Schoeffter, P., Dion, R. & Godfraind, T. (1988). Modulatory role of the vascular endothelium in the contractility of human isolated internal mammary artery. *Br. J. Pharmacol.*, **95**, 531–43.

Schulz, J.B., Huang, P.L., Matthews, R.T. et al. (1996). Striatal malonate lesions are attenuated in neuronal nitric oxide synthase knockout mice. *J. Neurochem.*, **67**, 430–3.

Scott-Burden, T. & Vanhoutte, P.M. (1993). The endothelium as a regulator of vascular smooth muscle proliferation. *Circulation*, **87** (Suppl. V), V51–5.

Shaul, P.W., Smart, E.J., Robinson, L.J. et al. (1996). Acylation targets endothelial nitric-oxide synthase to plasmalemmal caveolae. *J. Biol. Chem.*, **271**, 6518–22.

Shears, L.L., Kibbe, M.R., Murdock, A.D. et al. (1998). Efficient inhibition of intimal hyperplasia by adenovirus-mediated inducible nitric oxide synthase gene transfer to rats and pigs in vivo. *J. Am. Coll. Surg.*, **187**, 295–306.

Shesely, E.G., Maeda, N., Kim, H.S. et al. (1996). Elevated blood pressures in mice lacking endothelial nitric oxide synthase. *Proc. Natl Acad. Sci. U.S.A.*, **93**, 13176–81.

Shimasaki, Y., Yasue, H., Yoshimura, M. et al. (1998). Association of the missense Glu298Asp variant of the endothelial nitric oxide synthase gene with myocardial infarction. *J. Am. Coll. Cardiol.*, **31**, 1506–10.

Shimokawa, H, & Vanhoutte, P.M. (1989). Impaired endothelium-dependent relaxation to aggregating platelets and related vasoactive substances in porcine coronary arteries in hyper-cholesterolemia and atherosclerosis. *Circ. Res.*, **64**, 900–14.

Shimokawa, H., Yasutake, H., Fujii, K. et al. (1996). The importance of the hyperpolarizing mechanism increases as the vessel size decreases in endothelium-dependent relaxations in rat mesenteric circulation. *J. Cardiovasc. Pharmacol.*, **28**, 703–11.

Shinozaki, K., Kashiwagi, A., Nishio, Y. et al. (1999). Abnormal biopterin metabolism is a major cause of impaired endothelium-dependent relaxation through nitric oxide/O₂-imbalance in insulin-resistant rat aorta. *Diabetes*, **48**, 2437–45.

Smits, P., Kapma, J.-A., Jacobs, M.-C., Lutterman, J. & Thien, T. (1993). Endothelium-dependent vascular relaxation in patients with type 1 diabetes. *Diabetes*, **42**, 148–53.

Solzbach, U., Hornig, B., Jeserich, M. & Just, H. (1997). Vitamin C improves endothelial dysfunction of epicardial coronary arteries in hypertensive patients. *Circulation*, **96**, 1513–19.

Stamler, J.S., Loh, E., Roddy, M.A., Currie, K.E. & Creager, M.A. (1994). Nitric oxide regulates systemic and pulmonary vascular resistance in healthy humans. *Circulation*, **89**, 2035–40.

Stampfer, M.J., Hennekens, C.H., Manson, J.E. et al. (1993). Vitamin E consumption and the risk of coronary disease in women. *N. Engl. J. Med.*, **328**, 1444–9.

Steinberg, H.O., Brechtel, G., Johnson, A., Fineberg, N. & Baron, A.D. (1994). Insulin-mediated skeletal muscle vasodilation is nitric oxide dependent. A novel action of insulin to increase nitric oxide release. *J. Clin. Invest.*, **94**, 1172–9.

Steudel, W., Ichinose, F., Huang, P.L. et al. (1997). Pulmonary vasoconstriction and hypertension in mice with targeted disruption of the endothelial nitric oxide synthase (NOS 3) gene. *Circ. Res.*, **81**, 34–41.

Stroes, E., Kastelein, J., Cosentino, F. et al. (1997). Tetrahydrobiopterin restores endothelial function in hypercholesterolemia. *J. Clin. Invest.*, **99**, 41–6.

Suffredini, A.F., Fromm, R.E., Parker, M.M. et al. (1989). The cardiovascular response of normal humans to the administration of endotoxin. *N. Engl. J. Med.*, **321**, 280–7.

Sun, D., Huang, A., Smith, C.J. et al. (1999). Enhanced release of prostaglandins contributes to flow-induced arteriolar dilation in eNOS knockout mice. *Circ. Res.*, **85**, 288–93.

Taddei, S., Virdis, A., Mattei, P. & Salvetti, A. (1993). Vasodilation to acetylcholine in primary and secondary forms of human hypertension. *Hypertension*, **21**, 929–33.

Takahashi, M., Ikeda, U., Masuyama, J. et al. (1996). Nitric oxide attenuates adhesion molecule expression in human endothelial cells. *Cytokine*, **8**, 817–21.

Tesfamariam, B. & Cohen, R.A. (1992). Free radicals mediate endothelial cell dysfunction caused by elevated glucose. *Am. J. Physiol.*, **263**, H321–6.

Thom, S., Hughes, A., Martin, G. & Sever, P.S. (1987). Endothelium-dependent relaxation in isolated human arteries and veins. *Clin. Sci.*, **73**, 547–52.

Ting, H.H., Timimi, F.K., Boles, K.S. et al. (1996). Vitamin C improves endothelium-dependent vasodilatation in patients with non-insulin dependent diabetes mellitus. *J. Clin. Invest.*, **97**, 22–8.

Ting, H.H., Timimi, F.K., Haley, E.A. et al. (1997). Vitamin C improves endothelium-dependent vasodilatation in forearm resistance vessels of humans with hypercholesterolaemia. *Circulation*, **95**, 2617–22.

Tousoulis, D., Davies, G. & Toutouzas, P. (1999). Vitamin C increases nitric oxide availability in coronary atheroselerosis. *Ann. Intern. Med.*, **131**, 156–7.

Tsao, P.S., Theilmeier, G., Singer, A.H., Leung, L.L. & Cooke, J.P. (1994). L-arginine attenuates platelet reactivity in hypercholesterolemic rabbits. *Arterioscler. Thromb.*, **14**, 1529–33.

Tunctan, B., Uluda, O., Altu, S. & Abacio, N. (1998). Effects of nitric oxide synthase inhibition in lipopolysaccharide-induced sepsis in mice. *Pharmacol. Res.*, **38**, 405–11.

Ueda, S., Matsuoka, H., Miyazaki, H. et al. (2000). Tetrahydrobiopterin restores endothelial function in long-term smokers. *J. Am. Coll. Cardiol.*, **35**, 71–5.

Uematsu, M., Ohara, Y., Navas, J.P. et al. (1995). *Am. J. Physiol.*, **269**, C1371–8.

Vallance, P. (1999). Nitric oxide in human hypertension – up, down or unaffected? *Clin. Sci.*, **97**, 343–4.

Vallance, P., Collier, J. & Moncada, S. (1989a). Effects of endothelium-derived nitric oxide on peripheral arterial tone in man. *Lancet*, **ii**, 997–1000.

Vallance, P., Collier, J. & Moncada, S. (1989b). Nitric oxide synthesised from L-arginine mediates endothelium-dependent dilatation in human veins in vivo. *Cardiovasc. Res.*, **23**, 1053–7.

Vallance, P., Leone, A., Calver, A., Collier, J. & Moncada, S. (1992a). Endogenous dimethylarginine as an inhibitor of nitric oxide synthesis. *J. Cardiovasc. Pharmacol.*, **20** (Suppl. 12), S60–2.

Vallance, P., Leone, A., Calver, A., Collier, J. & Moncada, S. (1992b). Accumulation of an endogenous inhibitor of nitric oxide synthesis in chronic renal failure. *Lancet*, **339**, 572–5.

Vallance, P., Patton, S., Bhagat, K. et al. (1995). Direct measurement of nitric oxide in human beings. *Lancet*, **346**, 153–4.

Vanhoutte, P.M. (1974). Inhibition by acetylcholine of adrenergic neurotransmission in vascular smooth muscle. *Circ. Res.*, **34**, 317–26.

Varenne, O., Pislaru, S., Gillijns, H. et al. (1998). Local adenovirus-mediated transfer of human endothelial nitric oxide synthase reduces luminal narrowing after coronary angioplasty in pigs. *Circulation*, **98**, 919–26.

von der Leyden, H.E., Gibbons, G.H., Morishita, R. et al. (1995). Gene therapy inhibiting neointimal vascular lesion: in vivo transfer of endothelial cell nitric oxide synthase gene. *Proc. Natl Acad. Sci. U.S.A.*, **92**, 1137–41.

Waldron, G.J., Ding, H., Lovren, F., Kubes, P. & Triggle, C.R. (1999). Acetylcholine-induced relaxation of peripheral arteries isolated from mice lacking endothelial nitric oxide synthase. *Br. J. Pharmacol.*, **128**, 653–8.

Wang, Y. & Marsden, P.A. (1995). Nitric oxide synthases: biochemical and molecular regulation. *Curr. Opin. Nephrol. Hypertens.*, **4**, 12–22.

Wang, B.Y., Singer, A.H., Tsao, P.S. et al. (1994a). Dietary arginine prevents atherogenesis in the coronary artery of the hypercholesterolemic rabbit. *J. Am. Coll. Cardiol.*, **23**, 452–8.

Wang, P., Ba, Z.E. & Chaudry, I.H. (1994b). Administration of tumour necrosis factor-alpha in vivo depresses endothelium-dependent relaxation. *Am. J. Physiol.*, **266**, H2535–41.

Wang, X.L., Sim, A.S., Badenhop, R.F., McCredie, R.M. & Wilcken, D.E. (1996). A smoking-dependent risk of coronary artery disease associated with a polymorphism of the endothelial oxide synthase gene. *Nat. Med.*, **2**, 41–5.

Wang, X.L., Mahaney, M.C., Sim, A.S. et al. (1997). Genetic contribution of the endothelial constitutive nitric oxide synthase gene to plasma nitric oxide levels. *Arterioscler. Thromb. Vasc. Biol.*, **17**, 3147–53.

Wei, X.Q., Charles, I.G., Smith, A. et al. (1995). Altered immune responses in mice lacking inducible nitric oxide synthase. *Nature*, **375**, 408–11.

Weisbrod, R.M., Brown, M.L. & Cohen, R.A. (1993). Effect of elevated glucose on cyclic GMP and eicosanoids produced by porcine aortic endothelium. *Arterioscler. Thromb.*, **13**, 915–23.

Wennmalm, A., Benthin, G. & Petersson, A.-S. (1992). Dependence of metabolism of nitric oxide (NO) in healthy human whole blood on the oxygenation of its red cell haemoglobin. *Br. J. Pharmacol.*, **106**, 507–8.

Werns, S.W., Walton, J.A., Hsia, H.H. et al. (1989). Evidence of endothelial dysfunction in angiographically normal coronary arteries of patients with coronary artery disease. *Circulation*, **79**, 287–91.

Wheeler, M.A., Smith, S.D., Garcia-Gardena, G. et al. (1997). Bacterial infection induces nitric oxide synthase in human neutrophils. *J. Clin. Invest.*, **99**, 110–16.

White, R.P., Vallance, P., Deane, C. & Markus, H.S. (1997). Maintenance of human basal cerebral blood flow in nitric oxide dependent. In: *New Trends in Cerebral Hemodynamics*, ed. Klingelhofer, J. et al., pp. 1–5. London: Elsevier.

Whittle, B.J., Lopez-Belmonte, J. & Rees, D.D. (1989). Modulation of the vasodepressor actions of acetylcholine, bradykinin, substance P and endothelin in the rat by a specific inhibitor of nitric oxide formation. *Br. J. Pharmacol.*, **98**, 646–52.

Williams, S.B., Goldfine, A.B., Timimi, F.K. et al. (1998). Acute hyperglycaemia attenuates endothelium-dependent vasodilation in humans in vivo. *Circulation*, **97**, 1695–701.

Wolf, A., Zalpour, C., Theilmeier, G. et al. (1997). Dietary L-arginine supplementation normalizes platelet aggregation in hypercholesterolaemic humans. *J. Am. Coll. Cardiol.*, **29**, 479–85.

Wolfe, T.A. & Dasta, J.F. (1995). Use of nitric oxide synthase inhibitors as a novel treatment for septic shock. *Annu. Pharmacother.*, **29**, 36–46.

Wolin, M.S. (1996). Reactive oxygen species and vascular signal transduction mechanisms. *Microcirculation*, **3**, 1–17.

Wong, J.M. & Biliar, T.R. (1995). Regulation and function of inducible nitric oxide synthase during sepsis and acute inflammation. *Adv. Pharmacol.*, **34**, 155–70.

Wu, G. & Morris, S.M. Jr. (1998). Arginine metabolism: nitric oxide and beyond. *Biochem. J.*, **336**, 1–17.

Xu, W., Charles, I.G., Moncada, S. et al. (1994). Mapping of the genes encoding human inducible and endothelial nitric oxide synthase (NOS_2 and NOS_3) to the pericentric region of chromosome 17 and to chromosome 7, respectively. *Genomics*, **21**, 419–22.

Yang, Z., Von Segesser, L., Bauer, E. et al. (1991). Different activation of the endothelial-L-arginine and cyclooxygenase pathway in the human internal mammary artery and saphenous vein. *Circ. Res.*, **68**, 52–60.

Yasue, H., Matsuyama, K., Okumura, K., Morikami, Y. & Ogawa, H. (1990). Responses of angiographically normal human coronary arteries to intracoronary injection of acetylcholine by age and segment. Possible role of early coronary atherosclerosis. *Circulation*, **81**, 482–90.

Yoshida, H., Nakamura, M., Akatsu, T., Arakawa, N. & Hiramori, K. (1998). Effects of nitric oxide inhibition on basal forearm blood flow in patients with nonischaemic chronic heart failure. *Heart Vessels*, **13**, 142–6.

Yoshimura, M., Yasue, H., Nakayama, M. et al. (1998). A missense Glu298Asp variant in the endothelial nitric oxide synthase gene is associated with coronary spasm in the Japanese. *Hum. Genet.*, **103**, 65–9.

Yu, X.J., Li, Y.J. & Xiong, Y. (1994). Increase of an endogenous inhibitor of nitric oxide synthesis in serum of high cholesterol fed rabbits. *Life Sci*, **54**, 753–8.

Zeiher, A.M., Drexler, H., Wollschlager, H. & Just, H. (1991). Endothelial dysfunction of coronary microvasculature is associated with impaired coronary blood flow regulation in patients with early atherosclerosis. *Circulation*, **84**, 1984–92.

Zenere, B.M., Arcaro, G., Saggiani, F. et al. (1995). Noninvasive detection of functional alterations of the arterial wall in IDDM patients with and without microalbuminuria. *Diabetes Care*, **18**, 975–82.

Zoche, M., Beyermann, M. & Koch, K.W. (1997). Introduction of a phosphate at serine (741) of the calmodulin-binding domain of the neuronal nitric oxide synthase (NOS-I) prevents binding of calmodulin. *Biol Chem*, **378**, 851–7.

11

Magnetic resonance imaging in vascular biology

Alan R. Moody

Department of Academic Radiology, Queens Medical Centre, Nottingham

Introduction

For any individual the way in which his or her vascular system responds in health and disease is unique. The ability to visualize the normal and abnormal processes of vascular biology on an individual basis is therefore of paramount importance. It is clear that the vascular system is much more than a passive conduit for the transport of blood, so the means by which it is imaged must respond by providing information relevant to its function and dysfunction. The ideal imaging technique would be one that is noninvasive and repeatable, thus allowing longitudinal study without influencing the system under investigation. It should provide localized information about normal morphology and physiology as well as being able to detect early abnormalities and overt disease states. By so doing, imaging has the potential to reveal normal vascular biology within an individual at a specific anatomical site; provide a means by which early dysfunction can be detected, i.e. screening for disease; and be an accurate technique for the detection and characterization of established disease. Conventional imaging techniques have concentrated on visualizing the lumen of blood vessels, defining the resultant narrowing or occlusion brought about by disease. In an attempt to understand better the process of vascular disease it is necessary to visualize the site of disease and the interacting processes that occur there, and imaging techniques must respond to this challenge.

Imaging

Catheter angiography

Catheter angiography allows great access to the vascular system, providing detailed information regarding the lumen of vessels (Figure 11.1). Unfortunately, the

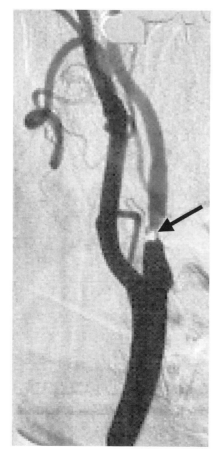

Figure 11.1 Conventional carotid angiography has high spatial resolution for defining tight stenoses (arrow).

technique is invasive, requiring vessel wall puncture and contrast injection, thus precluding practical longitudinal study requiring frequent repeated imaging. While the images provided are adequate for the detection of established vascular disease which results in luminal narrowing, the presence and extent of vessel wall disease can only be inferred from these studies as no direct visualization of the vessel wall itself is achieved. Physiological information with reference to blood flow is also not routinely available, though some estimate of the blood supply to endorgans can be obtained from imaging during the capillary phase of contrast enhancement.

CT scanning

A completely different approach to the visualization of vessels was achieved with the advent of cross-sectional imaging techniques. The greater contrast generated by computed tomography (CT) scanning, in combination with higher spatial

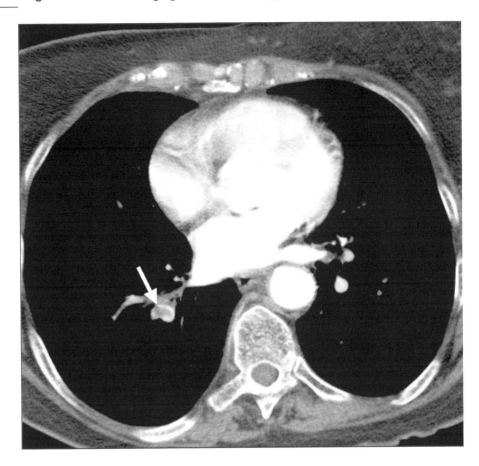

Figure 11.2   Contrast enhanced spiral computed tomography scan demonstrating a pulmonary embolus in the right lower-lobe artery (arrow).

resolution in three dimensions, has resulted in a technique that can visualize not only the vascular lumen but also the vessel wall itself. Rapid imaging techniques (spiral or volumetric scanning or multislice imaging) allow the acquisition of a large volume of data in a short (breath-hold) imaging time. This therefore overcomes movement artefact that occurs during more prolonged scanning but, importantly, also allows a compact, high-concentration bolus of contrast medium to be delivered during scanning, resulting in high vascular contrast (Rydberg et al., 2000; Figure 11.2).

CT scanning has the same fundamental contrast-generating capability as plain radiography, being dependent on the absorption of X-rays by the tissue under study. Tissue characterization is therefore limited. CT scanning is particularly good at detecting calcium. (Figure 11.3). Scoring the presence of calcium within the coronary arteries has been used as a surrogate marker of atherothrombotic

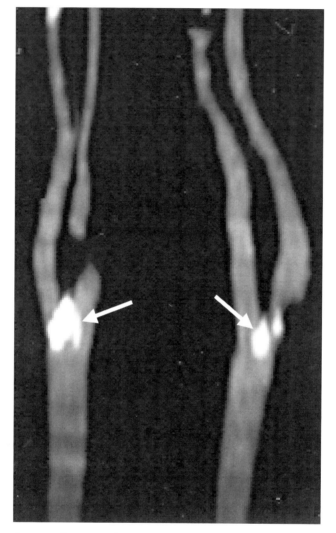

Figure 11.3 Computed tomography angiography of the carotid arteries is capable of defining calcific atheromatous plaque (arrows).

disease. It has been shown that those patients with high coronary artery calcium scores are prone to cardiac and, for that matter, other vascular events, such as stroke (Becker et al., 1999; Rabin et al., 2000). This technique therefore acts as a test of global vascular disease rather than identifying local at-risk regions within a single vascular bed. Being dependent on ionizing radiation for image generation, the technique is not ideal. The image acquisition plane is relatively fixed and postprocessing to produce angiographic-type effects can be lengthy; while calcium is easily detected on nonenhanced scans, the addition of contrast makes calcium identification difficult and may result in artefactual appearances.

Ultrasound scanning

Ultrasound scanning is a more versatile cross-sectional imaging technique that has many attractive features for the investigation of vascular biology. Images are dependent on the reflection of ultrasound waves from, and transmission through, tissues, providing an alternative means of generating tissue contrast. Of great benefit is the fact that image generation does not involve ionizing radiation and this is therefore a highly repeatable technique. The imaging plane is also completely variable, allowing optimal imaging conditions, though this degree of flexibility is also a disadvantage as the resultant image is often highly dependent upon the operator and interpretation of static images from complex investigations is often difficult by anyone other than the operator. One of the great disadvantages of ultrasound is its inability to gain access to various anatomical sites as a result of tissues and their contents (such as bone or gas). These do not allow the ultrasound beam to pass through, thus obscuring deeper structures. Superficial vessels are, however, accessible to ultrasound scanning and their superficial nature allows the use of high-resolution scanning techniques. The morphological information allows measurement of the vessel wall layers of larger-sized vessels providing a measure of abnormal thickening (intima media thickness). It has been shown that this measurement can also be used as a surrogate marker of more generalized vascular disease (Baldassarre et al., 2000). Because of its contrast-generating capabilities in association with high-resolution images, imaging of sites such as the carotid vessels is feasible such that characterization of individual lesions is possible. The application of ultrasound Doppler techniques also provides another essential element in the imaging of vascular biology – the detection and measurement of blood flow. Vessel wall abnormalities can then be investigated in conjunction with measurements of the resultant local blood flow. Measurement of changes in vessel diameter and blood flow also allows dynamic assessment of endothelial function in response to endogenous or exogenous nitric oxide and the effect of circulating substances on the vessel wall (Poredos et al., 1999).

Magnetic resonance imaging

The most recent addition to the armamentarium of imaging techniques to investigate vascular biology is magnetic resonance imaging (MRI). The first clinical use of MRI was largely confined to the neuroaxis and joints, body areas that could be immobilized for extended periods, which was necessary because of the prolonged imaging times. Imaging of vessels was largely ignored and signal generated from flowing blood was generally considered to be an artefact. With the advent of shorter acquisition times, imaging of areas of the body which were previously inaccessible to MRI, because of excessive physiological movement, such as the abdomen and chest, became feasible. The advantage of MRI lies in its lack of ionizing radiation and multiplanar imaging capability. Image contrast manipulation is far greater than with other simple 'transmission' techniques as the MRI signal is generated within the tissue, and reflects the molecular environment from which it has arisen. Alteration of the scanning acquisition parameters will therefore generate morphological images representing data dependent on the make-up of the tissue. The scans can be sensitized to flow that may provide a morphological image or data relating to direction and velocity of flow. Additional techniques measuring perfusion, diffusion, metabolism (spectroscopy) and tissue enhancement can all be applied to the investigation of vascular biology, making MRI potentially the most comprehensive imaging technique in this field. In light of the present and future capabilities of MRI, this chapter will address the MRI techniques for the investigation of vascular biology and disease.

MRI techniques

Morphology: established disease
Vessel lumen: MR angiography (MRA)

Time-of-flight angiography
The relatively uniform movement of flowing blood through a slice or volume of tissue generates information that can be interrogated to provide information about the vascular system. Most techniques in the field of MRA attempt to generate bright blood images akin to conventional angiograms. Using gradient echo imaging, stationary tissues within the imaged region will undergo repeated measurements with insufficient time for the tissues to recover, resulting in a reduced MR signal intensity. However, blood that flows into the MR imaging volume will continually refresh the vascular compartment, resulting in increased signal intensity within the vessel lumen (known as a time-of-flight effect). The combination of reduced background and increased intraluminal signal therefore results in an image depicting flowing blood, i.e. an MR angiogram. This technique therefore mimics conventional angiography demonstrating stenosis or occlusion (Figure 11.4).

The technique is attractive compared to conventional angiography as it is noninvasive, requiring no arterial catheter access or contrast agents. The application of further pulses to the MR sequence result in the signal from flow in certain directions being removed, resulting in the selection of predominantly arterial flow, being cardiofugal, and venous, cardiopetal. Drawbacks to this technique are the artefacts that can arise which mimic reduced or absent flow. Blood which travels within the plane of an imaging slice, rather than through it, experiences an increased number of measurements, causing an overall decrease in signal. Similarly, turbulent flow will cause a permanent loss of MR signal, resulting in apparent loss of flow.

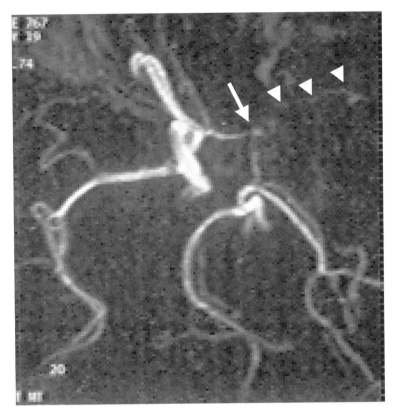

Figure 11.4 Time-of-flight magnetic resonance angiography shows complete occlusion of the left
internal carotid (arrow) and middle cerebral arteries (arrowheads).

Contrast-enhanced angiography

Many of the problems experienced using time-of-flight angiography can be
overcome using the combination of very rapidly acquired data in conjunction
with a small bolus of contrast agent. The rapidly acquired three-dimensional
imaging technique results in significant background suppression of stationary
tissues. The technique, however, is extremely sensitive to intravascular contrast
which produces high signal. The high intravascular signal and low background
signal result in high-definition angiograms. This technique is much less sensitive
to flow, because of the presence of contrast agent within the blood, and therefore is
not prone to the same artefacts as time-of-flight MRA. This results in greater
anatomical coverage and more accurate definition of tortuous or stenotic vessels.
Because of the natural timing of blood flow there is a reasonably well-defined
arterial and venous phase. By manipulation of these phases it is possible to image
selectively either the arterial or venous systems from the same acquisition (Figure
11.5).

(a)   (b)

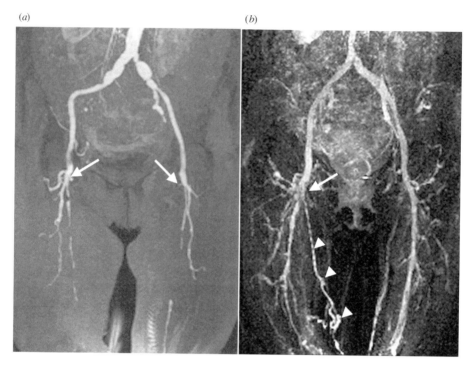

Figure 11.5 Contrast-enhanced angiography. Early phase (*a*) demonstrating the arterial phase which shows bilateral femoral artery occlusions (arrows). Late venographic phase (*b*) demonstrates a chronic right-sided occlusion of the femoral vein (arrow) with prominent superficial collaterals (arrowheads).

Phase contrast angiography

A further technique that is highly dependent on the presence of blood flow is phase contrast angiography. MR signal is produced by the changes in magnetic field produced within the blood travelling along the magnetic gradients present within the scanner itself. The more rapidly the blood moves, so the blood will experience a greater change in magnetic gradient strength. This information can be translated into the velocity at which the blood is travelling and also the direction. Phase contrast angiography is therefore a useful noninvasive means of acquiring information not only about vessel morphology but also blood velocity.

Vessel wall

Broadly speaking, inflammation accounts for much vessel wall pathology. Virchow first pointed out the importance of vessel wall disease and its relationship with thrombosis. This may be in the acute setting when inflammatory change within the vessel wall results in mural thrombosis, perhaps to be followed by complete luminal thrombotic occlusion. In the chronic setting inflammatory disease is now thought to be a major component of atherothrombotic disease. The origin of both of these conditions lies in the loss of normal endothelial function whose normal role is antithrombotic, antiinflammatory and to maintain blood flow.

Acute: thrombosis

Sudden cessation of blood flow due to vessel thrombosis, either arterial or venous, is a medical emergency. Ideally, diagnostic techniques should be able to confirm the diagnosis of acute thrombosis and define the extent of the problem. Application of conventional angiography in this setting is limited as the column of contrast within the patent lumen merely defines one end of the thrombosed vessel without visualizing the total extent. This can be overcome using ultrasound provided there is access to the vessel under examination. However, adequate views are not always possible, as in detecting deep vein thrombosis within the pelvis, where access is often obscured by bowel gas.

MR techniques may overcome some of these problems. However, time-of-flight MRA has similar drawbacks to conventional studies as it too is reliant on detecting flow, or its absence, rather than the causative pathology, i.e. the mural/occlusive thrombus. The use of contrast-enhanced techniques can help. When imaging venous thrombosis the upper extent of the thrombus is often defined, as the technique is not reliant on direct injection of contrast into a vein but utilizes the natural circulation of contrast agent into the venous system. By this means there is far better enhancement of the vessels distal to an occluding thrombus (Figure 11.6). Being a luminal technique, however, no information regarding the thrombus itself is acquired.

Conventional imaging is problematic when attempting to differentiate between acute and chronic thrombotic venous occlusion. Having suffered a thrombosis, resolution is commonly incomplete, to the extent that the vessel may remain completely occluded or significantly stenosed due to the organized thrombus. This may then result in continuing signs and symptoms that mimic the original acute disease. Patients, however, who have sustained one thrombosis are at increased risk of suffering further thrombosis at the same site. Attempts to differentiate between residual chronic disease and fresh acute thrombosis rely on the morphology of the filling defects using conventional venography and on the echotexture of the clot with ultrasound, both of which tend to be unreliable.

New techniques in MRI have attempted to overcome many of these problems. It has been known for some time that, as blood clots, it passes through a number of predictable stages, as the blood contains oxy- then deoxy- and then methaemoglobin. The MRI signal characteristics of each of these can be exploited to produce different appearances. Methaemoglobin causes a reduction in T1 similar to

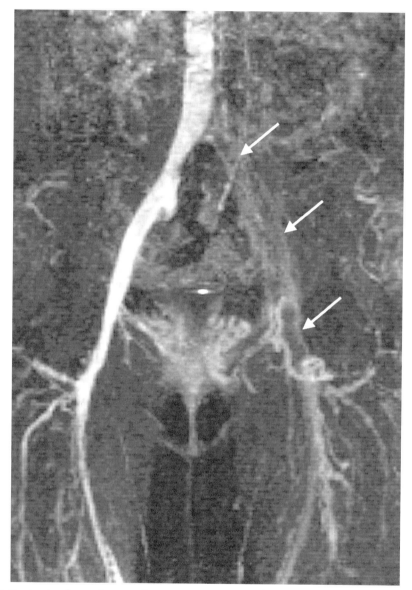

Figure 11.6 Contrast-enhanced magnetic resonance venogram demonstrating a large left sided filling defect due to a large deep vein thrombosis (arrows).

intravenous MRI contrast agents, so that it appears bright on T1-weighted image sequences. Clinical studies have suggested that blood passes through the oxy- and deoxy-phases of haemoglobin rapidly and that the methaemoglobin component persists thereafter for a number of weeks (Moody et al., 1998). This therefore provides a natural in vivo contrast agent that acts as a marker for acute thrombus.

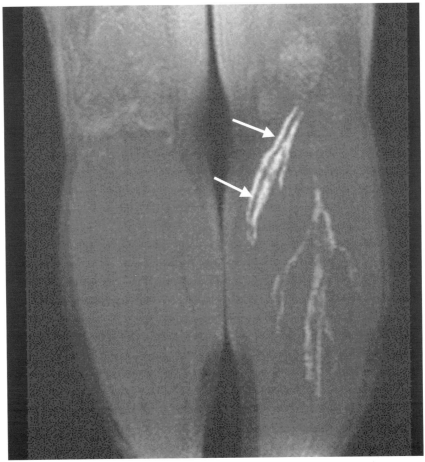

Figure 11.7   Direct clot image of below-knee deep vein thrombosis involving the gastrocnemius veins (arrows).

This technique allows the complete visualization of the thrombus as it is imaged directly (Figure 11.7). Because the generated signal is reliant on the age of the clot itself, it is possible to discriminate between acute/subacute clot and long-standing chronic clot, which is no longer of bright signal.

This technique has been applied in the setting of acute deep vein thrombosis (DVT). Diagnosis in this group can be difficult. Venography requires venous access and the injection of iodinated contrast media. Visualization of the pelvic vessels can be poor due to dilution of contrast in these larger vessels. Commonly, only the inferior aspect of the clot is visualized with no definition of the upper end of the clot. Ultrasonography has limitations in the calf vessels and, as stated previously, the pelvic vessels may be obscured by bowel gas. In the largest study of MR direct thrombus imaging to date, the technique had an overall sensitivity of

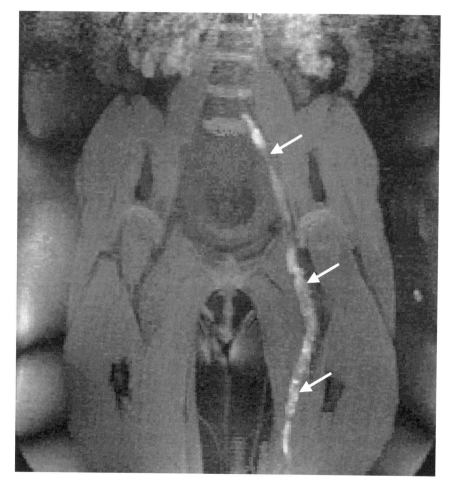

Figure 11.8 Large left-sided deep vein thrombosis (arrows) in a pregnant woman.

96% and specificity of 90% when compared with conventional venography. This degree of accuracy was maintained in all anatomical areas, i.e. below- and above-knee and pelvic. In addition to identifying clot within the symptomatic deep venous system the technique also detects disease within the asymptomatic deep veins and within the superficial system. This highlights the advantage of this technique, which has bilateral coverage from ankle to inferior vena cava and visualizes both the deep and superficial venous systems.

Because of the noninvasive nature of the technique, it can be repeated if necessary to follow disease progress or its treatment. Similarly, this technique is particularly useful in situations in which ionizing radiation and contrast media are to be avoided, such as pregnancy (Figure 11.8). Ultrasound may also provide a diagnosis but the reliance on demonstrating flow in vessels that may be compressed by the gravid uterus is less than ideal.

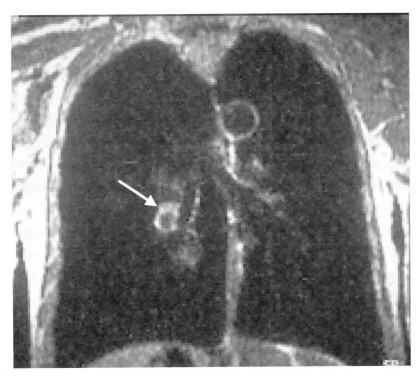

Figure 11.9   Direct embolus imaging demonstrates a large proximal right sided pulmonary embolus (arrow).

The danger of DVT is if it embolizes to the chest. The embolus is made up of the same thrombus that is in the leg and therefore should have the same MRI characteristics. Exploiting these characteristics allows the demonstration of pulmonary emboli as high signal material within the vessels of the chest. This technique can be combined with the DVT imaging at the same imaging session, thus providing a comprehensive diagnostic technique (Moody et al., 1997; Figure 11.9). Using these combined techniques it is possible to show that, in patients with DVT, the larger the volume of leg clot, or the closer it is to the inferior vena cava, then the greater the chance of embolization. Clots of greater than 60 ml volume or extending into the inferior vena cava were all found to embolize to the chest.

While the constituents of thrombus may differ between the arterial and venous systems there is still sufficient methaemoglobin within arterial clot to allow direct thrombus imaging within arteries. This will usually present as an ischaemic emergency and intervention depends on the extent of thrombosis and the age of the obstructing lesion. When combined with MRA it has been possible to define how much of the occlusion is due to recent thrombus and how much due to underlying chronic disease (Figure 11.10). This type of information may have a bearing on the type of intervention undertaken, i.e. thrombolysis.

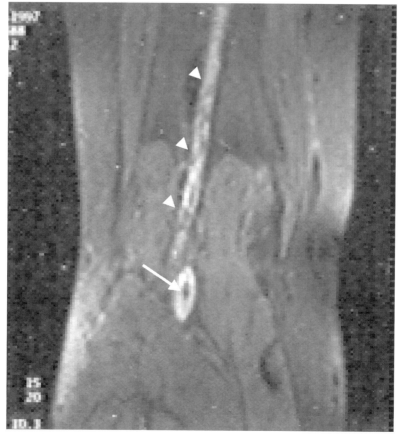

Figure 11.10 Direct thrombus imaging of the lower leg confirms arterial thrombosis (arrowheads) but also detects asymptomatic venous thrombosis (arrow).

Chronic: atherothrombosis

One of the biggest causes of mortality and morbidity today is atherothrombotic disease. In the heart this results in cardiac ischaemia with angina and myocardial infarction while in the brain it causes, transient ischaemic attacks and stroke. In the peripheral vessels this results in narrowing or occlusion with intermittent claudication and potentially amputation. Conventional techniques have again concentrated on the residual vessel lumen as the marker of disease severity. This requires disease to be sufficiently established to cause a luminal abnormality, which means that disease may be missed at its earlier stages and the opportunity for very early disease detection or screening is lost.

Ultrasound has been used to characterize vessel wall disease. Established disease can be recognized and the components within the plaque defined, i.e. calcification and hypoechoic plaque contents. Knowing that the earliest stages of atheromatous disease result in generalized thickening of the vessel wall, the intima media thickness has been used as an indicator of early disease and can be used to predict the likelihood of vascular events throughout the vascular system.

The ability of MRI to generate high tissue contrast is particularly useful in defining the individual components of atheromatous plaque. In vitro high-resolution imaging has the capacity to define accurately the significant disease components, with clear definition of the fibrous cap, shoulders of the plaque and the lipid contents (Toussaint et al., 1996). In vivo imaging has as yet to achieve similar spatial resolution, though similar components can be recognized in vessels with gross disease (Hatsukami et al., 2000). Most studies have so far been restricted to observation of the plaque morphology; further longitudinal studies into the relevance of these appearances and symptomatology are awaited. Improvements in scanning techniques (speed, resolution and contrast generation) coupled with hardware advances in surface coil design will lead to further improvements in these techniques that will allow their utilization beyond the research setting.

In addition to accepted morphological markers of risk such as cap thickness and lipid content, a marker of disease is the presence of intraplaque haemorrhage, defining the plaque as complex. Identification of intraplaque haemorrhage is possible using the same MRI techniques of direct thrombus imaging (Figure 11.11). High signal within the carotid vessel wall has been associated with patients suffering stroke and transient ischaemic attacks (Moody et al., 1999). A significant proportion of these patients have asymptomatic contralateral disease, the significance of which remains to be proven. Identification of patients with complex plaque may therefore allow selection of patients, otherwise unsuitable for surgical intervention, who may benefit from aggressive maximal medical therapy. The noninvasive nature of the MRI technique lends itself to follow-up of these patients, looking for signs of disease regression.

One area in which similar MRI techniques are being applied is in the coronary vessels. These vessels obviously hold the biggest challenge because of their size and the degree of physiological movement that occurs. Recent images, however, have shown that imaging of coronary vessel wall is becoming a reality. These techniques will therefore provide a means of not only diagnosing established disease but also detecting early at-risk disease, enabling intervention which can be followed using these noninvasive methods (Fayad et al., 2000).

Inflammation

Not only can MRI detect the endresult of chronic inflammation within the vessel wall, but recent work has shown that the inflammatory process itself can be detected, potentially providing a means of monitoring disease activity and its response to intervention. Macrophages play a pivotal role in the inflammatory

(a)

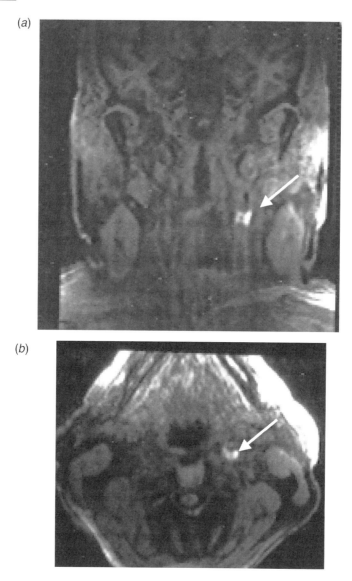

(b)

Figure 11.11 Coronal (*a*) and axial (*b*) direct clot image shows high signal within the left internal carotid artery (arrows).

response, migrating from the circulation through the vessel wall to within the plaque. Labelling of the macrophages while in the circulation can be achieved using ultrasmall particles of iron oxide (USPIO). These particles are taken up within the macrophages. Because of the magnetic effects of the iron, local magnetic homogeneity is lost, causing destruction of the MR signal and creating an area of low signal. Wherever there is a high concentration of USPIO-laden macrophages they will be detected as regions of low signal within the tissue. In the experimental setting increased accumulation of USPIO was detected within the endothelial cells and macrophages of rabbits pretreated with USPIO contrast agent and particularly in areas of early atheromatous formation (Schmitz et al., 2000).

Hyper/neovascularity

Part of the inflammatory response to perimural thombosis is the hypervascularity that occurs within the wall of the vessel. Some researchers have suggested that this finding may be useful in differentiating between acute and chronic thrombosis, as the latter does not display this appearance (Londy et al., 1999). This can readily be detected using MR contrast agents, which result in an intense increase in vessel wall signal at the site of thrombosis.

A similar microvascular response has been noted in the chronic setting within the wall of atheromatous vessels. New vessels arise from the vasa vasorum and permeate the thickened vessel wall. These vessels are tortuous and fragile, and may act as a source of intraplaque haemorrhage (Barger and Beeuwkes, 1990). The hypervascularity caused by these neovessels can be visualized by the injection of MRI contrast agent into the blood stream, causing an increase in MR signal at the site of high-density vessels. This therefore potentially provides another means by which the process of local inflammation and plaque formation can be monitored and the effect of modifying drugs upon the vessel wall such as vascular endothelial growth factor can be measured (Aoki et al., 1999).

Physiology: disease prediction/prevention?

Many, if not all of the imaging techniques used in clinical practice aim at detecting changes in tissue morphology which result from disease that is already established. The vasculature is extremely dynamic, responding to changes in its local and global environment. Numerous defence mechanisms exist within the lumen and the wall itself to protect the vessel from these changes. When stressed, there are a number of changes that occur which could be used to detect and monitor disease when it is still at a treatable, reversible phase. The time scale of these changes is also sufficiently protracted that there is sufficient opportunity for detection and intervention. Many of the changes are reflected in the local physiology, or resultant pathophysiology, and while these tests may not find their way into clinical usage, may be applicable in the research setting when investigating the development of early vascular disease.

Vessel lumen

The aim of the normal blood vessel is to maintain flow to the tissues. Complete occlusion of the vessel with cessation of flow will compromise the viability of that tissue. Lesser degrees of disturbed flow may be able to provide sufficient supply to the tissues but will have an effect on the local intravascular environment to which the vessel wall will respond. Turbulent flow is one such change in the blood flow. This will result in changes both to the direction and velocity of flow. Common sites for turbulent flow are at vessel bifurcations, and this accounts for the high incidence of vascular disease at these sites. We have already seen how the image of blood travelling within a vessel has the capacity to carry information regarding speed and direction (phase contrast angiography). The application of similar phase-mapping techniques to blood, which is turbulent, can also produce images reflecting the degree of complex flow and the effects of the vessel morphology upon these flow patterns.

Shear stress

Further manipulation of this data can provide specific information regarding the effects of flowing blood at the lumen–wall interface. The shear stress upon the vessel's endothelial surface has a direct effect on the endothelial response, with increased shear stress resulting in increased endothelial activity, nitric oxide production and vasodilation. Mapping of localized vessel wall shear stress is possible throughout the cardiac cycle and thus the effects of normal and turbulent flow on specific areas of vessel wall can be studied (Stokholm et al., 2000).

Vessel wall

Abnormalities within the vessel, either the constituents of the blood itself or the flow characteristics, will have a significant effect upon the vessel wall. The wall itself is capable of responding to these changes which will initially act to protect the vessel but will eventually result in structural changes, manifest as vessel wall disease.

Vasodilatation

Nitric oxide acts as one of the main regulators of endothelial homeostasis, being antiinflammatory, antiplatelet and bringing about local vasodilatation. The ability of the endothelium to produce these effects can be tested in a number of ways. Shear stress will have a profound effect on the endothelial response. Increase in shear stress, detected by the endothelium, results in increased nitric oxide production and subsequent vasodilation (endothelium-dependent). This can be brought about by initially causing a reduction in flow to a tissue by reducing arterial flow by way of a tourniquet. Following removal of the tourniquet and reconstitution of flow, there is an endothelially driven vasodilatation. Alternatively, the effect of nitric oxide on the vessel can be tested without local nitric oxide production by providing an nitric oxide precursor such as glyceryl trinitrate (endothelium-independent). Whichever technique is used, the endresult is vasodilatation. Measurement of vessel wall diameter or luminal area before and after such manoeuvres will allow the measurement of this vasodilatory response. Ultrasound has been used successfully to monitor this response using the brachial or femoral arteries. MRI also has the capability of measuring the same response as part of a multimodal approach to imaging of vascular function (Sorensen et al., 1999).

Compliance

Abnormalities in the vessel wall will cause increased stiffness such that there is a decrease in expansion of the vessel in response to systole, i.e. compliance of the vessel wall is reduced. The ability of MRI to be gated to the cardiac cycle allows the acquisition of images at different time-points within the cardiac cycle, i.e. end-diastole and end-systole. Knowing the pulse pressure during the acquisition of these images, the compliance of the vessel wall can be calculated. Using the aorta as the vessel of choice, reproducible results can be obtained (Forbat et al., 1995). Comparison of different patient populations, such as those with coronary artery disease, normal volunteers and elite athletes, results in significant differences in the measured aortic compliance between the groups (Mohiaddin et al., 1989).

Endorgan effects

A major advantage of MRI is its ability to image not only the vasculature but also the endorgans supplied by those vessels. It is therefore possible to construct an imaging algorithm that will include investigation of a complete vascular organ system visualizing the local pathology within the vessel and distant effects within the endorgan.

Tissue ischaemia and irreversible damage

Myocardial infarction

Rupture of an atheromatous plaque within a large coronary artery can trigger a train of events which will result in luminal thrombosis and occlusion. In this acute setting collateral blood supply is minimal and the territory supplied by this vessel will rapidly become ischaemic and undergo infarction. MR cardiac imaging is technically challenging because of the normal physiological motion (respiratory, cardiac, vascular) that exists. This can be overcome by gating the image acquisition to the same phase of each cardiac cycle. Respiratory motion is overcome by using sequences that are sufficiently short that the whole of the image acquisition can be achieved in suspended respiration. In the acute phase of myocardial ischaemia, MR imaging can differentiate between regions of irreversible tissue infarction and at-risk tissue (Fieno et al., 2000). Furthermore, perfusion imaging can depict the region of the heart which has lost its blood supply (Bluemke and Halefoglu, 1999). In the chronic phase myocardial tissue will be lost and the muscle wall will become thinned. Because of the ability to detect morphology these changes can be accurately depicted.

Cerebral infarction

While the underlying vascular abnormality in cerebral infarction is the same as myocardial infarction – rupture of an atheromatous plaque – the means by which this has an effect on the endorgan, the brain, is different. Cerebral infarction is most commonly secondary to vascular disease within the carotid vessels in the neck. Because of the collateral vascular networks that exist within the brain via the vessels of the circle of Willis, thrombotic occlusion of a carotid vessel does not necessarily bring about symptomatic brain disease as blood supply can still be maintained. Global reduction in flow, secondary to carotid occlusion, can produce transient symptoms or intermittent reduction in cerebral blood flow, though the latter is rare. The most common aetiology of cerebral infarction secondary to carotid disease is due to thromboembolic disease which can be as a result of occlusion, but more commonly arises from nonocclusive, stenotic carotid disease. As with myocardial ischaemia, the cause for acute onset of symptoms is plaque rupture which acts as a focus for the production of thrombus emboli. When one of these emboli travel into the cerebral circulation they will impact, occlude and then bring about ischaemia. Just as the precipitating event within the carotid vessel has a number of different outcomes, this variability continues within the brain because of its extensive collateral blood supply which exists at a number of different levels. Firstly, the circle of Willis, if intact, can overcome a proximal carotid obstruction by stealing blood flow from the contralateral carotid, posterior or external carotid circulations. Above the circle of Willis these circulations are no longer accessible but collateral supply can still be achieved via the leptomeningeal plexus which connects all three cerebral arterial territories and allows relatively free cross-communication. The response to a carotid or cerebral artery occlusion is therefore quite variable. The clinical presentation can also be misleading and there is a dynamic environment in which vessels may further thrombose or spontaneously recanalize. Clinical assessment of these patients is therefore difficult (Allder et al., 1999). The ability of MRI to define the site of causative vascular lesion and endorgan damage is therefore a great advantage.

Routine MRI techniques will depict areas of damaged brain by the presence of excess water within the tissues. This may be within the acute phase (6–12 h) or in the chronic phase when the resultant brain damage can be visualized. Recent technical advances however have resulted in MRI techniques that can detect cerebral ischaemia within minutes of its onset. Diffusion-weighted sequences are

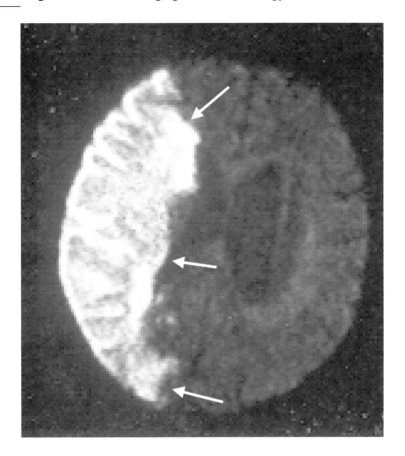

Figure 11.12 Diffusion-weighted magnetic resonance imaging rapidly detects acute cerebral ischaemia in the right middle cerebral artery territory (arrows).

able to detect the normal random diffusion of water molecules within the brain. Following ischaemia, the cell membrane pumps are inactivated, resulting in cellular influx of fluid. This restricted fluid no longer undergoes random diffusion and therefore becomes apparent on this sequence as an area of high signal intensity (Figure 11.12). This appears to be a highly sensitive technique for the detection of infarction in its earliest stages (Albers, 1998). To this technique further methods of better defining the endresult of vascular occlusion can also be added, including MR cerebral angiography and perfusion (Fisher et al., 1995).

Organ function

Cardiac

Having made the diagnosis of myocardial infarction, the most important question is: what effect has the loss of that region of viable myocardium had upon cardiac function? This can be measured in a number of ways, which include stroke

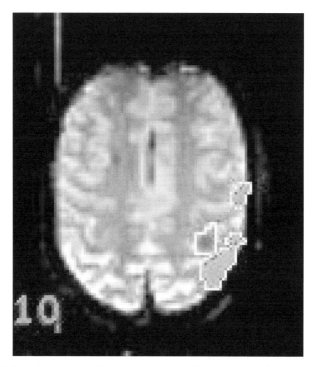

Figure 11.13 Functional magnetic resonance imaging demonstrating motor and sensory activation.

volume, ejection fraction and cardiac output. These parameters rely on the measurement of the maximum volume of blood within the ventricle (at diastole) and the minimum volume (at systole). Subtraction of the two will give the volume of blood expelled from the cardiac chamber per heart beat (stroke volume); multiplied by the heart rate, this gives the cardiac output. The speed of MRI allows breath-hold imaging and the ability to acquire data during the same part of the cardiac cycle using electrocardiograph gating results in images of high spatial resolution. Visualization of the cardiac chambers through the cardiac cycle can be achieved, and the appropriate volume measurements can be derived. From the same images it is also possible to calculate wall thickening and global myocardial mass. By magnetically tagging the myocardium the distortion of regions within the ventricle wall can also be visualized (Pettigrew et al., 1999).

Brain

The effect of vascular brain damage is usually assessed using neurological or psychometric tests. Recent advances in MRI have resulted in techniques that allow the depiction of cerebral activation. These techniques are reliant on detecting the changes in the cerebral microcirculation. During brain activation blood flow to the activated region increases. There is however dissociation between the resultant oxygen supply and oxygen extraction such that there is an excess of oxygenated blood in the tissue circulation. Because the MRI characteristics of blood alter in changing from oxy- to deoxyhaemoglobin, it is possible to detect the alteration in signal when a task is performed. This will be represented by an increase in signal intensity during the task and will be localized to the area undergoing activation (Welch et al., 2000; Figure 11.13).

REFERENCES

Albers, G.W. (1998). Diffusion-weighted MRI for evaluation of acute stroke. *Neurology*, **51** (suppl. 3): S47–9.

Allder, S.J., Moody, A.R., Martel, A.L. et al. (1999). Limitations of clinical diagnosis in acute stroke (letter). *Lancet*, **354**, 1523.

Aoki, S., Aoki, K., Ohsawa, S. et al. (1999). Dynamic MR imaging of the carotid wall. *J. Magn. Reson. Imaging*, **9**, 420–7.

Baldassarre, D., Amato, M., Bondioli, A., Sirtori, C.R. & Tremoli, E. (2000). Carotid artery intima-media thickness measured by ultrasonography in normal clinical practice correlates well with atherosclerosis risk factors. *Stroke*, **31**, 2426–30.

Barger, A.C. & Beeuwkes, R.D. (1990). Rupture of coronary vasa vasorum as a trigger of acute myocardial infarction. *Am. J. Cardiol.*, **66**, 41G–3G.

Becker, C.R., Knez, A., Jakobs, T.F. et al. (1999). Detection and quantification of coronary artery calcification with electron-beam and conventional CT. *Eur. Radiol.*, **9**, 620–4.

Bluemke, D.A. & Halefoglu, A.M. (1999). Cardiac disease in the adult: MR evaluation. *Crit. Rev. Diagn. Imaging*, **40**, 203–49.

Fayad, Z.A., Fuster, V., Fallon, J.T. et al. (2000). Noninvasive in vivo human coronary artery lumen and wall imaging using black-blood magnetic resonance imaging. *Circulation*, **102**, 506–10.

Fieno, D.S., Kim, R.J., Chen, E.L. et al. (2000). Contrast-enhanced magnetic resonance imaging of myocardium at risk: distinction between reversible and irreversible injury throughout infarct healing. *J. Am. Coll. Cardiol.*, **36**, 1985–91.

Fisher, M., Prichard, J.W. & Warach, S. (1995). New magnetic resonance techniques for acute ischemic stroke. *J.A.M.A.*, **274**, 908–11.

Forbat, S.M., Mohiaddin, R.H., Yang, G.Z., Firmin, D.N. & Underwood, S.R. (1995). Measurement of regional aortic compliance by MR imaging: a study of reproducibility. *J. Magn. Reson. Imaging*, **5**, 635–9.

Hatsukami, T.S., Ross, R., Polissar, N.L. & Yuan, C. (2000). Visualization of fibrous cap thickness and rupture in human atherosclerotic carotid plaque in vivo with high-resolution magnetic resonance imaging. *Circulation*, **102**, 959–64.

Londy, F.J., Kadell, A.M., Wrobleski, S.K. et al. (1999). Detection of perivenous inflammation in a rat model of venous thrombosis using MRV. *J. Invest. Surg.*, **12**, 151–6.

Mohiaddin, R.H., Underwood, S.R., Bogren, H.G. et al. (1989). Regional aortic compliance studied by magnetic resonance imaging: the effects of age, training, and coronary artery disease. *Br. Heart J.*, **62**, 90–6.

Moody, A.R., Liddicoat, A. & Krarup, K. (1997). Magnetic resonance pulmonary angiography and direct imaging of embolus for the detection of pulmonary emboli. *Invest. Radiol.*, **32**, 431–40.

Moody, A.R., Pollock, J.G., O'Connor, A.R. & Bagnall, M. (1998). Lower-limb deep venous thrombosis: direct MR imaging of the thrombus. *Radiology*, **209**, 349–55.

Moody, A.R., Allder, S., Lennox, G., Gladman, J. & Fentem, P. (1999). Direct magnetic resonance imaging of carotid artery thrombus in acute stroke (letter). *Lancet*, **353**, 122–3.

Pettigrew, R.I., Oshinski, J.N., Chatzimavroudis, G. & Dixon, W.T. (1999). MRI techniques for cardiovascular imaging. *J. Magn. Reson. Imaging.*, **10**, 590–601.

Poredos, P., Orehek, M. & Tratnik, E. (1999). Smoking is associated with dose-related increase of intima-media thickness and endothelial dysfunction. *Angiology*, **50**, 201–8.

Rabin, D.N., Rabin, S. & Mintzer, R.A. (2000). A pictorial review of coronary artery anatomy on spiral CT. *Chest*, **118**, 488–91.

Rydberg, J., Buckwalter, K.A., Caldemeyer, K.S. et al. (2000). Multisection CT: scanning techniques and clinical applications. *Radiographics*, **20**, 1787–806.

Schmitz, S.A., Coupland, S.E., Gust, R. et al. (2000). Superparamagnetic iron oxide-enhanced MRI of atherosclerotic plaques in Watanabe hereditable hyperlipidemic rabbits. *Invest Radiol.*, **35**, 460–71.

Sorensen, M., Ong, P., Hayward, C. et al. (1999). Gradient echo magnetic resonance imaging of the brachial artery: a novel method for assessing vascular reactivity. *Circulation*, (suppl): 248.

Stokholm, R., Oyre, S., Ringgaard, S. et al. (2000). Determination of wall shear rate in the human carotid artery by magnetic resonance techniques. *Eur. J. Vasc. Endovasc. Surg.*, **20**, 427–33.

Toussaint, J.F., LaMuraglia, G.M., Southern, J.F., Fuster, V. & Kantor, H.L. (1996). Magnetic resonance images lipid, fibrous, calcified, hemorrhagic, and thrombotic components of human atherosclerosis in vivo. *Circulation*, **94**, 932–8.

Welch, K.M., Cao, Y. & Nagesh, V. (2000). Magnetic resonance assessment of acute and chronic stroke. *Prog. Cardiovasc. Dis.*, **43**, 113–34.

Part III

Clinical practice

12

Vascular biology of hypertension

Michael Schachter

Department of Clinical Pharmacology, Imperial College School of Medicine, St Mary's Hospital, London

Introduction

What does the title of this chapter actually mean? It has to be said at the outset that it sounds more comprehensive than it can possibly be within the constraints of space and the reader's patience. In other words, it has to represent the author's selective interests and prejudices. In this case this will wholly exclude from consideration the role of large arteries and their mechanical properties, apart from one brief mention. Instead the focus will be on the following main questions:

- Is there endothelial dysfunction in hypertension?
  - If so, what is its severity?
  - How does it occur?
  - Is it influenced and even corrected by antihypertensive drugs?
  - Is this clinically important?
- What determines peripheral vascular resistance, especially in terms of the structure of the vessels concerned?

As one might expect, these are contentious issues despite, or rather because of, intensive research. The reader, as always, will have to make up his or her own mind and should note that in some cases reviews have been cited in order to keep the number of references within manageable limits.

Endothelial dysfunction in hypertension

Is there endothelial dysfunction in hypertension?

The dynamic nature of the endothelium is now very much a truism, though it would have surprised most vascular biologists 30 or even 20 years ago. Table 12.1 lists some of the vasoconstrictor and vasodilator substances produced by the endothelium. Though this list is likely to grow it is also probable that the most important factors have now been identified. Of course, the one that has attracted by far the most attention is nitric oxide (NO), as we know the original

Table 12.1 Vasoactive substances produced by the endothelium

Constrictors	Dilators
Endothelins[a]	Nitric oxide
Endoperoxides/thromboxanes	Prostacyclin
Superoxide/free radicals	EDHF(s)[b]

[a] Note that endothelins may also stimulate endothelial nitric oxide release.
[b] EDHF(s), endothelium-derived hyperpolarizing factor(s). Not discussed in text.

'endothelium-derived relaxant factor'. We also know that its physiological and pathological role extends far beyond the vasculature. The term 'endothelial dysfunction' is now mostly a synonym for impaired endothelium-dependent vasodilatation. This is convenient, and will largely be followed in this chapter, but is only a part of the possible spectrum of endothelial pathophysiology in hypertension and other cardiovascular diseases. In particular, this includes abnormal balance between clotting and fibrinolysis and increased platelet–endothelium interaction (Lip and Li-Saw-Hee, 1998).

Endothelial dysfunction has been investigated in several of the commonly used animal models of hypertension. The general consensus is that there is impairment of endothelium-dependent vasodilatation whether tested in isolated vessels or in vascular beds (Boulanger, 1999). In most cases acetylcholine has been the stimulus used, but in some instances this has not produced a definitely abnormal response while other agents (e.g. bradykinin) have been more conclusive. This indicates that the mechanism of the dysfunction can vary widely in different models

In human hypertension too, the majority of researchers agree that endothelium-dependent relaxation is abnormal, even though there are a few dissenting findings (Taddei et al., 1998; John and Schmieder, 2000). In fact, these relate less to the fundamental observation than to its relationship with cholinergic muscarinic receptors. This once again raises the question: what is the actual mechanism of this abnormality?

What is wrong with endothelium-dependent vasodilatation in hypertension?

If it is accepted that an abnormality is present, one can envisage several levels at which it can occur:

- abnormal muscarinic receptor function (itself a composite of several potential defects
- reduced substrate availability of the endothelial nitric oxide synthase (eNOS or NOS-III)
- reduced expression or activity of the enzyme itself

- increased degradation of the NO that is generated, possibly at a normal rate
- increased release of an endothelial vasoconstrictor, or vasoconstrictors, which does not directly interact with NO but functionally antagonizes its effects
- reduced sensitivity of the smooth muscle cell to normal levels of NO (this too may have several components)

Clearly there are many possible processes in which dysfunction can occur and they are not necessarily mutually exclusive. The overall result in any case is reduced bioavailability of NO. It is hardly surprising that dissecting out exactly what is wrong is not straightforward, even in animals, where it has to be acknowledged that the available models are not accurate parallels of essential hypertension. The evidence quoted in this chapter will in fact focus largely on human hypertension.

Are receptors or their signalling mechanisms abnormal?

Hypertensive patients show impaired endothelium-dependent vasodilatation in response not only to acetylcholine but also to the peptides substance P and bradykinin (Panza et al., 1995). However, even though these are distinct receptors, they are members of the G protein-linked superfamily with similar signal transduction mechanisms (Figure 12.1). It is therefore still possible that postreceptor mechanisms are abnormal in these individuals. To some extent, this is supported by the finding that isoprenaline-induced vasodilatation is not impaired in hypertensive subjects (Cardillo et al., 1998). This too is endothelium-dependent, but in this instance the signal for increased NO synthase activity is increased intracellular cyclic adenosine monophosphate rather than calcium, as is the case with the other three agonists.

Is there a deficiency of the substrate for endothelial NO synthase?

Apparently not. The vasodilator response to acetylcholine is not enhanced by increased availability of substrate, the amino acid L-arginine (Taddei et al., 1997). However $N^G N^G$-dimethyl-L-arginine (ADMA), which is an endogenous circulating inhibitor of NO synthase, may be increased in the plasma of patients with hypertension (Surdacki et al., 1999).

Is there reduced expression or activity of NO synthase?

This *may* be the case in preeclampsia (Brennecke et al., 1997; Napolitano et al., 2000) but evidence is even less decisive in other types of human hypertension (and in animal models). On the other hand, inhibitors of NO synthase, such as N^G-monomethyl-L-arginine (L-NMMA), cause less vasoconstriction in hypertensive individuals under basal conditions (Calver et al., 1992) and also fail to modify the response to acetylcholine (Taddei et al., 1997). This tends to support the view that reduced synthesis of NO is part of the endothelial defect in hypertension, as

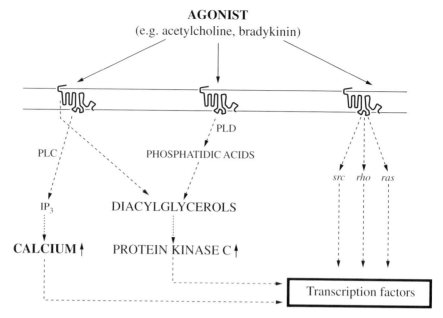

Figure 12.1 Highly simplified scheme of the effects of G protein-linked agonists involved in nitric oxide release. Note that some cholinergic receptors have other transduction mechanisms. PLC, phospholipase C; PLD, phospholipase D; IP$_3$, inositol trisphosphate; *src, rho, ras*: protooncogenes.

do reduced circulating levels of nitrite and nitrate, the endproducts of NO metabolism (Forte et al., 1997).

Is there increased degradation of nitric oxide?

This is proving to be perhaps the most interesting area of research in the whole field of endothelial dysfunction in hypertension. There is increasing evidence that the reduced bioavailability of NO is largely determined by its increased inactivation. The main agent of this inactivation is the superoxide anion (Boulanger, 1999; de Artiñano and Gonzalez, 1999; Kojda and Harrison, 1999). This has a high affinity for NO and the reaction between the two, which produces the peroxynitrite anion, is very rapid. Peroxynitrite is itself a powerful oxidant (Beckman and Koppenol, 1996) but may also spontaneously generate the hydroxyl radical under physiological conditions (Figure 12.2). It can act either as a vasodilator or vasoconstrictor and may interfere with endothelium dependent dilatation pro duced by other agents. The key issue therefore is the source and quantity of superoxide that is likely to be present in the vasculature. This will be discussed separately.

$$O_2 \cdot^- \ + \ NO \ = \ ONOO^-$$
Superoxide   *Nitric oxide*   *Peroxynitrite*

$$ONOO^- \ + \ H^+ \ = \ ONOOH$$
Peroxynitrous acid

$$ONOOH \ = \ NO_2 \cdot \ + \ OH \cdot$$

Figure 12.2 Formation of peroxynitrite ($ONOO^-$) and some of its breakdown products, including the nitrogen dioxide and hydroxyl radicals.

Is there a vasoconstrictor (or several) generated by the endothelium?

This question cannot be wholly separated from the previous one. The neutralization of a vasodilator is clearly potentially vasoconstrictor. But in fact there may be more direct vasoconstrictors generated by the endothelium. The most plausible candidates are prostanoids generated by cyclooxygenase (COX), specifically the COX-1 form of the enzyme, and the endothelins. Endothelium-dependent vasodilatation is facilitated in patients treated with indometacin (Taddei et al., 1997). The opposing effects of L-arginine and L-NMMA are both restored after indometacin treatment, implying that cyclooxygenase-derived compounds are reducing NO bioavailability. The exact nature of these compounds is not known but may in fact include superoxide.

Endothelin-1 is well-known as an extremely potent vasoconstrictor, although it must be remembered that it can also stimulate endothelial NO release. Although there are reports of increased plasma levels of endothelin in some groups of hypertensive patients (John and Schmieder, 2000), this is not universally accepted (Boulanger, 1999) and in any case it is uncertain whether it would be haemodynamically relevant. However, a nonselective endothelin receptor antagonist has been shown to reduce blood pressure in patients with essential hypertension (Krum et al., 1998).

What are the possible sources of superoxide?

The superoxide anion, while not strictly a free radical, is none the less highly reactive with other biological molecules and is also the precursor of genuine free radicals of greater reactivity (Figure 12.3). Where does it come from? In fact, there are several possible sources in the vascular wall apart from the cyclooxygenase already mentioned:

1. 'leakage' from the mitochondrial electron chain, which is never of course 100% efficient

$$\overset{Fe^{2+}}{O_2 \cdot^- + H_2H_2 = O_2 + OH\cdot + OH^-}$$

Superoxide anion   Hydrogen peroxide   Hydroxyl radical   Hydroxyl anion

Figure 12.3 The Fenton reaction, catalysed by trace metals such as divalent iron or copper.

2. xanthine oxidase, which generates superoxide during the process of purine oxidation
3. endothelial NO synthase
4. nicotin amide-adenine dinucleotide phosphate (NADPH)-dependent oxidases in vascular cells, similar to those found in phagocytic blood cells

The first of these sources is not thought to be of major significance. The others are of greater interest. Increased superoxide production, primarily but not exclusively from the endothelium, has been described in several animal models of hypertension (de Artiñano and Gonzalez, 1999). Angiotensin II is one of the stimulants for this process and appears to act mainly through the NADPH oxidase system (Griendling et al., 1994; Zhang et al., 1999; Berry et al., 2000). Endothelial NO synthase is perhaps a more surprising source. The purified enzyme was known to generate superoxide in the absence of the cofactor tetrahydrobiopterin (BH_4), which is required for NO production (Wang et al., 2000). These effects of BH_4 are also apparently relevant for constitutive NO synthase in the spontaneously hypertensive rat and in humans with smoking-induced endothelial dysfunction (Cosentino et al., 1998; Ueda et al., 2000). It has since been shown that this apparently aberrant pathway can occur in cultured cells, again in association with deficiency of BH_4. The importance of xanthine oxidase as a source of superoxide is less clearly established, but it has been reported that the xanthine oxidase inhibitor allopurinol largely reversed endothelial dysfunction in patients with type 2 diabetes and mild hypertension, even though it did not affect blood pressure (Butler et al., 2000).

Endothelial dysfunction and therapy

It is clearly important to know whether current and potential antihypertensive therapies have an impact on endothelial function, even if we do not yet know the significance of this in terms of clinical outcome. The drugs with the best-documented effect in this regard are the angiotensin converting enzyme (ACE) inhibitors (Mombouli and Vanhoutte, 1999; Ruschitzka et al., 1999). These have a dual action, not only reducing the generation of angiotensin II and therefore reducing its constrictor activity, but also increasing levels of the peptide bradykinin, a stimulator of endothelial NO release. Understandably, there is much less information on the activity of the angiotensin II receptor antagonists selective for the angiotensin II type 1 (AT1) receptor, but it seems that they too might improve endothelial dysfunction (Schiffrin et al., 2000). Calcium channel blockers also appear to have beneficial effects during chronic administration (Ruschitzka et al., 1999). Several mechanisms have been proposed: they may counteract the cellular action vasoconstrictors such as the endothelins and cyclooxygenase products. They may also enhance the effects of endothelium-dependent vasodilators, though it is not clear how this takes place. The novel vasopeptidase inhibitors, which inhibit ACE and also neutral endopeptidase (which inactivates natriuretic peptides) can also increase endothelium-dependent vasodilatation but have complex actions since neutral endopeptidase is also involved in the degradation of vasoconstrictors such as endothelin-1 (Ruschitzka et al., 1999). It is worth noting, of course, that several major classes of antihypertensive drugs, notably diuretics and conventional β-blockers, do not directly improve endothelial dysfunction: some β-blockers (celiprololol and nebivolol; Dawes et al., 1999) have ancillary NO-releasing properties.

Resistance vessels in hypertension

Hypertension is characterized by increased total systemic peripheral resistance. This is not strictly true for isolated systolic hypertension (systolic blood pressure ≥ 160 mmHg, diastolic blood pressure < 90 mmHg), which is believed to be primarily the consequence of increased stiffness in medium to large arteries (Kocemba et al., 1998). The increased resistance can be partly attributed to changes in the structure of small arteries and arterioles (luminal diameter $< 300\,\mu$m). It is at this point in the circulation that the largest pressure drop occurs (Figure 12.4). The structural properties will be discussed in much greater detail below. The other factor relates to the microvasculature, that is to say, vessels that are even smaller, particularly capillaries. In many vascular beds (e.g. skin and conjunctiva), there is a reduction in the total number of such vessels (Struijker Boudier et al., 1992). This of course is functionally equivalent to increasing the total resistance of the vascular bed concerned. As one might expect, there is considerable controversy over whether these changes are causative or secondary adaptations to sustained rises in blood pressure. This will not be discussed here in detail except to comment that firstly, there is some evidence that, even if not causative, the microvascular changes occur very early in the evolution of hypertension (Antonios et al., 1999); and secondly, a related point is that the apparent 'underdevelopment' of the microvasculature has been linked to what is now known as the Barker hypothesis. This proposes, to put it very simplistically, that hypertension is related to fetal growth retardation and relative placental insufficiency (Barker, 1997).

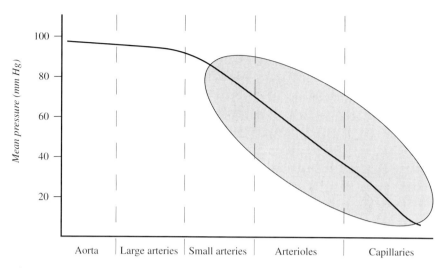

Figure 12.4 Schematic illustration of the pressure gradient on the arterial side of the systemic circulation. See text for discussion.

Small-vessel structure in hypertension

The characteristic change in these vessels, often described as resistance arteries, is a decrease in the lumen and usually an increase in the thickness of the media, resulting in an increased media-to-lumen ratio: this is recognized as the crucial characteristic of small-vessel structural change in hypertension (Mulvany and Aalkjaer, 1990). The increase in media-to-lumen ratio can occur in up to three ways (Heagerty et al., 1993; Mulvany, 1999; Figure 12.5). In animal models of hypertension the predominant processes are hyperplasia (often in small to medium arteries) and hypertrophy (in the aorta). In the first instance there is proliferation of medial smooth muscle cells; in the second the total mass of the media increases but largely by increase in the size of individual cells rather than their number. It appears that hypertrophy does occur in small arteries in patients with secondary hypertension, for instance in renovascular disease (Rizzoni et al., 2000). In the much more frequent circumstance of primary (essential) hypertension the usual change in resistance arteries is eutrophic remodelling. Here there is no change in cell size and number but instead a smaller lumen is formed by rearrangement of cells unchanged in number and size by a process which is not clearly understood. The exact role of this remodelling remains unclear and the experimental procedures from which these data are derived are very laborious and time-consuming.

It is important at this point to note two fundamental concepts which are relevant regardless of the exact nature of the structural change:

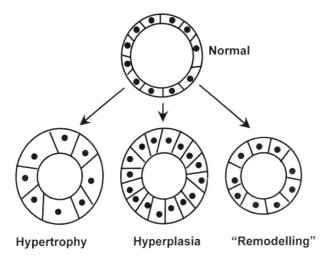

Figure 12.5   Possible structural changes in small arteries and arterioles in hypertension. See text.

1. relatively small changes in luminal diameter will have a major impact on resistance since, in accordance with Poiseuille's law,

   flow $\propto r^4$

2. resistance should not be regarded as a static state but as a dynamic one, since in the altered vessel – by whatever mechanism that change may come about – the vasodilator capacity is reduced and the sensitivity to vasoconstriction is generally enhanced (Folkow, 1982).

Small vessels and the amplifier hypothesis

Folkow in Sweden and Lever in the UK have developed a hypothesis for the pathophysiology of hypertension that is often described as the *amplifier hypothesis* (Lever and Harrap, 1992; Folkow, 1995; Wright and Angus, 1999). This has two basic elements. Firstly, as mentioned above, there is the increased response to vasoconstrictors (Figure 12.6). Secondly, they have put forward a scheme which takes in to account the structural changes noted in small vessels in animal and human hypertension and links them to genetic factors and the activity of trophic substances such angiotensin II (Figure 12.7). These concepts of the pathogenesis of hypertension are widely but certainly not universally accepted (Izzard et al., 1999), or at least are recognized as a useful basis for discussion and research (Folkow, 2000). Clearly, it is difficult to prove the validity of these schemes, particularly the latter, but one can look at the endresult in two ways: firstly, what happens to vascular structure and blood pressure in animals when there is

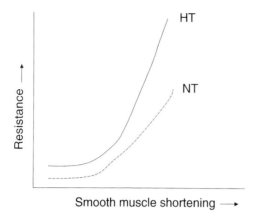

Figure 12.6 Schematic illustration of the different responses of hypertensive (HT) and normotensive (NT) resistance arteries. In the hypertensive vessels, with greater media-to-lumen ratios, there is greater increase in resistance for a given degree of smooth muscle contraction.

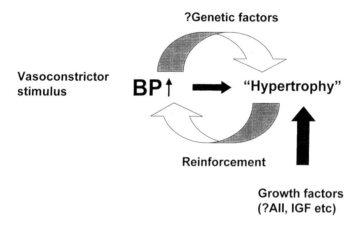

Figure 12.7 Simplified scheme of the hypothesis for the pathogenesis of hypertension proposed by Folkow, Lever and their coworkers. The nature of the initiating vasoconstrictor stimulus is generally speculative, but in some cases may be sympathetic overactivity. 'Hypertrophy' in this context refers to all the processes illustrated in Figure 12.6. BP, blood pressure; AII, angiotensin II; IGF, insulin-like growth factors.

interference with growth of resistance (and other) arteries? Secondly, what happens to the structure of human arteries when raised blood pressure is successfully treated?

Inhibition of vascular growth in hypertension

This approach is a consequence of the following question: if the (presumably largely adaptive; Ueno et al., 2000) growth response of small arteries is inhibited

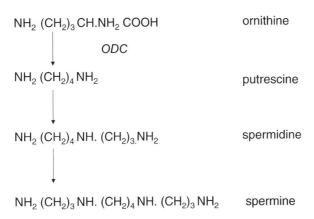

Figure 12.8 Synthetic pathway of the polyamines. Note that cycling occurs, so that spermine to spermidine conversion may take place. ODC, ornithine decarboxylase (rate-limiting enzyme of the pathway).

during the development of hypertension, will the rise in blood pressure be abolished or attenuated? In practical terms one needs to find some means of influencing vascular growth that does not directly affect haemodynamics and has low toxicity. Several groups, including our own, have chosen to inhibit polyamine synthesis to achieve these objectives. Polyamines are essential intracellular cations and in almost all circumstances in all cells growth-promoting stimuli cause increases in polyamine concentrations (Igarashi and Kashigawi, 2000; Wallace, 2000). The rate-limiting enzyme for polyamine synthesis is ornithine decarboxylase (Figure 12.8) and highly selective inhibitors of this enzyme have been developed, such as α-difluoromethyornithine (eflornithine) which is of low toxicity and has been used in the chemotherapy of protozoal infections. This agent has been used in several animal models of hypertension, including the spontaneously hypertensive rat (Soltis et al., 1994), aortic coarctation (Lipke et al., 1997), deoxycorticosterone acetate-salt induced hypertension (Soltis et al., 1991) and chronic low-dose angiotensin II infusion (Ibrahim et al., 1996). Eflornithine reduced vascular polyamine levels, modified the characteristic changes in vascular structure and reduced the expected rise in blood pressure as compared to controls. Not surprisingly, analogous experiments have not been carried out in hypertensive patients, but these studies do support the validity of a pathophysiological link between vascular structure and blood pressure.

Reversibility of vascular structural changes in hypertension

It is a well-established observation, frustrating for both patients and clinicians, that in the majority of cases patients do not remain normotensive after withdrawal of antihypertensive drugs, even after years of successful blood pressure control (Jennings et al., 1995; Froom et al., 1997; Aylett et al., 1999). This is a surprisingly poorly studied field, and the reasons for this problem are largely conjectural. However, it is reasonable to assume that changes in vascular structure at least contribute to this situation and that it is relevant to assess the reversibility of these changes. A few groups have examined this question since the introduction by Mulvany and Halpern of the microvascular myograph, which allows structural and functional studies on vessels with internal diameters as small as $100\,\mu m$ (Froom et al., 1997). Human clinical investigations have used arteries obtained from biopsies of subcutaneous fat and of course this always raises the issue of how far this is representative of the whole circulation (Warshaw et al., 1979). Nevertheless, the data have been informative. Patients treated with thiazide diuretics, conventional β-blockers, α-blockers and short- to medium-acting calcium channel blockers show partial or no regression of structural abnormalities in subcutaneous vessels. On the other hand, long-acting ACE inhibitors, selective AT1 antagonists and long-acting calcium channel blockers did show structural regression (Schiffrin et al., 1995, 2000; Thybo et al., 1995; Rizzoni et al., 1997; Schiffrin, 1998). The reasons for these discrepancies are not known but appear to be unrelated to differential effects on pulse pressure, as has been suggested (Schiffrin and Deng, 1999). On the other hand, it is striking that the same drugs that improve endothelial function also promote the partial normalization of small-artery structure. This is potentially an extremely important link and it is tempting once again to attribute a pivotal role to the renin–angiotensin system.

Summary and conclusions

We know a great deal about the vascular biology of hypertension, as this brief review must indicate without even touching on the biology of larger vessels. At the same time, there are obvious gaps in our understanding. The consensus can be summarized as follows. In hypertensive individuals small vessels (from small arteries to capillaries, with internal diameters $< 500\,\mu m$), differ from those of controls in number, structure and function. That is to say:

1. in some vascular beds at least, the number and density of capillaries is reduced (rarefaction).
2. in small arteries the media-to-lumen ratio is generally increased, mostly by eutrophic remodelling, where the configuration of the blood vessel is altered, without any change in the mass of the vascular wall.
3. endothelium-dependent relaxation is impaired in most small (and large) vessels.

Some further issues arise from this: is there any unifying mechanism underlying

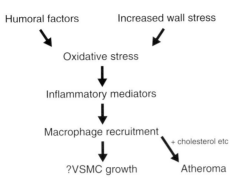

Figure 12.9 Scheme of possible roles of oxidative stress and inflammation in the pathogenesis of hypertension. VSMC, vascular smooth muscle cell.

these changes? What is their relevance in the wider context of cardiovascular disease, particularly atherosclerosis?

The 'chicken and egg' questions about vascular structure and function remain largely unresolved in primary essential hypertension, mainly because of our very incomplete understanding of the aetiology of this condition. For the moment it may be best to avoid too much immersion in such questions. Instead, it may be interesting to focus on two issues that appear to be interrelated: oxidative stress and angiotensin II. As earlier discussion has indicated, angiotensin II is a promoter of free radical generation in the vasculature (Romero and Reckelhoff, 1999). In addition to the direct and indirect vasconstrictor effects that this produces, it is also possible that the overall increase in cellular oxidative stress may have other consequences (Chakraborti et al., 1998; Kunsch and Medford, 1999) which may include vascular smooth muscle cell proliferation (Griendling and Ushio-Fukai, 1998; Viedt et al., 2000). It is hardly likely that angiotensin II is the sole stimulus for such processes. Increased wall stress is another likely candidate (Howard et al., 1997), as are circulating lipoproteins, particularly oxidized low-density lipoprotein (Andalibi et al., 1993; Galle et al., 1999). This therefore forms one point of convergence between the vascular abnormalities related to high blood pressure and those attributed to raised levels of plasma lipids. Although atherosclerosis is usually characterized as a disease of medium and large arteries, it is now well established that functional endothelial abnormalities also encompass smaller vessels (Cooper and Heagerty, 1998). One way of looking at hypertension and hyperlipidaemia may be as promoters of oxidative stress (Kojda and Harrison, 1999; Dhalla et al., 2000), and indeed of inflammation (Taylor, 1999; Figure 12.9). There is also a further link to angiotensin II. Hypercholesterolaemia induces

expression of angiotensin AT1 receptor and these can be downregulated by lowering cholesterol with hydroxymethyl glutaryl coenzyme A reductase inhibitors (Nickenig et al., 1999). A picture is therefore emerging of the totality of the vascular biology of human disease, of which hypertension is a critical component.

REFERENCES

Andalibi, A., Liao, F., Imes, S., Fogelman, A.M. & Lusis, A.J. (1993). Oxidized lipoproteins influence gene expression by causing oxidative stress and activating the transcription factor NF-kappa B. *Biochem. Soc. Trans.*, **21**, 651–5.

Antonios, T.F.T., Singer, D.R.J., Markandu, N.D., Mortimer, P.S. & McGregor, G.A. (1999). Rarefaction of skin capillaries in borderline essential hypertension suggests an early structural abnormality. *Hypertension*, **34**, 655–8.

Aylett, M., Creighton, P., Jachuck, S., Newrick, D. & Evans, A. (1999). Stopping drug treatment of hypertension: experience in 18 British general practices. *Br. J. Gen. Pract.*, **49**, 977–80.

Barker, D.J. (1997). Fetal nutrition and cardiovascular disease in later life. *Br. Med. Bull.*, **53**, 96–108.

Beckman, J.S. & Koppenol, W.H. (1996). Nitric oxide, superoxide and peroxynitrite: the good, the bad and the ugly. *Am. J. Physiol.*, **271**, C1424–37.

Berry, C., Hamilton, C.A., Brosnan, M.J. et al. (2000). Investigation into the sources of superoxide in human blood vessels: angiotensin II increases superoxide production in human internal mammary arteries. *Circulation*, **101**, 2206–12.

Boulanger, C.M. (1999). Secondary endothelial dysfunction: hypertension and heart failure. *J. Mol. Cell Cardiol.*, **31**, 39–49.

Brennecke, S.P., Gude, N.M., Di Iulio, J.L. & King, R.G. (1997). Reduction of placental nitric oxide synthase activity in pre-eclampsia. *Clin. Sci. (Colch.)*, **93**, 51–5.

Butler, R., Morris, A.D., Belch, J.J., Hill, A. & Struthers, A.D. (2000). Allopurinol normalizes endothelial dysfunction in type 2 diabetics with mild hypertension. *Hypertension*, **35**, 746–51.

Calver, A., Collier, J., Moncada, S. & Vallance, P. (1992). Effect of local intra-arterial N^G-monomethyl-L-arginine in patients with hypertension: the nitric oxide dilator mechanism appears abnormal. *J. Hypertens.*, **10**, 1025–31.

Cardillo, C., Kilcoyne, C.M., Quyyumi, A.A., Cannon, R.O. III & Panza, J.A. (1998). Selective defect in nitric oxide synthesis may explain the impaired endothelium-dependent vasodilatation in patients with essential hypertension. *Circulation*, **97**, 851–6.

Chakraborti, T., Ghosh, S.K., Michael, J.R., Batabyal, S.K. & Chakraborti, S. (1998). Targets of oxidative stress in cardiovascular system. *Mol. Cell. Biochem.*, **187**, 1–10.

Cooper, A. & Heagerty, A.M. (1998). Endothelial dysfunction in human intramyocardial small arteries in atherosclerosis and hypercholesterolemia. *Am. J. Physiol.*, **275**, H1482–8.

Cosentino, F., Patton, S., d'Uscio, L.V. et al. (1998). Tetrahydrobiopterin alters superoxide and nitric oxide release in prehypertensive rats. *J. Clin. Invest.*, **101**, 1530–7.

Dawes, M., Brett, S.E., Chowienczyk, P.J., Mant, T.G. & Ritter, J.M. (1999). The vasodilator action of nebivolol in forearm vasculature of subjects with essential hypertension. *Br. J. Clin. Pharmacol.*, **48**, 460–3.

de Artiñano, A.A. & Gonzalez, V.L.-M. (1999). Endothelial dysfunction and hypertensive vasoconstriction. *Pharmacol. Res.*, **40**, 113–24.

Dhalla, N.S., Temsah, R.M. & Netticadan, T. (2000). Role of oxidative stress in cardiovascular diseases. *J. Hypertens.*, **18**, 655–73.

Folkow, B. (1982). Physiological aspects of primary hypertension. *Physiol. Rev.*, **62**, 340–504.

Folkow, B. (1995). Hypertensive structural changes in systemic precapillary resistance vessels: how important are they for *in vivo* haemodynamics? *J. Hypertens.*, **13**, 1546–59.

Folkow, B. (2000). The debate on the 'amplifier hypothesis' – some comments. *J. Hypertens.*, **18**, 375–8.

Forte, P., Copland, M., Smith, L.M. et al. (1997). Basal nitric oxide synthesis in essential hypertension. *Lancet*, **349**, 837–42.

Froom, J., Trilling, J.S., Yes, S.S. et al. (1997). Withdrawal of antihypertensive medications. *J. Am. Board. Fam. Pract.*, **10**, 249–58.

Galle, J., Schneider, R., Heinloth, A. et al. (1999). Lp(a) and LDL induce apoptosis in human endothelial cells and in rabbit aorta: role of oxidative stress. Kidney Int., **55**, 1450–61.

Griendling, K.K. & Ushio-Fukai, M. (1998). Redox control of vascular smooth muscle proliferation. *J. Lab. Clin. Med.*, **132**, 9–15.

Griendling, K.K., Minieri, C.A., Ollerenshaw, J.D. & Alexander, R.W. (1994). Angiotensin II stimulates NADH and NADPH oxidase activity in cultured smooth muscle cells. *Circ. Res.*, **74**, 1141–8.

Heagerty, A.M., Aalkjaer, C., Bund, S.J., Korsgaard, N. & Mulvany, M.J. (1993). Small artery structure in hypertension. Dual processes of remodeling and growth. *Hypertension*, **21**, 391–7.

Howard, A.B., Alexander, R.W., Nerem, R.M., Griendling, K.K. & Taylor, W.R. (1997). Cyclic strain induces an oxidative stress in endothelial cells. *Am. J. Physiol.*, **272**, C421–7.

Ibrahim, J., Hughes, A.D., Schachter, M. & Sever, P.S. (1996). Depletion of resistance vessel polyamines attenuates angiotensin II induced blood pressure rise in rats. *Clin. Exp. Hypertens.*, **18**, 811–30.

Igarashi, K. & Kashigawi, K. (2000). Polyamines: mysterious modulator of cellular functions. *Biochem. Biophys. Res. Commun.*, **271**, 559–64.

Izzard, A.S., Heagerty, A.M. & Leenan, F.H.H. (1999). The amplifier hypothesis: permission to dissent? *J. Hypertens.*, **17**, 1667–9.

Jennings, G.L., Reid, C.M., Sudhir, K., Laufer, E. & Korner, P.I. (1995). Factors influencing the success of withdrawal of antihypertensive drug therapy. *Blood Press. Suppl.*, **2**, 99–107.

John, S. & Schmieder, R.E. (2000). Impaired endothelial function arterial hypertension and hypercholesterolemia: potential mechanism and differences. *J. Hypertens.*, **18**, 363–74.

Kocemba, J., Kawecka-Jaszcz, K., Gryglewska, B. & Grodzicki, T. (1998). Isolated systolic hypertension: pathophysiology, consequences and therapeutic benefits. *J. Hum. Hypertens.*, **12**, 621–6.

Kojda, G. & Harrison, D. (1999). Interactions between NO and reactive oxygen species: pathophysiological importance in atherosclerosis, hypertension, diabetes and heart failure. *Cardiovasc. Res.*, **43**, 562–71.

Krum, H., Viskoper, R.J., Lacourciere, Y., Budde, M. & Charlon, V. (1998). The effect of an endothelin-receptor antagonist, bosentan, on blood pressure in patients with essential hypertension. Bosentan hypertension investigators. *N. Engl. J. Med.*, **338**, 784–90.

Kunsch, C. & Medford, R.M. (1999). Oxidative stress as a regulator of gene expression in the vasculature. *Circ. Res.*, **85**, 753–66.

Lever, A.F. & Harrap, S.B. (1992). Essential hypertension: a disorder of growth with origins in childhood? *J. Hypertens.*, **10**, 101–20.

Lip, G.Y.H. & Li-Saw-Hee, F.L. (1998). Does hypertension confer a hypercoagulable state? *J. Hypertens.*, **16**, 913–16.

Lipke, D.W., Newman, P.S., Tofiq, S., Aziz, S.M. & Soltis, E.E. (1997). Eflornithine alters changes in vascular responsiveness associated with coarctation hypertension. *Clin. Exp. Hypertens.*, **19**, 297–312.

Mombouli, J.-V. & Vanhoutte, P.M. (1999). Endothelial dysfunction: from physiology to therapy. *J. Mol. Cell Cardiol.*, **31**, 61–74.

Mulvany, M.J. (1999). Vascular remodelling of resistance vessels: can we define this? *Cardiovasc. Res.*, **41**, 9–13.

Mulvany, M.J. & Aalkjaer, C. (1990). Structure and function of small arteries. *Physiol. Rev.*, **70**, 921–61.

Napolitano, M., Miceli, F., Calce, A. et al. (2000). Expression and relationship between endothelin-1 messenger ribonucleic acid (mRNA) and inducible/endothelial nitric oxide synthase mRNA isoforms from normal and preeclamptic placentas. *J. Clin. Endocrinol. Metab.*, **85**, 2318–23.

Nickenig, G., Baumer, A.T., Temur, Y. et al. (1999). Statin-sensitive dysregulated AT1 receptor function and density in hypercholesterolemic men. *Circulation*, **100**, 2131–4.

Panza, J.A., Garcia, C.E., Kilcoyne, C.M., Quyyumi, A.A. & Cannon, R.O. III (1995). Impaired endothelium-dependent vascular relaxation in patients with essential hypertension. Evidence that nitric oxide abnormality is not localized to a single signal transduction pathway. *Circulation*, **91**, 1732–8.

Rizzoni, D., Muiesan, M.L., Porteri, E. et al. (1997). Effects of long-term antihypertensive treatment with lisinopril on resistance arteries in hypertensive patients with left ventricular hypertrophy. *J. Hypertens.*, **15**, 197–204.

Rizzoni, D., Porteri, E., Guefi, D. et al. (2000). Cellular hypertrophy in subcutaneous small arteries of patients with renovascular hypertension. *Hypertension*, **35**, 931–5.

Romero, J.C. & Reckelhoff, J.F. (1999). Role of angiotensin and oxidative stress in essential hypertension. *Hypertension*, **34**, 943–9.

Ruschitzka, F., Corti, R., Noll, G. & Lüscher, T.F. (1999). A rationale for the treatment of endothelial dysfunction in hypertension. *J. Hypertens.*, **17** (suppl. 1), S25–35.

Schiffrin, E.L. (1998). Vascular remodelling and endothelial function in hypertensive patients: effects of antihypertensive therapy. *Scand. Cardiovasc. J. Suppl.*, **47**, 15–21.

Schiffrin, E.L. & Deng, L.Y. (1999). Relationship between small-artery structure and systolic, diastolic and pulse pressure in essential hypertension. *J. Hypertens.*, **17**, 381–7.

Schiffrin, E.L., Deng, L.Y. & Larochelle, P. (1995). Progressive improvement in the structure of resistance arteries of hypertensive patients after 2 years of treatment with an angiotensin

I-converting enzyme inhibitor: comparison with effects of a beta-blocker. *Am. J. Hypertens.*, **8**, 229–36.

Schiffrin, E.L., Park, J.B., Intengan, H.D. & Touyz, R.M. (2000). Correction of arterial structure and endothelial dysfunction in human essential hypertension by the angiotensin receptor antagonist losartan. *Circulation*, **101**, 1653–9.

Soltis, E.E., Newman, P.S. & Olson, J.W. (1991). Polyamines, vascular smooth muscle, and deoxycorticosterone acetate-salt hypertension. *Hypertension*, **18**, 85–92.

Soltis, E.E., Newman, P.S. & Olson, J.W. (1994). Eflornithine treatment in SHR: potential role of vascular polyamines and ornithine decarboxylase in hypertension. *Clin. Exp. Hypertens.*, **16**, 595–610.

Struijker Boudier, H.A., le Noble, J.L., Messing, M.W. et al. (1992). The microcirculation and hypertension. *J. Hypertens.*, **10** (suppl.), S147–56.

Surdacki, A., Nowicki, M., Sandmann, J. et al. (1999). Reduced urinary excretion of nitric oxide metabolites and increased plasma levels of asymmetric dimethylarginine in men with essential hypertension. *J. Cardiovasc. Pharmacol.*, **33**, 652–8.

Taddei, S., Virdis, A., Ghiadoni, L., Magagna, A. & Salvetti, A. (1997). Cyclooxygenase inhibition restores nitric oxide activity in essential hypertension. *Hypertension*, **29**, 274–9.

Taddei, S., Virdis, A., Ghiadoni, L. & Salvetti, A. (1998). Endothelial dysfunction in hypertension: fact or fancy? *J. Cardiovasc. Pharmacol.*, **32** (suppl 3), S41–7.

Taylor, W.R. (1999). Hypertensive vascular disease and inflammation: mechanical and humoral mechanisms. *Curr. Hypertens. Rep.*, **1**, 96–101.

Thybo, N.K., Stephens, N., Cooper, A. et al. (1995). Effect of antihypertensive treatment on small arteries of patients with previously untreated essential hypertension. *Hypertension*, **25**, 474–81.

Ueda, S., Matsuoka, H., Miyazaki, H. et al. (2000). Tetrahydrobiopterin restores endothelial function in long-term smokers. *J. Am. Coll. Cardiol.*, **35**, 71–5.

Ueno, H., Kanellakis, P., Agrotis, A. & Bobik, A. (2000). Blood flow regulates the development of vascular hypertrophy, smooth muscle cell proliferation, and endothelial cell nitric oxide synthase in hypertension. *Hypertension*, **36**, 89–96.

Viedt, C., Soto, U., Krieger-Bauer, H.I. et al. (2000). Differential activation of mitogen-activated protein kinases in smooth muscle cells by angiotensin II: involvement of p22[phox] and reactive oxygen species. *Arteriscler. Thromb. Vasc. Biol.*, **20**, 940–8.

Wallace, H.M. (2000). The physiological role of polyamines. *Eur. J. Clin. Invest.*, **30**, 1–3.

Wang, W., Wang, S., Yan, L. et al. (2000). Superoxide production and reactive oxygen species signalling by endothelial nitric-oxide synthase. *J. Biol. Chem.*, **275**, 16899–903.

Warshaw, D.M., Mulvany, M.J. & Halpern, W. (1979). Mechanical and morphological properties of arterial resistance vessels in young and old spontaneously hypertensive rats. *Circ. Res.*, **45**, 250–9.

Wright, C.E. & Angus, J.A. (1999). Enhanced total peripheral vascular responsiveness in hypertension accords with amplifier hypothesis. *J. Hypertens.*, **17**, 1687–96.

Zhang, H., Schmeisser, A., Garlichs, C.D. et al. (1999). Angiotensin II-induced superoxide anion generation in human vascular endothelial cells: role of membrane-bound NADH-/NADPH-oxidases. *Cardiovasc. Res.*, **44**, 215–22.

13

Atherosclerosis

James H. F. Rudd and Peter L. Weissberg

School of Clinical Medicine, University of Cambridge, Cambridge

Introduction

Atherosclerosis continues to be a leading cause of mortality and morbidity throughout the world. It has until recently been thought of as a degenerative disease, affecting predominantly older people, with progression over several decades, and eventually leading to symptoms through its mechanical effects on blood flow, particularly in the small-calibre arteries supplying the myocardium and brain. Because of the perceived insidious and relentless nature of its development, there has been a somewhat pessimistic view of the potential to modify its progression by medical therapy, and treatment has instead been dominated by interventional revascularization approaches, targeting the largest and most visible or symptomatic lesions with angioplasty or bypass surgery. There has been little emphasis on the diagnosis and quantification of subclinical disease, or the treatment of high-risk, asymptomatic patients. Recently, this defeatist view of the pathogenesis and progression of atherosclerosis has begun to change, firstly, because careful descriptive studies of the underlying pathology of atherosclerosis have revealed that atherosclerotic plaques differ in their cellular composition, and that the cell types predominating in the plaque can determine the risk of a fatal clinical event such as myocardial infarction or stroke. Secondly, cellular and molecular biological studies, particularly involving transgenic mice, have emphasized the importance of inflammatory cells and inflammatory mediators in the pathogenesis of atherosclerosis. The third and most important reason is because several recent large-scale clinical studies have shown that drugs, in particular the statin group of lipid-lowering agents, can reduce clinical events in patients with established atherosclerosis without necessarily reducing the size of flow-limiting lesions. Taken together, this evidence has shown that, rather than being an irreversible, inevitably progressive disease, atherosclerosis is a dynamic, inflammatory process that is potentially modifiable with medical therapy. Understanding the cellular and molecular interactions that determine the development and

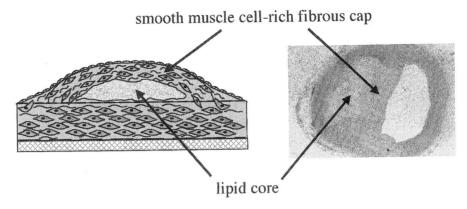

smooth muscle cell-rich fibrous cap

lipid core

Figure 13.1   Stable atherosclerotic lesion. This lesion has a low risk of rupture. There are numerous vascular smooth muscle cells in a uniformly thick fibrous cap, with relatively few inflammatory cells present.

progression of atherosclerosis brings with it opportunities to develop novel therapeutic agents targeting key molecular and cellular interactions in its aetiology. In addition, the recognition that the outcome of atherosclerotic disease depends much more on plaque composition than plaque size also argues for a new diagnostic approach dominated less by determining plaque size, as in angiography, and focused more on plaque cellular content and activity.

The pathogenesis of atherosclerosis

The normal artery consists of a tube of vascular smooth muscle cells (VSMCs) with their associated extracellular matrix (the media), lined by a single layer of endothelial cells on the luminal surface (the intima), and surrounded by connective tissue containing blood vessels and nerves on the outside (the adventitia). In normal arteries, the luminal diameter of the vessel can be altered by contraction and relaxation of the VSMCs, in response to a variety of local and circulating signals.

Histologically, the earliest lesion in atherosclerosis is a subendothelial accumulation of lipid-laden monocyte-derived foam cells and associated T lymphocytes which form a nonstenotic fatty streak. Fatty streaks are asymptomatic and are present in most people in the western world by the second decade of life. With progression, the core of the plaque becomes necrotic, containing cellular debris, crystalline cholesterol and inflammatory cells, particularly macrophage foam cells. This core is bounded on its luminal aspect by an endothelialized fibrous cap containing VSMCs embedded in an extensive collagenous extracellular matrix (Figure 13.1). Inflammatory cells are also present in the fibrous cap, particularly in the 'shoulder' regions, where T cells, mast cells and especially macrophages have a tendency to accumulate. In advanced lesions, there are also deposits of calcium hydroxyapatite, which make the lesions less compressible and therefore more prone to rupture. There are also numerous immature new blood vessels that facilitate further recruitment of inflammatory cells and tend to predispose to intraplaque haemorrhage. Thus, the composition of atherosclerotic lesions is variable and complex, and it is the interaction between the various cell types within a plaque that determines the progression, complications and outcome of the disease.

The endothelium

Over the last few years, it has become clear that the endothelium plays a crucial role in vascular biology and the development of vascular disease by producing a number of vasoactive and antithrombotic molecules, in particular prostacyclin and nitric oxide (NO). NO is a potent vasodilator, but is also involved in inhibition of platelet aggregation, inhibition of VSMC proliferation, inhibition of inflammation and, depending on concentration, either scavenging or production of potentially destructive oxygen free radicals, in particular peroxynitrite (Anggard, 1994; Bhagat and Vallance, 1996; Hobbs et al., 1999). Physiologically, the earliest detectable manifestation of atherosclerosis is reduced production or bioavailability of NO in response to pharmacological or haemodynamic stimuli (Ross, 1999). This is demonstrable even in children with hypercholesterolaemia (Sorensen et al., 1994) where there is reduced brachial artery dilatation in response to increased forearm blood flow. This is consistent with the hypothesis that high circulating levels of atherogenic lipoproteins cause endothelial dysfunction and (by unknown mechanisms) subendothelial lipid accumulation. Importantly, drugs that have been shown to improve the outcome of vascular disease, including statins and angiotensin-converting enzyme inhibitors, also improve endothelial function.

Crucially, endothelial cells in atherosclerosis also express surface-bound selectins and adhesion molecules, such as P-selectin, intercellular adhesion molecule-1 (ICAM-1) and vascular cell adhesion molecule-1 (VCAM-1) that attract and capture circulating inflammatory cells and facilitate their migration into the subendothelial space (Ross, 1999). Their importance in the development of atherosclerosis is clearly demonstrated by experiments using genetic knockout mice which lack their expression. The animals developed smaller lesions with lower lipid content and fewer inflammatory cells than control mice when fed a high-cholesterol diet (Nakashima et al., 1998). These animal models clearly demonstrate the importance of inflammatory cell recruitment to the pathogenesis of atherosclerosis, but since inflammatory cells are never seen in the intima in the absence of lipid, the results are consistent with the underlying premise that lipid accumulation is the trigger to the development of an atherosclerotic plaque. The tendency for atherosclerosis to occur preferentially at particular sites in the arterial tree may be due to subtle differences in endothelial function, induced particularly by alterations in local shear stress, which is known to influence expression of a number of endothelial cell genes, including ICAM-1 and endothelial cell nitric oxide synthase (eNOS; Topper et al., 1996; Resnick et al., 1997).

Inflammatory cells

The accumulation of subendothelial lipid, particularly if oxidized, is thought to stimulate the local inflammatory reaction that initiates and maintains activation of overlying endothelial cells. This results in their continued expression of selectins and adhesion molecules and the expression of chemokines, in particular monocyte chemoattractant proteins-1 (MCP-1; Boring et al., 1998). Chemokines are proinflammatory cytokines that are responsible for chemoattraction, migration and activation of leukocytes. Mice lacking MCP-1 develop smaller atherosclerotic lesions than mice expressing MCP-1 when fed an atherogenic diet (Gosling et al., 1999). Under the influence of activated endothelial cells, appropriate chemokines and adhesion molecules, inflammatory cells migrate into the subendothelial space where they become activated. Monocytes differentiate into macrophages and express the scavenger receptors that allow them to ingest modified, particularly oxidized, lipids and develop into macrophage foam cells, the predominant cell in an early atherosclerotic lesion. In early atherosclerosis at least, the macrophage can be thought of as performing a predominantly beneficial role in 'neutralizing' potentially harmful lipid components in the vessel wall. However, activated inflammatory cells also express a variety of proinflammatory cytokines and growth factors that contribute both beneficially and detrimentally to the evolution of the plaque. Some of these factors are chemoattractant, for example osteopontin (Liaw et al., 1994; Shanahan et al., 1994), and growth-enhancing, for example, platelet-derived growth factor (PDGF) for VSMCs. These cytokines induce VSMCs firstly to migrate from the media to the intima. In addition, activated macrophages may undergo apoptosis, and release their lipid content into the core of the plaque, thereby contributing to its enlargement. It is now generally recognized that the progression and consequences of atherosclerosis are determined by dynamic interactions between inflammatory cells recruited in response to subendothelial lipid accumulation and the local reparative 'wound-healing' response of surrounding VSMCs.

The role of vascular smooth muscle cells

VSMCs reside mostly in the media of adult arteries where their role is to regulate vascular tone. Thus, medial VSMCs contain large amounts of contractile proteins. Continued expression of this 'contractile' phenotype is maintained by the influence of the extracellular proteins in the vessel media acting via integrins in the VSMC membrane. However, on migration from the media to the intima of atherosclerotic arteries, VSMCs undergo a phenotypic change characterized by a reduction in content of contractile proteins and a large increase in the number of synthetic organelles. The migration of VSMCs from the media to the intima and consequent change from a 'contractile' to a 'synthetic' phenotype was once thought to enhance or even initiate the development of an atherosclerotic lesion (Ross and Glomset, 1976). However, it has recently been recognized that intimal VSMCs in atherosclerotic plaques bear a remarkable similarity to VSMCs in the early developing blood vessel (Shanahan and Weissberg, 1998), suggesting that intimal VSMCs may be performing a reparative rather than a destructive role in atherosclerosis. By adopting a synthetic 'repair' phenotype, VSMCs become well adapted to perform this role. Thus, they are able to express the proteinases that they require to break free from their surrounding basement membrane and allow them to migrate to the site of inflammation or injury in response to inflammatory cell chemokines. They are also capable of producing growth factors and their receptors that act in an autocrine loop to facilitate their proliferation at the site of injury. Finally, and most importantly, they produce large quantities of matrix proteins, in particular collagens and elastin, necessary to repair the plaque. Indeed, it is only by changing phenotype and expressing a new repertoire of genes that VSMCs are uniquely able to form and maintain the fibrous cap over the lipid core of an atherosclerotic plaque. The fibrous cap separates the highly thrombogenic lipid-rich core from circulating platelets and the proteins of the coagulation cascade and confers structural stability to the atherosclerotic lesion. And since the VSMC is the only cell capable of synthesizing the cap, it follows that VSMCs play a pivotal role in maintaining plaque stability and protecting against the potentially fatal thrombotic consequences of atherosclerosis (Libby, 1995).

Cellular interactions and plaque stability

Most adult males in the developed world have atherosclerosis to a greater or lesser extent, but females do not usually develop atherosclerosis until after the menopause. Although the precise reasons for this marked gender difference remain uncertain, beneficial effects of female hormones on lipoprotein profiles and endothelial function are likely to bear a strong influence. Early atherosclerosis in

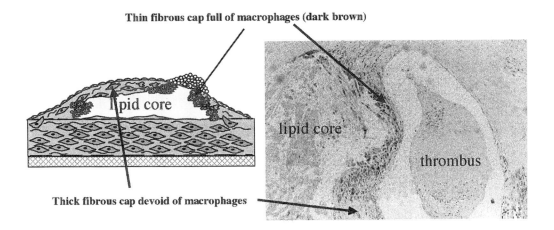

Figure 13.2   Unstable atherosclerotic lesion. A complicated atherosclerotic plaque, with an area of thrombus overlying a fibrous cap rupture.

either sex progresses without symptoms until a lesion manifests itself by one of two mechanisms. With time, macrophage foam cells undergo apoptosis and the remnants become part of an enlarging lipid-rich core. This results in an enlarging plaque, which may limit blood flow at times of increased demand, resulting in reversible ischaemia, as in chronic stable angina. Alternatively, the fibrous cap of a plaque may suddenly rupture or erode, leading to exposure of the thrombogenic lipid core. This is likely to result in subsequent platelet accumulation, fibrin deposition, intravascular thrombosis and consequent tissue necrosis, as in myocardial infarction.

The degree of stenosis, which is the angiographic measure of atherosclerosis, does not necessarily reflect the size of a particular lesion. This is because arteries can remodel to accommodate an expanding atherosclerotic lesion and thus maintain a normal, or near normal, lumen diameter (Glagov et al., 1987). Thus, large atherosclerotic lesions may be, and often are, clinically silent and angiographically insignificant. This is an important and frequently overlooked consideration in the clinical evaluation of atherosclerosis.

Plaques with a large lipid pool and a thin fibrous cap are prone to rupture, whereas those with a thick cap are more able to resist local mechanical stresses and therefore less likely to rupture. The most important determinant of the structure and integrity of the fibrous cap is its cellular composition. Plaques containing a heavy inflammatory cell infiltrate and relatively few VSMCs are at highest risk of rupture (Davies, 1996). If the inflammatory process instigated by the inflammatory cells in the cap predominates over the repairing, stabilizing effects of the VSMCs, there will be fibrous cap destruction (Figure 13.2).

Inflammatory cells act synergistically to promote plaque rupture by a number of different mechanisms. Firstly, by producing proinflammatory cytokines, such as interferon-γ (IFN-γ), they directly inhibit VSMC proliferation (Warner et al., 1989) and collagen synthesis (Amento et al., 1991). Secondly, inflammatory cytokines, in particular interleukin-1β (IL-1β), tumour necrosis factor-α (TNF-α) and IFN-γ, are synergistically cytotoxic for VSMCs, causing depletion in cell number by apoptosis (Geng et al., 1996). Thirdly, it has been demonstrated in cell culture experiments that activated macrophages can induce VSMC apoptosis by direct cell–cell contact (Boyle et al., 1998). Finally, and probably most importantly, macrophages secrete a variety of matrix metalloproteinases that degrade the matrix components of the fibrous cap by proteolytic cleavage of its protein components (Libby, 1995). In combination with these detrimental inflammatory cell actions, VSMCs themselves within the fibrous cap of a mature plaque have a reduced ability to proliferate (Ross et al., 1984; Bennett et al., 1998) and an enhanced susceptibility to apoptosis (Bennett et al., 1997). Thus, inflammatory cells can destroy the fabric of the fibrous cap, and resident VSMCs are poorly equipped to compensate, particularly in the presence of inhibitory inflammatory cytokines. Importantly, all these features can be present in small, haemodynamically insignificant plaques that are clinically silent and angiographically invisible. Thus, plaque composition is far more important than plaque size in determining outcome.

Consequences of plaque rupture

The collagen-rich extracellular matrix that makes up the fibrous cap contains large amounts of tissue factor which, along with the lipid core, is highly thrombogenic. Therefore rupture of the fibrous cap leads invariably to local platelet accumulation and activation. This may result in triggering of the clotting cascade, thrombus formation and, if extensive, complete vessel occlusion. However, plaque rupture does not invariably lead to vessel occlusion and an acute coronary syndrome. Up to 70% of plaques causing high-grade stenosis contain histological evidence of previous subclinical plaque rupture and subsequent repair (Davies, 1995). This is particularly likely to occur if high blood flow through the vessel prevents the accumulation of a large occlusive thrombus. A platelet-rich thrombus contains chemokines and mitogens, in particular PDGF and thrombin, that induce migration and proliferation of VSMCs from the arterial wall (McNamara et al., 1996). It is also a rich source of transforming growth factor-β (TGF-β; Grainger et al., 1995), the most potent stimulator of VSMC matrix synthesis. Thus, nonocclusive plaque rupture induces formation of a new fibrous cap over the organizing thrombus which restabilizes the lesion, but at the expense of increasing its size.

Since this occurs suddenly, there is little opportunity for adaptive remodelling of the artery and the healed lesion may now impede flow sufficiently to produce ischaemic symptoms. This explains why patients who have previously had normal exercise tolerance may suddenly develop symptoms of stable limiting angina. It also follows that, if lesions can grow as a consequence of repeated episodes of silent rupture and repair, inhibition of plaque rupture will reduce progression of atherosclerosis. In summary, therefore, atheromatous plaques may become larger by two methods: the first is a gradual increase in size as a consequence of the apoptotic death of macrophage foam cells and their incorporation into an enlarging necrotic lipid-laden plaque core. The second is a stepwise increase in size because of repeated, often silent episodes of plaque rupture with subsequently excessive VSMC-driven repair.

Implications for clinical evaluation of atherosclerosis

Risk factor assessment

The realization that atherosclerosis is essentially an inflammatory process has prompted the evaluation of circulating markers of inflammation to predict plaque rupture and risk of clinical events. These markers may reflect levels of macrophage activation. Circulating levels of serum amyloid A (SAA), C-reactive protein (CRP) and TNF-α all correlate with risk of a coronary event, but they are nonspecific and may be elevated as a consequence of many inflammatory processes. A major advance in this field has been the development of a highly sensitive assay to measure levels of CRP (hs-CRP) that are below the limit of detection of assays used routinely. This revealed a strong correlation between CRP level and future risk of myocardial infarction and stroke in the Physicians Health Study (Ridker et al., 1997) where it was also demonstrated that subjects with the highest CRP levels (albeit within the conventional normal range) derived most benefit from prophylactic aspirin therapy. The CARE study (a secondary prevention study comparing effects of pravastatin with placebo in patients after myocardial infarction with only mildly elevated cholesterol levels) not only confirmed the association between risk of a vascular event and CRP (and SAA) levels, but also demonstrated that, whilst the CRP level rose over 5 years in the placebo group, it fell in association with risk of an event in the active treatment group, and this reduction was not correlated with the magnitude of the decrease in serum lipids in the treated group (Ridker et al., 1998b). It has also been demonstrated recently that hs-CRP levels in apparently healthy postmenopausal women are also strongly predictive of future coronary events (Ridker et al., 2000). Interestingly, there was no association between the degree of cardiovascular risk or hs-CRP level and the titres of immunoglobulin G antibodies to *Chlamydia pneumoniae*, *Helicobacter pylori*, herpes simplex virus or cytomegalovirus. Levels of more specific markers of vascular inflammation, such as ICAM-1 and VCAM-1, also correlate with risk of vascular events, but their role in clinical practice also remains to be established. Ridker et al. demonstrated a relationship between levels of soluble ICAM-1 in apparently healthy men and the risk of future myocardial infarction, with levels in the highest quartile conferring an increased risk of 80% compared to those with values in the lowest quartile (Ridker et al., 1998a). These results provide powerful support for the theory that atherosclerosis is an inflammatory process and they suggest that biochemical measures of inflammation can be used, in combination with conventional risk factors, to refine risk prediction and help select high-risk patients for primary prevention therapy and to monitor their progress. They also add weight to the idea that statin therapy has an antiinflammatory plaque-stabilizing effect, which could be independent of its lipid-lowering action.

Atherosclerosis imaging

Although plaque composition is more important than size in determining clinical outcome, contrast angiography remains the gold standard diagnostic test in vascular disease. This technique allows high-resolution definition of the site and severity of luminal obstructions. Angiography, however, is not an ideal investigation for predicting risk of plaque rupture and therefore clinical events. Firstly, it only detects lesions that impinge significantly on the lumen, and is unable to image the vessel wall. It cannot therefore give any information about the composition or inflammatory state of plaques. Secondly, it is invasive and involves a finite degree of risk and is therefore usually only performed on patients who already have symptoms of ischaemia. Thirdly, most of the lesions that cause myocardial infarction produce less than a 50% stenosis (Falk et al., 1995), explaining why myocardial infarction occurs so commonly in patients who have experienced no previous symptoms. Thus, despite its continued importance in the evaluation and management of symptomatic coronary disease, angiography has little to offer in terms of risk prediction or therapeutic monitoring, particularly in the asymptomatic population.

Intravascular ultrasound provides much more information than angiography on the extent and composition of targeted plaques but, like angiography, is invasive and expensive and is therefore unsuitable for large-scale evaluation of coronary disease. The extent of coronary calcification, as quantified by electron beam computed tomography, has been shown to predict clinical events, and the technique has a high negative predictive value, with a low calcium score making significant atherosclerotic disease unlikely (Budoff et al., 1998). However, the precise relationship between calcification and plaque progression remains to be

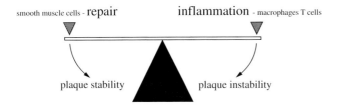

smooth muscle cells - repair   inflammation - macrophages T cells

plaque stability   plaque instability

Figure 13.3   A balancing act. The plaque cell content determines the balance between plaque stability and plaque instability.

determined and monitoring calcification as a surrogate marker of atheroma load will only be of value if, as recently suggested (Callister et al., 1998), it proves to be reversible.

The most promising emerging imaging techniques are magnetic resonance imaging (MRI) and positron emission tomography (PET). MRI can differentiate different plaque components in animal models and human vessels (Toussaint et al., 1996). In addition, it is possible to image plaque progression, regression and rupture (Skinner et al., 1995; McConnell et al., 1999). However, image resolution and movement artefact remain substantial obstacles to its use in diagnosis or monitoring of coronary artery disease. In addition, whilst it may provide some anatomical detail, MRI is unlikely to provide information on inflammatory activity within plaques. In contrast, PET provides no anatomical information but may be able to measure plaque inflammatory cell content and activity. It has been shown that macrophages avidly accumulate the positron-emitting tracer, the glucose analogue 18-fluoro-deoxyglucose ([^{18}F]FDG; Kubota et al., 1994). Early animal studies using [^{18}F]FDG-PET to measure plaque metabolism in balloon-injured hypercholesterolaemic rabbits have been encouraging, with intense uptake noted in the aorta (Vallabhajosula et al., 1996; Vallabhajosula, 1999). However, as with MRI, there are a number of technical obstacles to overcome before its place in clinical evaluation of atheroma (if any) can be established. There is an urgent need to develop new imaging technologies to evaluate plaque composition and inflammatory state, in order to help determine risk of plaque rupture.

The balance of atherosclerosis: therapeutic implications

Atherosclerosis is a dynamic process in which the balance between the destructive influence of inflammatory cells and the reactive, stabilizing effects of VSMCs determines outcome (Figure 13.3). The balance is tipped in favour of plaque rupture by factors such as an atherogenic lipoprotein profile, extent of lipid oxidation and local free radical generation, and genetic variability in expression and activity of the inflammatory molecules involved. For example, a correlation has been described between plaque progression and a polymorphism in the stromelysin-1 gene promoter (Ye et al., 1996). In addition, it is plausible that infective organisms may exacerbate the inflammatory reaction within the plaque. Whilst earlier reported associations between *H. pylori* infection and cardiac events appear to be spurious (Danesh and Peto, 1998), *C. pneumoniae* remains a plausible candidate pathogen, particularly since it can be found within plaque macrophages (Kol et al., 1998). However, currently, the association between infection and coronary events remains hypothetical and the results of ongoing antibiotic treatment clinical trials are awaited with interest.

The balance can be tipped towards plaque stability by a reduction in plaque inflammation and/or an increase in VSMC-driven repair. Lipid reduction, by whatever means, reduces clinical events. Evidence that this may be due to a plaque-stabilizing effect comes from animal studies which showed that statins reduced inflammatory cell and increased VSMC content of plaques (Shiomi et al., 1995), changes that would be expected to enhance stability. More importantly, however, evidence from human clinical studies also points to a plaque-stabilizing effect of statins. Angiographic studies have shown that statins produce a small, haemodynamically insignificant reduction in progression of established stenoses (Investigators, 1994; Jukema et al., 1995; Pitt et al., 1995). They also reduce new lesion formation and, importantly, the number of new vessel occlusions. These arise when a plaque ruptures, and an occlusive thrombus occurs in the context of a well-collateralized myocardial circulation. This seems to imply that statins are stabilizing plaques by reducing rupture rate. This conclusion is supported by the results of all the large primary and secondary prevention studies, which have demonstrated that statins (pravastatin, simvastatin and lovastatin) produce a major reduction in events such as myocardial infarction and stroke, due to plaque rupture (Scandinavian Simvastatin Surival Study, 1994; Shepherd et al., 1995; Sacks et al., 1996; Downs et al., 1998; LIPID Study Group, 1998). Since statins have only a modest effect on plaque size, but cause profound reductions in number of clinical events, these results argue strongly that the statins have a beneficial effect on plaque stability, in addition to effects on lipid lowering. They also highlight the inadequacy of angiography for the prediction of clinical events.

Statin drugs may help stabilize plaques by a variety of different means. It is known that they can exert direct effects on endothelial cell function, inflammatory cell activity, VSMC proliferation, platelet aggregation and thrombus formation (Lacoste et al., 1995; Treasure et al., 1995; Negre-Aminou et al., 1997; Katznelson et al., 1998; Rosenson and Tangney, 1998). Evidence that non-lipid-lowering effects may be important in vivo comes from animal studies in which pravastatin caused beneficial changes in plaque composition (but not size), even when lipid levels were maintained at pretreatment levels (Williams et al., 1998), and from the

WOSCOPS study, in which the outcome benefit from pravastatin therapy was greater than predicted by the achieved reduction in low-density lipoprotein cholesterol. These observations point to potentially important effects of statins that are poorly understood and still have to be defined, but also imply that, since the statins may not exert uniform effects on the biological events contributing to plaque progression and rupture, it is possible that some may afford more or less protection than others for an equivalent lipid-lowering effect.

The notion that plaque stability may be enhanced by directly targeting specific lipid-independent events in the pathogenesis of atherosclerosis has paved the way for the development of new therapies to try to achieve this. Possible therapeutic targets include endothelial NO and adhesion molecule production, the matrix metalloproteinases and inflammatory cytokines and their receptors. Stimulation of VSMC repair is also a potential therapeutic aim. This is currently best achieved by balloon angioplasty which stimulates a vigorous VSMC response to create a matrix-rich neointima. Although this may combine with other factors, most notably arterial recoil and remodelling, to cause restenosis, the resulting lesion rarely, if ever, precipitates an acute coronary event, even when the original target lesion was unstable. It is feasible therefore that regulators of VSMC behaviour, in particular modulators of TGF-β-driven matrix production, may lead to new therapies aimed at enhancing and maintaining the fibrous cap.

Summary

Plaque composition reflects the dynamic balance between lipid-driven inflammatory cell mediated inflammation and the stabilizing, reparative influence of the surrounding VSMCs, and is more important than plaque size in determining outcome in atherosclerosis. This argues for new diagnostic strategies that rely less on angiographic appearances in symptomatic patients and more on potential measures of vascular inflammation and plaque activity in asymptomatic patients with subclinical disease. Results of recent clinical trials have shown that atherosclerosis is a dynamic and therefore potentially reversible process, and have paved the way for new approaches to treatment based on understanding of the underlying biological interactions that determine plaque stability.

Acknowledgements

James Rudd is a British Heart Foundation Clinical Research Fellow. Peter Weissberg is the British Heart Foundation Professor of Cardiovascular Medicine.

REFERENCES

Amento, E.P., Ehsani, N., Palmer, H. & Libby, P. (1991). Cytokines and growth factors positively and negatively regulate interstitial collagen gene expression in human vascular smooth muscle cells. *Arterioscler. Thromb.*, **11**, 1223–30.

Anggard, E. (1994). Nitric oxide: mediator, murderer, and medicine. *Lancet*, **343**, 1199–206.

Bennett, M.R., Littlewood, T.D., Schwartz, S.M. & Weissberg, P.L. (1997). Increased sensitivity of human vascular smooth muscle cells from atherosclerotic plaques to p53-mediated apoptosis. *Circ. Res.*, **81**, 591–9.

Bennett, M.R., Macdonald, K., Chan, S.W., Boyle, J.J. & Weissberg, P.L. (1998). Co-operative interactions between RB and p53 regulate cell proliferation, cell senescence, and apoptosis in human vascular smooth muscle cells from atherosclerotic plaques. *Circ. Res.*, **82**, 704–12.

Bhagat, K. & Vallance, P. (1996). Nitric oxide 9 years on. *J. R. S. Med.*, **88**, 667–73.

Boring, L., Gosling, J., Cleary, M. & Charo, I.F. (1998). Decreased lesion formation in CCR2-/- mice reveals a role for chemokines in the initiation of atherosclerosis. *Nature*, **394**, 894–7.

Boyle, J., Bennett, M., Proudfoot, D., Bowyer, D. & Weissberg, P. (1998). Human monocyte/macrophages induce human vascular smooth muscle cell apoptosis in culture. *J. Pathol.*, **184**, A13.

Budoff, M.J., Shavelle, D.M., Lamont, D.H. et al. (1998). Usefulness of electron beam computed tomography scanning for distinguishing ischemic from non-ischemic cardiomyopathy. *J. Am. Coll. Cardiol.*, **32**, 1173–8.

Callister, T.Q., Raggi, P., Cooil, B., Lippolis, N.J. & Russo, D.J. (1998). Effect of HMG-CoA reductase inhibitors on coronary artery disease as assessed by electron-beam computed tomography. *N. Engl. J. Med.*, **339**, 1972–8.

Danesh, J. & Peto, R. (1998). Risk factors for coronary heart disease and infection with *Helicobacter pylori*: meta-analysis of 18 studies. *Br. Med. J.*, **316**, 1130–2.

Davies, M.J. (1995). Acute coronary thrombosis – the role of plaque disruption and its initiation and prevention. *Eur. Heart J.*, **16** (suppl. L), 3–7.

Davies, M.J. (1996). Stability and instability: two faces of coronary atherosclerosis. *Circulation*, **94**, 2013–20.

Downs, J.R., Clearfield, M., Weis, S. et al. (1998). Primary prevention of acute coronary events with lovastatin in men and women with average cholesterol levels. *J.A.M.A.*, **279**, 1615–22.

Falk, E., Shah, P. & Fuster, V. (1995). Coronary plaque disruption. *Circulation*, **92**, 657–71.

Geng, Y., Wu, Q., Muszynski, M., Hansson, G. & Libby, P. (1996). Apoptosis of vascular smooth muscle cells induced by in vitro stimulation with interferon-gamma, tumor necrosis factor-alpha, and interleukin-1 beta. *Arterioscl. Thromb. Vasc. Biol.*, **16**, 19–27.

Glagov, S., Weisenberg, E., Zarius, C., Starkunavicius, R. & Kolletis, G. (1987). Compensatory enlargement of human atherosclerotic coronary arteries. *N. Engl. J. Med.*, **316**, 371–5.

Gosling, J., Slaymaker, S., Gu, L. et al. (1999). MCP-1 deficiency reduces susceptibility to atherosclerosis in mice that overexpress human apolipoprotein. *J. Clin. Invest.*, **103**, 773–8.

Grainger, D.J., Wakefield, L., Bethell, H.W., Farndale, R.W. & Metcalfe, J.C. (1995). Release and activation of platelet latent TGF-beta in blood clots during dissolution with plasmin. *Nat. Med.*, **1**, 932–7.

Hobbs, A.J., Higgs, A. & Moncada, S. (1999). Inhibition of nitric oxide synthase as a potential therapeutic target. *Annu. Rev. Pharmacol. Toxicol.*, **39**, 191–220.

Investigators (1994). Effect of simvastatin on coronary atheroma: the Multicentre Anti-Atheroma Study (MAAS). *Lancet*, **334**, 633–8.

Jukema, J.W., Bruschke, A.V., van Boven, A.J. et al. (1995). Effects of lipid lowering by pravastatin on progression and regression of coronary artery disease in symptomatic men with normal to moderately elevated serum cholesterol levels. The Regression Growth Evaluation Statin Study (REGRESS). *Circulation*, **91**, 2528–40.

Katznelson, S., Wang, X.M., Chia, D. et al. (1998). The inhibitory effects of pravastatin on natural killer cell activity in vivo and on cytotoxic T lymphocyte activity in vitro. *J. Heart Lung Transplant*, **17**, 335–40.

Kol, A., Sukhova, G. K., Lichtman, A.H. & Libby, P. (1998). Chlamydial heat shock protein 60 localizes in human atheroma and regulates macrophage tumor necrosis factor-alpha and matrix metalloproteinase expression. *Circulation*, **98**, 300–7.

Kubota, R., Kubota, K., Yamada, S. et al. (1994). Active and passive mechanisms of [fluorine-18] fluorodeoxyglucose uptake by proliferating and prenecrotic cancer cells in vivo: a micro-autoradiographic study. *J. Nucl. Med.*, **35**, 104–12.

Lacoste, L., Lam, J.Y., Hung, J. et al. (1995). Hyperlipidemia and coronary disease. Correction of the increased thrombogenic potential with cholesterol reduction. *Circulation*, **92**, 3172–7.

Liaw, L., Almeida, M., Hart, C.E., Schwartz, S.M. & Giachelli, C.M. (1994). Osteopontin promotes vascular cell adhesion and spreading and is chemotactic for smooth muscle cells in vitro. *Circ. Res.*, **74**, 214–24.

Libby, P. (1995). Molecular bases of the acute coronary syndromes. *Circulation*, **91**, 2844–50.

LIPID Study Group (1998). Prevention of cardiovascular events and death with pravastatin in patients with coronary heart disease and a broad range of initial cholesterol levels. The long-term intervention with pravastatin in ischaemic disease. *N. Engl. J. Med.*, **339**, 1349–57.

McConnell, M.V., Aikawa, M., Maier, S.E. et al. (1999). MRI of rabbit atherosclerosis in response to dietary cholesterol lowering. *Arterioscl. Thromb. Vasc. Biol.*, **19**, 1956–9.

McNamara, C.A., Sarembock, I.J., Bachhuber, B.G. et al. (1996). Thrombin and vascular smooth muscle cell proliferation: implications for atherosclerosis and restenosis. *Semin. Thromb. Hemost.*, **22**, 139–44.

Nakashima, Y., Raines, E., Plump, A., Breslow, J. & Ross, R. (1998). Upregulation of VCAM-1 and ICAM-1 at atherosclerosis-prone sites on the endothelium in the ApoE-deficient mouse. *Arterioscl. Thromb.*, **18**, 842–51.

Negre-Aminou, P., van Vliet, A., van Erck, M. et al. (1997). Inhibition of proliferation of human smooth muscle cells by various HMG-CoA reductase inhibitors; comparison with other human cell types. *Biochim. Biophys. Acta*, **1345**, 259–68.

Pitt, B., Mancini, G.B., Ellis, S.G. et al. (1995). Pravastatin limitation of atherosclerosis in the coronary arteries (PLAC I): reduction in atherosclerosis progression and clinical events. PLAC I investigation. *J. Am. Coll. Cardiol.*, **26**, 1133–9.

Resnick, N., Yahav, H., Khachigian, L.M. et al. (1997). Endothelial gene regulation by laminar shear stress. *Adv. Exp. Med. Biol.*, **430**, 155–64.

Ridker, P., Cushman, M., Stampfer, M., Tracy, R. & Hennekens, C. (1997). Inflammation, aspirin, and the risk of cardiovascular disease in apparently healthy men. *N. Engl. J. Med.*, **336**, 973–9.

Ridker, P.M., Hennekens, C.H., Roitman-Johnson, B., Stampfer, M.J. & Allen, J. (1998a). Plasma concentration of soluble intercellular adhesion molecule 1 and risks of future myocardial infarction in apparently healthy men. *Lancet*, **351**, 88–92.

Ridker, P.M., Rifai, N., Pfeffer, M.A. et al. (1998b). Inflammation, pravastatin, and the risk of coronary events after myocardial infarction in patients with average cholesterol levels. Cholesterol and Recurrent Events (CARE) investigators. *Circulation*, **98**, 839–44.

Ridker, P.M., Hennekens, C., Buring, J.E. & Rifai, N. (2000). C-reactive protein and other markers of inflammation in the prediction of cardiovascular disease in women. *N. Engl. J. Med.*, **342**, 836–43.

Rosenson, R.S. & Tangney, C.C. (1998). Antiatherothrombotic properties of statins: implications for cardiovascular event reduction. *J.A.M.A.*, **279**, 1643–50.

Ross, R. (1999). Atherosclerosis – an inflammatory disease. *N. Engl. J. Med.*, **340**, 115–26.

Ross, R. & Glomset, J. (1976). The pathogenesis of atherosclerosis. *N. Engl. J. Med.*, **295**, 369–77.

Ross, R., Wight, T.N., Strandness, E. & Thiele, B. (1984). Human atherosclerosis. I. Cell constitution and characteristics of advanced lesions of the superficial femoral artery. *Am. J. Pathol.*, **114**, 79–93.

Sacks, F.M., Pfeffer, M.A., Moye, L.A. et al. (1996). The effect of pravastatin on coronary events after myocardial infarction in patients with average cholesterol levels. *N. Engl. J. Med.*, **335**, 1001–9.

Scandinavian Simvastatin Survival Study (1994). Randomised trial of cholesterol lowering in 4444 patients with coronary heart disease. *Lancet*, **344**, 1383–9.

Shanahan, C. & Weissberg, P. (1998). Smooth muscle cell heterogeneity: patterns of gene expression in vascular smooth muscle cells in vitro and in vivo. *Arteriosci. Thromb. Vasc. Biol.*, **18**, 333–8.

Shanahan, C.M., Cary, N.R., Metcalfe, J.C. & Weissberg, P.L. (1994). High expression of genes for calcification-regulating proteins in human atherosclerotic plaques. *J. Clin. Invest.*, **93**, 2393–402.

Shepherd, J., Cobbe, S., Ford, I. et al. (1995). Prevention of coronary heart disease with pravastatin in men with hypercholesterolemia. West of Scotland coronary prevention study group. *N. Engl. J. Med.*, **333**, 1301–7.

Shiomi, M., Ito, T., Tsukada, T. et al. (1995). Reduction of serum cholesterol levels alters lesional composition of atherosclerotic plaques. Effect of pravastatin sodium on atherosclerosis in mature WHHL rabbits. *Arteriosci. Thromb. Vasc. Biol.*, **15**, 1938–44.

Skinner, M.P., Yuan, C., Mitsumori, L. et al. (1995). Serial magnetic resonance imaging of experimental atherosclerosis detects lesion fine structure, progression and complications in. *Nat. Med.*, **1**, 69–73.

Sorensen, K.E., Celermajer, D.S., Georgakopoulos, D. et al. (1994). Impairment of endothelium-dependent dilation is an early event in children with familial hypercholesterolemia and is related to the lipoprotein(a) level. *J. Clin. Invest.*, **93**, 50–5.

Topper, J.N., Cai, J., Falb, D. & Gimbrone, M.A. Jr. (1996). Identification of vascular endothelial genes differentially responsive to fluid mechanical stimuli: cyclooxygenase-2, manganese superoxide dismutase, and endothelial cell nitric oxide synthase are selectively up-regulated by steady laminar shear stress. *Proc. Natl Acad. Sci. U.S.A.*, **93**, 10417–22.

Toussaint, J.F., LaMuraglia, G.M., Southern, J.F., Fuster, V. & Kantor, H.L. (1996). Magnetic resonance images lipid, fibrous, calcified, hemorrhagic, and thrombotic components of human atherosclerosis in vivo. *Circulation*, **94**, 932–8.

Treasure, C.B., Klein, J.L., Weintraub, W.S. et al. (1995). Beneficial effects of cholesterol-lowering therapy on the coronary endothelium in patients with coronary artery disease. *N. Engl. J. Med.*, **332**, 481–7.

Vallabhajosula, S. (1999) In: *The Vulnerable Atherosclerotic Plaque: Understanding, Identification, and Modification*, Ed. Fuster, V., pp. 213–29. New York: Futura.

Vallabhajosula, S., Machac, J., Knesaurek, K. et al. (1996). Imaging atherosclerosis macrophage density by positron emission tomography using F-18-fluorodeoxyglucose (FDG). *J. Nucl. Med.*, **37**, 38P.

Warner, S.J., Friedman, G.B. & Libby, P. (1989). Immune interferon inhibits proliferation and induces 2'-5'-oligoadenylate synthetase gene expression in human vascular smooth muscle cells. *J. Clin. Invest.*, **83**, 1174–82.

Williams, J.K., Sukhova, G.K., Herrington, D.M. & Libby, P. (1998). Pravastatin has cholesterol-lowering independent effects on the artery wall of atherosclerotic monkeys. *J. Am. Coll. Cardiol.*, **31**, 684–91.

Ye, S., Eriksson, P., Hamsten, A. et al. (1996). Progression of coronary atherosclerosis is associated with a common genetic variant of the human stromelysin-1 promoter which results in reduced gene expression. *J. Biol. Chem.*, **271**, 13055–60.

14

Abdominal aortic aneurysm

Janet T. Powell

Department of Vascular Surgery, Imperial College School of Medicine, London

Introduction

The aorta has to withstand the load imposed by arterial blood pressure for a lifetime. The microanatomy of the aorta reflects this burden and the media is thick, composed of numerous concentric lamellae of elastic connective tissue and smooth muscle cells. In youth and health elastin is the principal load-bearing component of the aorta with collagen fibres only being recruited at the highest loads (Burton, 1954). Other microfibrils, including fibrillin-rich fibrils, also contribute to load bearing. The abdominal aorta, distal to the renal arteries, is the aortic segment with least elastin and least nutrient vasa vasorum in the adventitia. With ageing this segment of the aorta is vulnerable to weakening and fusiform aneurysmal dilatation: abdominal aortic aneurysms (AAAs) are present in approximately 5% of men aged 65 years or older.

Definition of an abdominal aortic aneurysm

The normal diameter of the infrarenal aorta is 1.5–2.2 cm, with taller patients tending to have wider aortas. The infrarenal aorta is conveniently assessed by ultrasonography. A localized fusiform dilation is clearly evidenced when the proximal and distal aortic diameters are much smaller than the maximum diameter. One suggested definition of an AAA is when the ratio of maximum diameter to infrarenal diameter exceeds 1.5 cm. However, the resolution and visualization of the suprarenal aorta by ultrasonography are poor. A more convenient and widely accepted definition of an aneurysm is when the maximum anterior–posterior diameter exceeds 3 cm.

Clinical examination often fails to detect the smallest aneurysms (3 5 cm) but larger aneurysms are readily detected by clinical examination. The largest aneurysms may reach from 10 to 15 cm in diameter, but the larger the aneurysm, the higher the risk of catastrophic rupture.

Disease burden and epidemiology

Studies in three continents have indicated that the incidence of AAA is increasing (Fowkes et al., 1989). AAA was one of the outcomes documented in the Framingham study and has been associated strongly with smoking. Two other epidemiological studies have identified hypertension as a risk factor for AAA (Strachan, 1991; Reed et al., 1992). In Strachan's study diastolic blood pressure and the smoking of hand-rolled cigarettes were associated with a greatly increased risk of death from ruptured AAA. It is also the author's prejudice that AAA is usually a smoking-related disorder and the increasing incidence of AAA lags 30–40 years behind the rise of cigarette consumption (Henney et al., 1993). The recommended treatment option for all larger aneurysms (> 5.5 cm) is elective aortic graft replacement surgery or endovascular repair. The UK Small Aneurysm Trial, which was established to identify whether prophylactic surgery also provided the best management for smaller aneurysms, reported in 1998 (UK Small Aneurysm Trial Participants, 1998). Early prophylactic surgery had no benefit on long-term survival, minimal benefit on quality of life and increased health service costs. For these reasons, early surgery cannot be recommended for asymptomatic aneurysms < 5.5 cm in diameter. The focus must now be on developing medical therapies to limit the growth of small aneurysms. This emphasizes our need to know more about the biology of aneurysms. Aortic biopsy is readily available at the time of open surgery. Even though the number of elective aneurysm repairs performed each year grows rapidly, so too do the number of emergency operations for ruptured AAA. With the population of 65 + years expected almost to double by 2025, the burden of AAA on health resources is enormous.

Screening studies and clues to the aetiology of abdominal aortic aneurysm

Ultrasonographic screening studies of the general population > 65 years of age have demonstrated the presence of AAA in approximately 5% of men. The prevalence of AAA in women is much lower. The screening of particular groups has indicated predisposing risk factors (Table 14.1; Henney et al., 1993).

Screening hypertensive patients has provided a low yield of AAA but about 10% of patients with intermittent claudication have an AAA and approximately 25% of the brothers of patients with AAA also have an AAA detected on screening. Such studies indicate a strong familial tendency to AAA, although this may be environmental rather than genetic. These studies also indicate a common risk factor for peripheral atherosclerosis and AAA: smoking, dyslipidaemia and hypertension are possible common risk factors. Interestingly, AAA is rare amongst patients with type 2 diabetes.

Table 14.1 Screening for abdominal aortic aneurysm (AAA)

	Prevalence of AAA (%)
Population (> 65 years general practice)	2–6
Patients with hypertension	1
Patients with peripheral arterial disease	10–12
Brothers of patients with AAA	20–30

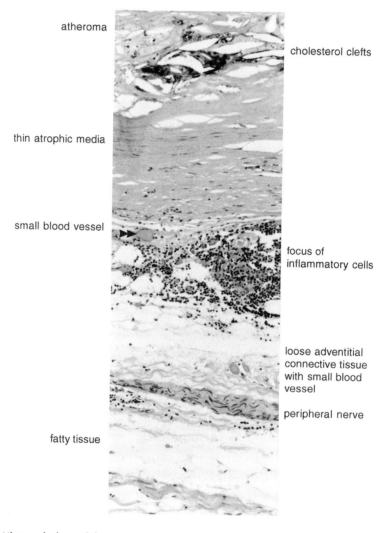

Figure 14.1   Histopathology of the aneurysm.

Histopathology

The aneurysm wall as observed at surgery is lined with laminated thrombus, which must act to deny luminal nutrition to the aortic wall. Underneath this extensive intimal atherosclerosis is the rule (Figure 14.1). Beneath this the media is very thin and atrophic, there is fibrous replacement with few smooth muscle cells being observed, with good evidence for smooth muscle cell apoptosis (Lopez-Candales et al., 1997). The medial connective tissue has become collagen-rich and the elastic fibres are very disrupted, with the elastin content being very reduced. The adventitia has undergone compensatory thickening and neovascularization. In larger aneurysms an extensive inflammatory infiltrate (mainly B cells and macrophages) in the adventitia is an important finding (Koch et al., 1990). Although the media thins and the elastin content is very low, there is compensatory increase in both adventitial collagen and thickness.

Biomechanical properties of the abdominal aorta

With ageing the elastic resilience of the aorta is gradually lost and this accords with a declining elastin content and increasing content of polar glycoproteins in the media. In youth the dry weight elastin content of the aortic wall is approximately 35% compared with about 25% at the age of 70 years and only 8–10% or less in an AAA wall. The aneurysmal wall also is very inelastic and stiff and the stiffness or loss of elasticity appears to depend upon both the elastin content and genetic variation in the type III collagen and fibrillin genes (MacSweeney et al., 1994).

Cell biology and biochemical perspectives

It is very difficult to propagate in culture smooth muscle cells isolated from the adult abdominal aorta. In contrast, cells isolated from the adult thoracic aorta can be passaged readily. It is these cells that, as the aorta develops, synthesize the load-bearing connective tissue components of the aortic media: elastin, types I, III, V collagen, microfibril-associated glycoproteins and fibrillin. Smooth muscle cells isolated from adult abdominal aortic media synthesize collagens type I and III but not elastin in culture.

The earliest theories about aneurysm formation came from experiments of the instillation of elastase into canine aorta in vivo or human vessels in vitro, which was sufficient to cause aneurysmal dilatation (Dobrin et al., 1984; Anidjar et al., 1990). Such aneurysms do not rupture unless collagenase also is installed. These experiments have given rise to a widely held hypothesis for aneurysmal dilatation in the aorta:

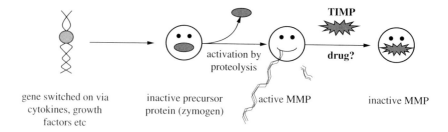

Figure 14.2 Control of matrix metalloproteinases (MMP). TIMP, tissue inhibitor of metalloprotease.

Elastinolysis → aortic dilatation

Collagenolysis → aneurysm rupture

Not surprisingly, many workers have identified increased elastase activity in both the blood and aortic wall of patients with AAA. Elastin is very resistant to both chemical and enzymic degradation and only a few enzymes are known to degrade elastin: these include leukocyte elastase (a serine protease), cathepsin S (a cysteine protease) and matrix metalloproteinases (MMPs), including gelatinases A and B (MMP-2 and MMP-9, respectively), matrilysin (MMP-7) and a metalloelastase (MMP-12). All these enzymes degrade insoluble elastin and, together with their inhibitors, are likely to contribute to the vascular remodelling in the AAA wall. All these enzymes are likely to be present in the aneurysm wall and all are under tight biological control. These enzymes are tightly regulated at both gene and protein level, and often secreted as inactive precursors (zymogens; Figure 14.2). Activation may be triggered by proteolytic cascades and each protease family is inhibited by a separate family of inhibitors: serpins (e.g. α_1-antitrypsin) inhibit the serine proteases, tissue inhibitors of metalloproteases (TIMPs) inhibit MMPs and cystatins inhibit the cysteine proteases MMPs.

As elastin peptides are known to be chemotatic for inflammatory cells, the scheme shown in Figure 14.3 accords with our current knowledge about aneurysmal dilatation. Inflammatory cells in the aneurysm wall, macrophages and lymphocytes, are rich sources of proteases, including MMP-2 and MMP-9.

Inflammation is an important feature of the aneurysm biopsy, with a variable infiltrate of chronic inflammatory cells (B cells and macrophages) in the adventitia; T cells commonly are found as a cuff around the neovasculature in the adventitia. There is no evidence that this inflammation is a response to specific antigens, although viral infection with cytomegalovirus has been suggested to have a pathogenic role in inflammatory aneurysms (Yonemitsu et al., 1996). These inflammatory aneurysms are defined clinically by the dense periaortic fibrosis, which makes surgical resection more difficult. Such inflammatory aneurysms are

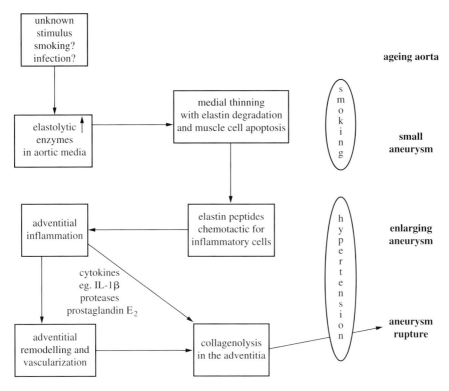

Figure 14.3 Pathogenesis of the abdominal aortic aneurysm. IL-1β, interleukin-1β

not common and in the most common form the chronic inflammation may be a response to hypoxia or a result of a unique stromal environment which favours inflammatory cell residence and proliferation. Irrespective of its origin, this influx of inflammatory cells will play a prominent part in connective tissue remodelling in the aortic wall through secretion of proteases, cytokines and other inflammatory mediators.

Inflammation and proteolysis are considered to be the two key pathological processes driving aneurysm over expansion (Shah, 1997). Hence these processes are attractive targets for therapeutic intervention, e.g. tetracycline derivatives to inhibit metalloprotease activity.

The genetics of AAA

The strong familial predisposition to AAA raises the question of an inherited disorder manifest late in life. Two well-characterized genetic disorders have been associated with aortic fragility (Ehlers–Danlos type IV syndrome) and aortic rupture (Marfan syndrome). These disorders are caused by mutations in the type

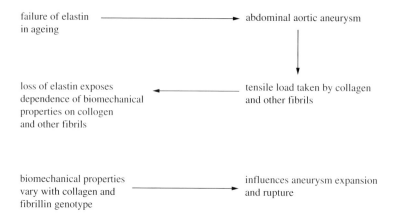

failure of elastin ——————————————→ abdominal aortic aneurysm
in ageing

loss of elastin exposes ←—————————— tensile load taken by collagen
dependence of biomechanical   and other fibrils
properties on collogen
and other fibrils

biomechanical properties ——————————→ influences aneurysm expansion
vary with collagen and   and rupture
fibrillin genotype

Figure 14.4 Abdominal aortic aneurysm: a genetic disorder of the elderly?

III collagen gene (chromosome 2) and the fibrillin-1 gene (chromosome 15), respectively. Both direct gene-sequencing studies and population molecular genetics have failed to demonstrate that mutations or genetic variation in either the fibrillin or type III collagen genes are a common cause of AAA. Similarly, variation in the elastin gene is not a common cause of AAA; however, variations in both the fibrillin and type III collagen gene have been associated with the biomechanical properties of the aneurysm wall (Figure 14.4). Several other candidate genes (e.g. TIMP-1) have been investigated, without any strong associations being observed.

The genetics of AAA remains an unsolved problem and several centres are collecting and pooling families enriched in AAA for a more systematic approach to this problem.

Animal and other models of aortic aneurysm

Dissection of the complex interactions between proteolysis and inflammation in driving aneurysm expansion would be facilitated by the availability of an appropriate animal model. Several animal species, including turkeys and mice (blotchy mice), may develop aneurysms. However, recent focus has been on the development of aneurysms in transgenic mice. The role of serine proteases, particularly plasminogen and its activators – tissue (t + PA) and urokinase (uPA) plasminogen activator – has been highlighted in the work of Carmeliet and colleagues (1997). They found that reduced activity of uPA protected apoE$^-$ mice from elastin destruction and aneurysm formation. These workers have suggested that uPA catalysed activation of plasmin results in the activation of MMPs which degrade elastin. Other workers are trying to evaluate the role of specific MMPs by following the development of elastase-induced aneurysms in transgenic mice (instillation of elastase via balloon catheter provokes elastin degradation and an inflammatory reaction). The role of specific cytokines and inflammatory mediators is also being followed in a rabbit model, where periarterial application of calcium chloride causes aneurysms. However, the mechanisms of the human disease appear to be more complex (Parks, 1999). For these reasons the human tissue explant models, developed by Walton et al. (1999), may prove more useful in identifying the role of the specific inflammatory mediators, e.g. interleukin-1β and prostaglandin E_2.

The cause of abdominal aortic aneurysm

In the past there have been two champion causes of AAA: atherosclerosis and inheritance. My personal viewpoint is that AAA is a multifactorial disorder with complex environmental–genetic interactions, stimulating an adventitital inflammatory response which is critical to the aortic remodelling. The theory that proteolysis and inflammation are the two processes pivotal to aneurysm formation and growth is gaining widespread acceptance. In those who develop AAA at a young age (< 60 years) the genetic contribution is stronger while the environmental contribution is greater for those developing AAA in the seventh and eighth decades. If we all lived to 120 years we might all develop AAA as the elastin in the abdominal aorta wears out and is not replaced.

REFERENCES

Anidjar, S., Salzmann, J.L., Genetric, D., Lagueau, P., Camilleri, J.-P. & Michel, J.-B. (1990). Elastase induced experimental aneurysms in rats. *Circulation*, **82**, 973–81.

Burton, A.C. (1954). Relationship of structure to function of the tissues of the wall of blood vessels. *Physiol. Rev.*, **34**, 619–42.

Carmeliet, P., Moons, L., Lijnen, R. et al. (1997). Urokinase-generated plastin activates matric metalloproteinases during aneurysm formation. *Nat. Guest.*, **17**, 439–44.

Dobrin, P.B., Baker, W.H. & Gley, W.C. (1984). Elastolytic and collagenolytic studies of arteries: implications for the mechanical properties of arteries. *Arch. Surg.*, **119**, 405–9.

Fowkes, F.G.R., MacIntyre, C.C.A. & Ruckley, C.V. (1989). Increasing incidence of aortic aneurysms in England and Wales. *Br. Med. J.*, **298**, 33–5.

Henney, A.M., Adeiseshiah, M., MaxSweeney, S.T.R. et al. (1993). Abdominal aortic aneurysm. *Lancet*, **341**, 215–20.

Koch, A.E., Haines, G.K., Rizzo, R.J. et al. (1990). Human abdominal aortic aneurysms. Immunophenotypic analysis suggesting an immune-medicated response. *Am. J. Pathol.*, **137**, 1199–312.

Lopez-Candales, A., Holmes, D.R., Liao, S. et al. (1997). Decreased vascular smooth muscle cell density in medical degeneration of human abdominal aortic aneurysms. *Am. J. Pathol.*, **150**, 993–1007.

MacSweeney, S.T.R., Powell, J.T. & Greenhalgh, R.M. (1994). The pathogenesis of abdominal aortic aneurysm: a review. *Br. J. Surg.*, **81**, 935–41.

Parks, W.C. (1999). Who are the proteolytic culprits in vascular disease? *J. Clin. Invest.*, **104**, 1167–8.

Reed, D., Reed, C., Stemmerman, G. & Hayashi, T. (1992). Are aortic aneurysms caused by atherosclerosis? *Circulation*, **85**, 205–11, comment, p. 378.

Shah, P.K. (1997). Inflammation, metalloproteinases and increased proteolysis: an emerging pathological paradigm in aortic aneurysm. *Circulation*, **96**, 2115–17.

Strachan, D.P. (1991). Predictors of death from aortic aneurysm among middle-aged men: the Whitehall study. *Br. J. Surg.*, **78**, 401–4.

UK Small Aneurysm Trial Participants (1998). Mortality results for randomised controlled trial of early elective surgery or ultrasonographic surveillance for small abdominal aortic aneurysms. *Lancet*, **352**, 1649–55.

Walton, L.J., Franklin, I.J., Bayston, T. et al. (1999). Inhibition of prostaglandin E_2 synthesis in abdominal aortic aneurysms. *Circulation*, **100**, 48–54.

Yonemitsu, Y., Nakagawa, K., Tanaka, S. et al. (1996). *In situ* detection of frequent and active infection of human cytomegalovirus in inflammatory abdominal aortic aneurysms: possible pathogenic role in sustained chronic inflammatory reaction. *Lab. Invest.*, **74**, 723–36.

15

The vasculature in diabetes

John E. Tooke,[1] Kah Lay Goh[2] and Angela C. Shore[2]

[1]Department of Vascular Medicine, Postgraduate Medical School, Exeter
[2]Department of Diabetes and Vascular Medicine Research Centre, Royal Devon &
Exeter Hospital (Wonford), Exeter

Introduction

Diabetes mellitus owes much of its morbidity and most of its mortality to the late
complications of the condition. These are predominantly vascular in origin and
include diabetic retinopathy, the commonest cause of blindness in people of
working age in our society, and diabetic nephropathy, an increasingly common
cause of renal failure as well as premature peripheral vascular, cerebrovascular and
coronary artery disease. The person with diabetes is approximately three times as
likely to suffer a heart attack, at least twice as likely to suffer a stroke and 20 times
as likely to have a limb amputated.

It is common to refer to the vascular disease associated with diabetes as either
microangiopathy (involving the microcirculation) or macroangiopathy, i.e. arterial disease. It is none the less likely that diabetes affects the whole circulation
although little work has been done on the impact of the condition on venous
function or lymphatic function. Macroangiopathy includes atherosclerosis which
is typified by its prematurity, its multisegmental and distal nature and by the fact
that women of premenopausal age are not spared as they commonly are in the
absence of diabetes. Macroangiopathy also includes arteriosclerosis and may be
regarded as a manifestation of accelerated ageing of the vasculature in diabetes.

Both micro- and macroangiopathy exhibit certain stages in their evolution.
Atherosclerosis goes through the normal stages observed in the nondiabetic
including the formation of the fatty streak, the development of atherosclerotic
plaque, eventually resulting in vessel stenosis and the symptom complexes of
angina and intermittent claudication; the major vascular events of stroke and
myocardial infarction represent the superimposition of thrombus on ruptured
plaque (Ross, 1993). See Chapter 13 for a detailed account of atherogenesis.
Clinical microangiopathy is preceded by functional changes in the microcirculation with later structural adaptation, including capillary basement membrane

thickening. In the kidney the mesangium around the glomerular capillary loops develops to excess. The eventual terminal event is the extinction of the glomerular capillary or closure of the retinal capillary; in the latter case (misplaced), reparative mechanisms result in neovascularization, the resultant new vessels being friable and hyperpermeable (Zatz and Brenner, 1986).

The term 'diabetic angiopathy' suggests that the pathological processes involved are uniform, irrespective of the type of diabetes. There is none the less emerging evidence that the pathophysiology of microangiopathy may differ between two major types, type 1 and type 2.

Type 1 diabetes is characterized by early increase in microvascular pressure and flow. It is thought that this leads to endothelial injury and resultant capillary basement membrane thickening and microvascular sclerosis. This in turn limits maximum hyperaemia and impairs autoregulatory capacity (Parving et al., 1983). In contrast, in type 2 diabetes, in the absence of hypertension microvascular pressure appears normal (Shore et al., 1992). There is however a profound early reduction in vasodilatory reserve and increasing evidence that this abnormality, which probably represents endothelial dysfunction, precedes the development of diabetes (Tooke and Goh, 1999). Indeed, it has been argued that impaired endothelium-dependent vasodilatation may be an intrinsic feature of the vasculature associated with the metabolic syndrome, the insulin-resistant state which almost invariably precedes the development of type 2 diabetes. Whether or not endothelial dysfunction is itself a cause of insulin resistance through impaired insulin-mediated vasodilatation of skeletal muscle remains contentious.

Diabetic angiopathy: a role for the endothelium

Given the location of the vascular endothelium and its multiplicity of roles in relation to the control of vascular function, it is little surprise that it is perceived as the tissue that orchestrates much of the expression of clinical microangiopathy. Evidence for endothelial dysfunction stems from three major sets of observations: firstly, the release of markers of endothelial activation damage into the circulation in diabetic subjects; secondly, evidence for impaired endothelium-dependent vasodilatation and thirdly, changes in vascular permeability.

Endothelial marker studies

Elevated levels of soluble adhesion molecules expressed by endothelial cells and von Willebrand factor have been demonstrated in the serum of patients with diabetes, particularly in the context of diabetic complications (Lim et al., 1999). In line with the concept of intrinsic endotheliopathy being part of the metabolic syndrome, elevated levels of adhesion molecules have also been observed in obese hypertensive subjects with normal glucose tolerance (Ferri et al., 1999). Despite these observations it is difficult to be certain whether the presence of such markers represents occult existing vascular disease or endothelial activation that precedes vascular pathology.

Impaired endothelium-dependent vasodilatation

Endothelial function has been assessed in a variety of vessels in vivo from conduit arteries to skin microvessels. The data for each will be reviewed. In addition, in an attempt to assess whether there is evidence of any change in endothelial function as the disease progresses, studies investigating subjects without clinical complications or with retinopathy only (since the majority will develop some degree of retinopathy as the disease progresses) will be compared with those assessing patients with microalbuminuria, a marker of diabetic renal disease, associated with the more malignant forms of angiopathy expression.

Vascular function in type 1 diabetes (Table 15.1)

In vivo studies

Conduit artery function   Using high-resolution ultrasound and wall-tracking software, conduit artery endothelial function has been assessed by monitoring the change in diameter to an increase in flow through usually the brachial artery (induced by a 5-minute inflation and subsequent release of a cuff around the lower forearm), so called flow-related vasodilatation or FRD (Joannides et al., 1995; see Chapter 3 for a detailed account of flow-related vasodilatation). The femoral, radial or carotid artery may also be used. Impairment in the hyperaemic response to cuff release could result in different stimuli being applied to different groups, thus this should be assessed in all cases. To dissect out whether any abnormalities seen are due to endothelial or smooth muscle dysfunction, endothelium-independent vasodilatation is assessed by the response to sublingual glyceryl trinitrate (GTN). The technique is difficult to use, requiring highly skilled operators to ensure reproducible responses. Flow-related vasodilatation has been shown to vary with resting vessel diameter, thus it is important to ensure groups are matched for basal artery diameter.

Patients with type 1 diabetes with normoalbuminuria may demonstrate an impaired response to both endothelium-dependent and independent responses (Zenere et al., 1995; Clarkson et al., 1996; Donaghue et al., 1997), an impaired FRD but normal GTN response (Lekakis et al., 1997; Meeking et al., 1999) or normal responses for both the endothelium-dependent and independent response (Lambert et al., 1996; Enderle et al., 1998). In the Meeking study endothelium-dependent vasodilatation was impaired but the GTN response showed a wide variability in all groups with a trend to be impaired in the diabetics which failed to

Table 15.1 Summary of vascular function in type 1 diabetes

Vascular bed	Stimulus	Response		
		Long duration/no complications	Normoalbuminuria	Microalbuminuria
Conduit artery	Increased flow	Normal	→	→
	Glyceryl trinitrite	Normal	→	→
Forearm blood vessels	ED agonist	Normal	Normal	Normal
	EI agonist	Normal	Normal	Normal
Skin microvessels	ED agonist	Normal	?	→
	EI agonist	Normal	?	Normal

ED, endothelium-dependent; EI, endothelium-independent

reach statistical significance. The reasons for the discrepancies are unclear. Patient characteristics may contribute: thus in patients of long disease duration, who have had lifelong good glycaemic control, have no clinical complications and have normal lipids, conduit artery function may be normal (Lambert et al., 1996; Enderle et al., 1998), whereas in those with poorer control and abnormal lipids, abnormalities have been reported (Clarkson et al., 1996; Meeking et al., 1999). However, this is unlikely to be the complete explanation as Donaghue et al. (1997) reported in adolescents with moderate/good control, shorter disease duration, normal lipids and minimal complications (retinopathy in 4/16) that both endothelium-dependent and independent function are impaired. Other factors such as smoking (passive and active), exercise levels, sex, insulin, current glycaemia may all influence the response, making interpretation difficult.

In the presence of microalbuminuria, conduit artery endothelial function is abnormal (Zenere et al., 1995; Lekakis et al., 1997; Meeking et al., 1999). The endothelium-independent response is also impaired, although in one of the studies the impairment failed to reach statistical significance (Meeking et al., 1999).

Forearm blood flow The response of the forearm resistance vasculature to the intraarterial administration of endothelium-dependent (acetylcholine, methacholine, carbachol, bradykinin, etc.) and independent (usually sodium nitroprusside but also verapamil) agonists may be assessed by venous occlusion plethysmography. The data should be presented as change in blood flow in the drug-infused arm compared to the control arm in order to take into account nondrug-related changes in blood flow. Differences in baseline blood flow may result in delivery of different concentrations of drugs between groups and thus basal blood flow should be measured. Due to concerns regarding effects of different ambient glucose levels or differences in basal blood flow, several studies have been carried out during euglycaemic clamps, although one could argue that this represents an unphysiological environment.

A large number of such studies have been carried out in type 1 patients without microalbuminuria. The overall summary of these data is that the response to an endothelium-dependent agonist is usually normal whether subjects are studied under normal conditions (Halkin et al., 1991; Calver et al., 1993; Smits et al., 1993; Khan et al., 1996) or during euglycaemic clamp (Elliott et al., 1993; Huvers et al., 1999). The exceptions to this are a study by Johnstone and colleagues (1993) in which the clinical complications of the patients were not described and which was carried out during blockade of prostaglandins, and a study using historical controls which were younger than the patients, a factor which may have contributed to their findings (O'Driscoll et al., 1997). The contribution of nitric oxide

(NO) to resting tone (as determined by infusion of the NO synthax inhibitor N^G-monomethyl-L-arginine (L-NMMA)) has been described as normal (Elliott et al., 1993; Makimattila et al., 1996) or reduced (Calver et al., 1993; Elliott et al., 1993) in this group. The endothelium-independent response was normal in all but two of these studies (Khan et al., 1996; Makimattila et al., 1996).

In patients with microalbuminuria the responses to endothelium-dependent and independent vasodilators were normal when studied under conditions of euglycaemic clamp (Huvers et al., 1999), although the contribution of NO to this vasodilatation was reduced, suggesting other vasodilators may play a greater role (Elliott et al., 1993). Makimattila and colleagues (1996) suggest that diabetic subjects with or without microalbuminuria may have impaired endothelial function in the presence of long-term poor control.

Hyperresponsiveness to both acetylcholine and sodium nitroprusside has been described in patients with macroalbuminuria but normal creatinine. It has been postulated that this is linked to the pronounced autonomic dysfunction in this group (Makimattila et al., 1997).

Skin microcirculation   Acetylcholine and sodium nitroprusside can be introduced into the skin using a technique called iontophoresis. This noninvasive technique uses an electric charge to deliver the charged substances to the skin and the resulting vasodilatation is measured by laser Doppler perfusion imaging technique. In subjects with long disease duration without clinical complications, the endothelium-dependent and independent responses are normal. In contrast, in those with microalbuminuria there is an impaired response to the endothelial vasodilator acetylcholine whilst the smooth muscle cell response was normal (Shore et al., 1997). In a group of young people with diabetes, Khan and Elhadd (1997) reported that the impairment in acetylcholine-induced vasodilatation was inversely related to duration of diabetes and glycaemia.

In vitro studies

Subcutaneous resistance arteries from the gluteal region, mounted on the Mulvany wire myograph, demonstrate reduced reactivity to acetylcholine but normal responses to bradykinin and sodium nitroprusside (McNally et al., 1994). It has been suggested that this reflects an acetylcholine receptor abnormality, although recent preliminary evidence using vessels from a similar group of patients has failed to confirm this (Malik et al., 1999).

Vascular function in type 2 diabetes (Table 15.2)

In vivo studies

Conduit artery studies   Ultrasound wall-tracking studies have demonstrated that

Table 15.2 Summary of vascular function in type 2 diabetes (in the absence of hypertension and peripheral vascular disease)

Vascular bed	Stimulus	Response
Conduit artery	Increased flow	↓
	Glyceryl trinitrate	Normal
Forearm blood vessels	ED agonist	↓
	EI agonist	Normal / ↓
Skin microvessels	ED agonist	↓
	EI agonist	↓

ED, endothelium-dependent; EI, endothelium-independent.

flow-related vasodilatation is impaired in this group although there is no evidence of abnormalities in smooth muscle cell function (Goodfellow et al., 1996; Enderle et al., 1998).

Forearm blood flow studies   Many studies have performed assessment of forearm resistance vessel function in patients with type 2 diabetes. The majority of studies report an impaired endothelium-dependent response (McVeigh et al., 1992; Ting et al., 1996; Watts et al., 1996; Williams et al., 1996; Hogikyan et al., 1998; Gazis et al., 1999). One study in a small group of uncomplicated normolipidaemic normotensive men with type 2 diabetes found no difference in endothelium-dependent or independent vasodilatation compared to a body mass index (BMI)-matched control group (Avogaro et al., 1997). The reason for this discrepancy is unclear but may relate to lack of power to detect a difference in this small study, or the complication-free nature of this patient group. Vasodilatation to sodium nitroprusside is more variable with normal (Avogaro et al., 1997; Hogikyan et al., 1998; Gazis et al., 1999) or reduced responses (McVeigh et al., 1992; Watts et al., 1996; Williams et al., 1996).

The contribution of NO to resting flow (Watts et al., 1996; Avogaro et al., 1997; Catalano et al., 1997) and acetylcholine-stimulated blood flow appears normal, as assessed by infusion of L-NMMA, or nitrite/nitrate production (McVeigh et al., 1992; Watts et al., 1996; Avogaro et al., 1997).

Improvement of the response to acetylcholine was achieved by oral administration of fish oils for 6 weeks (McVeigh et al., 1992) or by the acute administration of vitamin C intraarterially (Ting et al., 1996). In contrast, oral vitamin E supplementation for 8 weeks was without effect (Gazis et al., 1999).

Skin microcirculation   In patients with type 2 diabetes with minimal complications, Morris and colleagues (1995) demonstrated an impairment in both endothelium-dependent and endothelium-independent vasodilatation in the skin microcirculation.

In vitro studies

Studies in vitro in type 2 diabetes have used tissue obtained at operation. Cipolla and colleagues (1996) compared responsiveness of subcutaneous vessels obtained from the lower limbs of diabetic and nondiabetic subjects undergoing vascular surgery. In both groups vascular disease was evident, such as coronary artery disease, peripheral vascular disease, ulcers, angina and many subjects in both groups were on multiple medication. The authors argue that this approach will identify any differences due to diabetes per se rather than vascular disease or therapy. This study identified an enhanced vasoconstriction to noradrenaline (norepinephrine) in vessels from diabetic individuals and this was attributed to a lack of endothelial release of NO and subsequent attenuation of the vasoconstrictor response. In contrast, the NO response to acetylcholine was enhanced in the diabetic group, perhaps by an alteration at the receptor level. The vascular response to sodium nitropresside was normal.

Internal mammary artery and saphenous vein rings obtained from patients with and without type 2 diabetes at coronary artery bypass surgery were compared in organ chambers. The two groups of patients had similar age and BMI but the type 2 patients had greater triglycerides and blood pressure. All patients received multiple therapy. Endothelium-independent relaxations were not influenced by the presence of type 2 diabetes. However, type 2 diabetes caused a deficit in the vasorelaxant activity of the endothelium, leading to an increase in contractility of both mammary artery and saphenous vein to noradrenaline and endothelin due to lack of attenuation of the vasoconstrictor effect by endothelial-released vasodilators (Karasu et al., 1995).

Studies in prediabetic subjects

Conduit artery studies

Caballero et al. (1999) demonstrated that subjects with impaired glucose tolerance (IGT) according to World Health Organization criteria have reduced flow-related brachial artery vasodilatation compared to healthy controls, although a direct NO donor was not used in this study to exclude an impairment in endothelium-independent function. Notably, the IGT subjects had higher BMI, waist–hip ratio, systolic blood pressure, triglyceride, total cholesterol and fasting insulin levels compared to the healthy controls. In a separate study, subjects with fasting hyperglycaemia (fasting plasma glucose between 5.5 and 7.7 mmol/l, 11 subjects with normal glucose tolerance and 2 with IGT) were similarly found to have reduced flow-related vasodilatation but intact vasodilatory response to GTN in the brachial artery compared to age- and sex-matched control subjects (Lee et al., 1998).

Forearm blood flow studies

Impaired forearm blood flow response to intraarterial acetylcholine infusion (endothelium-dependent vasodilatation) has been reported in patients with impaired fasting glucose (fasting glucose between 6.1 and 7.0 mmol/l). The endothelium-independent function was found to be intact in these individuals (Vehkavaara et al., 1999).

Skin microcirculation

Caballero and colleagues (1999) also demonstrated that the IGT subjects have both reduced endothelium-dependent and endothelium-independent vasodilatory responses in the skin microcirculation. In contrast, Morris and colleagues (1996) found that subjects with fasting hyperglycaemia have impaired endothelium-dependent vasodilatation but the endothelium-independent function remains intact.

Changes in vascular permeability

Endothelial dysfunction in diabetes is not only characterized by an alteration in the endothelium-dependent vasodilatory function but may also involve changes in the vascular permeability. Interendothelial cell junctional region has been proposed as the major route of traffic for molecular substances. Other alternative pathways proposed included transcellular holes in the endothelial cell layer (pores) and vesicular/ caveola tranport. The interendothelial cell cleft consists of an adherence junctional zone in which tight and gap junctions are inserted according to the vascular segment. This transendothelial permeability is governed by specialized junctional proteins and adhesion molecules and disruption of the junctional complexes is one mechanism whereby vascular permeability is increased in diabetes. In vitro studies have shown that confluent monolayers of human umbilical vein endothelial cells in a high glucose medium result in reduced expression of platelet endothelial cell adhesion molecule, which has a regulatory role in the maintenance of endothelial cell junctions (Baumgartner-Parzer et al., 1995). Animal studies reveal that retinal occludin, a protein specific to the tight junction, is decreased in the diabetic state and blood–retinal permeability is increased (Antonetti et al., 1998). However, the role of the endothelium in the regulation of microvascular permeability in human diabetes is hampered by the lack of unambiguous techniques for measuring capillary permeability. In early stages of diabetes glycaemic control-dependent water and albumin flux is increased (Parving et al., 1976), which could represent an increase in capillary pressure that is related to glycaemic control rather than primary changes in the integrity of the endothelial layer. Alteration in the capillary filtration coefficient (Jaap et al., 1996) and capillary diffusion capacity (Trap-Jensen and Lassen, 1968) in the later course of the disease are likely to be related to changes in microvascular permeability.

Vascular smooth muscle changes

In type 2 diabetes, as well as there being evidence of impaired endothelium-dependent vasodilatation, there is also evidence of impaired endothelium-independent vasodilatation implicating changes in vascular smooth muscle. For example, as stated above, the iontophoresis of sodium nitroprusside through the skin (a direct nitro donor) results in a diminished microvascular vasodilatory response in subjects with type 2 diabetes compared with age- and sex-matched healthy control subjects (Morris et al., 1995). IGT subjects were also reported to have impaired endothelium-independent function in the skin microcirculation (Caballero et al., 1999). This contrasts with the situation in another study where subjects who have mildly raised fasting glucose but who are at risk of type 2 diabetes in whom vascular smooth muscle responses appear normal (Morris et al., 1996). The nature of such vascular smooth muscle changes in type 2 diabetes is poorly understood but advanced glycation endproduct accumulation has been implicated.

Extracellular matrix

The endothelium is responsible for the generation of extracellular matrix in response to pressure shear and changes in the metabolic environment (including hyperglycaemia). This results in the almost ubiquitous development of capillary basement membrane thickening involving reduplication of the basal laminae. The tertiary structure of the basement membrane network is altered by advanced glycation which in turn appears to alter the compressibility of the basement membrane and its permeability behaviour under pressure. In the kidney, stimulated by raised glomerular pressure and a high glucose environment, mesangial proliferation occurs, mediated by transforming growth factor β.

Diabetic angiopathy: molecular mechanisms

Diabetes is characterized by glucose intolerance and hyperglycaemia and the central role of glucose in the pathogenesis of diabetic complications has been confirmed by two landmark studies, the Diabetes Control and Complication trial in type 1 diabetes (Group DCCT, 1993) and the United Kingdom Prospective Diabetes Study of type 2 diabetic patients (Group UKPDS, 1998a). Both studies confirmed that strict glycaemic control retards the development of diabetic microangiopathy. There were hints but no absolute proof that improved glycaemic control may also reduce the risk of large-vessel events. The United Kingdom Prospective Diabetes Study also conclusively demonstrated that reduction in arterial blood pressure, regardless of whether the primary therapeutic agent was a β-blocker or an angiotensin-converting enzyme inhibitor, reduced the development of microangiopathy, adding further weight to the concept that microangiopathy is accelerated in the presence of both hyperglycaemia and raised capillary pressure (Group UKPDS, 1998b).

Although a central role of hyperglycaemia has thus been demonstrated beyond reasonable doubt, the actual mechanism(s) by which hyperglycaemia results in cellular dysfunction and the range of pathophysiological abnormalities demonstrable in diabetes is less clear. Hyperglycaemia increases oxidative stress through several different mechanisms, including the autooxidation of glucose, increased flux through the sorbitol pathway, resulting in consumption of nicotinamide-adenine dinucleotide phosphate, a crucial cofactor in the regeneration of the antioxidant glutathione, and also through the generation of advanced glycation endproducts. Increased oxidative stress can result in the inactivation of NO with the formation of the toxic species peroxynitrite. Advanced glycation endproducts can also quench NO in their own right as well as contributing to changes in both the biophysical properties of the extracellular matrix, cell constituents and their immunogenicity.

A further way in which hyperglycaemia may induce cellular pathology is through activation of protein kinase C. Hyperglycaemia results in the generation of diacyl glycerol which increases protein kinase C activity, with a number of relevant potentially adverse vascular cellular consequences, including increased permeability and extravascular matrix production. Evidence for a key role for protein kinase C comes from recent studies suggesting that selective inhibition of the vascular isoform of this enzyme may reduce the development of diabetic microangiopathy in animal models; human studies are currently under way (King et al., 1996). Recently, it has been proposed that activation of the mitogen-activated protein kinase pathway may provide a final common path through which both oxidative stress and hyperglycaemia affect vascular function (Tomlinson, 1999).

Following capillary closure in the retina, the release of a variety of growth factors occurs stimulated by the hypoxic environment. Crucial amongst these is vascular endothelial growth factor (VEGF) release, which can also be stimulated by the diacyl glycerol–protein kinase C pathway. VEGF is not only a potent angiogenic factor but can also increase microvascular permeability and thus possesses clear credentials as a mediator of proliferative diabetic retinopathy (Wautier and Guillausseau, 1998). In support of this hypothesis, elevated levels of VEGF have been demonstrated in the vitreous humour of patients undergoing vitrectomy for proliferative retinopathy (Aiello et al., 1994).

Conclusions

It is a sobering thought that nearly 80 years after the introduction of insulin, there are no specific pharmacological approaches to the prevention of diabetic microangiopathy other than reduction in elevated blood pressure and glycaemic control. The pathophysiological framework for the development of microangiopathy is becoming clearer, whereas the atherogenic process is essentially the same as that observed in nondiabetic subjects. Endothelial dysfunction appears to play a crucial role, particularly in those subjects most prone to the development of vascular disease. There are now emerging data providing clues on the cellular and molecular basis for these changes and it is likely that the development of protective therapy will be dependent upon their further elucidation. In most instances, normoglycaemia in a diabetic patient is impossible to achieve in practice and its pursuit is not without risk, notably from hypoglycaemia. Given the growing prevalence of diabetes, which is approaching worldwide epidemic proportions, a vascular biological solution to the angiopathic process is urgently required.

REFERENCES

Aiello, L., Avery, R., Arrigg, P. et al. (1994). Vascular endothelial growth factor in ocular fluid of patients with diabetic retinopathy and other retinal disorders. *N. Engl. J. Med.*, **331**, 1480–7.

Antonetti, D., Barber, A., Khin, S. et al. (1998). Vascular permeability in experimental diabetes is associated with reduced endothelial occludin content. *Diabetes*, **47**, 1953–9.

Avogaro, A., Piarulli, F., Valerio, A. et al. (1997). Forearm nitric oxide balance, vascular relaxation and glucose metabolism in NIDDM patients. *Diabetes*, **46**, 1040–6.

Baumgartner-Parzer, S.M., Wagner, L., Pettermann, M., Gessl, A. & Waldhausl, W. (1995). Modulation by high glucose of adhesion molecule expression in cultured endothelial cells. *Diabetologia*, **38**, 1367–70.

Caballero, A., Arora, S., Saouaf, R. et al. (1999). Microvascular and macrovascular reactivity is reduced in subjects at risk for type 2 diabetes. *Diabetes*, **48**, 1856–62.

Calver, A., Collier, J. & Vallance, P. (1993). Inhibition and stimulation of nitric oxide synthesis in the human forearm arterial bed of patients with insulin-dependent diabetes. *J. Clin. Invest.*, **90**, 2548–54.

Catalano, M., Carzaniga, G., Perilli, E. et al. (1997). Basal nitric oxide production is not reduced in patients with noninsulin-dependent diabetes mellitus. *Vasc. Med.*, **2**, 302–5.

Cipolla, M.J., Harker, C.T. & Porter, J.M. (1996). Endothelial function and adrenegic reactivity in human type-II diabetic resistance arteries. *J. Vasc. Surg.*, **23**, 940–9.

Clarkson, P., Celemajer, D.S., Donald, A.E. et al. (1996). Impaired vascular reactivity in insulin-dependent diabetes mellitus is related to disease duration and low density lipoprotein cholesterol levels. *J. Am. Coll. Cardiol.*, **28**, 573–9.

Donaghue, K.C., Robinson, J., McCredie, R. et al. (1997). Large vessel dysfunction in diabetic adolescents and its relationship to small vessel complications. *J. Pediatr. Endocrinol. Metabol.*, **10**, 593–8.

Elliott, T.G., Cockcroft, J.R., Groop, P.-H., Viberti, G.C. & Ritter, J.M. (1993). Inhibition of nitric oxide synthesis in forearm vasculature of insulin-dependent diabetic patients: blunted vasoconstriction in patients with microalbuminuria. *Clin. Sci.*, **85**, 687–93.

Enderle, M.-D., Benda, N., Schmuelling, R.-M., Haering, H.U. & Pfohl, M. (1998). Preserved endothelial function in IDDM patients but not in NIDDM patients, compared with healthy subjects. *Diabetes Care*, **21**, 271–7.

Ferri, C., Desideri, G., Valenti, M. et al. (1999). Early upregulation of endothelial adhesion molecules in obese hypertensive men. *Hypertension*, **34**, 568–73.

Gazis, A., White, D., Page, S. & Cockcroft, J. (1999). Effect of oral vitamin E (alpha-tocopherol) supplementation on vascular function in type 2 diabetes mellitus. *Diabetic Med.*, **16**, 304–11.

Goodfellow, J., Ramsey, M.W., Luddington, L.A. et al. (1996). Endothelium and inelastic arteries: an early marker of vascular dysfunction in non-insulin dependent diabetes. *Br. Med. J.*, **312**, 744–5.

Group DCCT (1993). The effect of intensive treatment of diabetes on the development and progression of long-term complications in insulin-dependent diabetes mellitus. *N. Engl. J. Med.*, **329**, 978–86.

Group UKPDS (1998a). Intensive blood glucose control with sulphonylureas or insulin compared with conventional treatment and risk of complications in patients with type 2 diabetes (UKPDS 33). *Lancet*, **352**, 837–53.

Group UKPDS (1998b). Tight blood pressure control and risk of macrovascular and microvascular complications in type 2 diabetes: UKPDS 38. *Br. Med. J.*, **317**, 703–13.

Halkin, A., Benjamin, N., Doktor, H.S. et al. (1991). Vascular responsiveness and cation exchange in insulin-dependent diabetes. *Clin. Sci.*, **81**, 223–32.

Hogikyan, R., Galecki, A., Pitt, B. et al. (1998). Specific impairment of endothelium-dependent vasodilation in subjects with type 2 diabetes independent of obesity. *J. Clin. Endocrinol. Metab.*, **83**, 1946–52.

Huvers, F., Leeuw, P.D., Houben, A. et al. (1999). Endothelium-dependent vasodilatation, plasma markers of endothelial function, and adrenergic vasoconstrictor responses in type 1 diabetes under near-normoglycaemic conditions. *Diabetes*, **48**, 1300–7.

Jaap, A.J., Shore, A,C. & Tooke, J.E. (1996). Differences in microvascular fluid permeability between long-duration type 1 (insulin-dependent) diabetic patients with and without significant microangiopathy. *Clin. Sci.*, **90**, 113–17.

Joannides, R., Haefeli, W., Linder, L. et al. (1995). Nitric oxide is responsible for flow-dependent dilatation of human periheral conduit arteries in vivo. *Circulation*, **91**, 1314–19.

Johnstone, M.T., Creager, S.J., Scales, K.M. et al. (1993). Impaired endothelium-dependent vasodilation in patients with insulin-dependent diabetes mellitus. *Circulation*, **88**, 2510–16.

Karasu, C., Soncul, H. & Altan, M. (1995). Effects of non-insulin dependent diabetes mellitus on the reactivity of human internal mammary artery and human saphenous vein. *Life Sci.*, **57**, 103–12.

Khan, F. & Elhadd, T.A. (1997). Endothelium-dependent and independent skin vascular responses in children, adolescents and young adults with insulin-dependent diabetes mellitus. *Circulation*, **96**, I–139.

Khan, F., Cohen, R.A., Ruderman, N.B., Chipkin, S.R. & Coffman, J.D. (1996). Vasodilator responses in the forearm skin of patients with insulin-dependent diabetes mellitus. *Vasc. Med.*, **1**, 187–93.

King, G., Kunisaki, M., Nishio, Y. et al. (1996). Biochemical and molecular mechanisms in the development of diabetic vascular complications. *Diabetes*, **45** (suppl. 3), S105–8.

Lambert, J., Aarsen, M., Donker, A.J.M. & Stehouwer, C.D.A. (1996). Endothelium-dependent and -independent vasodilation of large arteries in normoalbuminuric insulin-dependent diabetes mellitus. *Arterioscler. Thromb. Vasc. Biol.*, **16**, 705–11.

Lee, B., Stockman, A., Shore, A. & Tooke, J. (1998). Flow-related brachial artery dilatation is impaired in subjects with hyperglycaemia. *Diabetic Med.*, **15**, A33.

Lekakis, J., Papamichael, C., Anastasiou, H. et al. (1997). Endothelial dysfunction of conduit arteries in insulin-dependent diabetes mellitus without microalbuminuria. *Cardiovasc. Res.*, **34**, 164–8.

Lim, S.C., Caballero, A.E., Smakowski, P. et al. (1999). Soluble intercellular adhesion molecule, vascular cell adhesion molecule, and impaired microvascular reactivity are early markers of vasculopathy in type 2 diabetic individuals without microalbuminuria. *Diabetes Care*, **22**, 1865–70.

Makimattila, S., Virkamaki, A., Groop, P.-H. et al. (1996). Chronic hyperglycemia impairs endothelial function and insulin sensitivity via different mechanisms in insulin-dependent diabetes mellitus. *Circulation*, **94**, 1276–82.

Makimattila, S., Mantysaari, M., Groop, P.H. et al. (1997). Hyperreactivity to nitrovasodilators in forearm vasculature is related to autonomic dysfunction in insulin-dependent diabetes mellitus. *Circulation*, **95**, 618–25.

Malik, R., Paniagua, O., Shaw, L., Austin, C. & Heagerty, A. (1999). Resistance vessel function and structure in normotensive patients with type 1 diabetes. *Diabetologia*, **42** (suppl. 1), A75.

McNally, P.G., Watt, P.A.C., Rimmer, T. et al. (1994). Impaired contraction and endothelium-dependent relaxation in isolated resistance vessels from patients with insulin-dependent diabetes mellitus. *Clin. Sci.*, **87**, 31–6.

McVeigh, G.E., Brennan, G.M., Johnston, G.D. et al. (1992). Impaired endothelium-dependent and independent vasodilation in patients with type 2 (non-insulin-dependent) diabetes mellitus. *Diabetologia*, **35**, 771–6.

Meeking, D.R., Cummings, M.H., Thorne, S. et al. (1999). Endothelial dysfunction in type 1 diabetes subjects with and without microalbuminuria. *Diabetic Med.*, **16**, 841–7.

Morris, S., Shore, A. & Tooke, J. (1995). Response of the skin microcirculation to acetylcholine and sodium nitroprusside in patients with NIDDM. *Diabetologia*, **38**, 1337–44.

Morris, S.J., Jaap, A.J., Shore, A.C. & Tooke, J.E. (1996). Responses of the skin microcirculation to acetylcholine and sodium nitroprusside in subjects with fasting hyperglycaemia. *J. Physiol.*, **491.P**, 14P.

O'Driscoll, G., Green, D., Rankin, J. et al. (1997). Improvement in endothelial function by angiotensin converting enzyme inhibition in insulin-dependent diabetes mellitus. *J. Clin. Invest.*, **100**, 678–84.

Parving, H.-H., Noer, I., Deckert, T. et al. (1976). The effect of metabolic regulation on microvascular permeability to small and large molecules in short-term juvenile diabetics. *Diabetologia*, **12**, 161–6.

Parving, H.-H., Viberti, G.C., Keen, H., Christiansen, J.S. & Lassen, N.A. (1983). Hemodynamic factors in the genesis of diabetic microangiopathy. *Metabolism*, **32**, 943–9.

Ross, R. (1993). The pathogenesis of atherosclerosis: a perspective for the 1990s. *Nature*, **362**, 801–9.

Shore, A.C., Sandeman, D.D., Jaap, A.J., Sampson, K.J. & Tooke, J.E. (1992). Is capillary pressure elevated in patients with non-insulin dependent diabetes? *Int. J. Microcirc. Clin. Exp.*, **11** (suppl. 1), S210.

Shore, A., Morris, S. & Tooke, J. (1997). Impaired skin microvascular endothelial cell responses in IDDM patients with microalbuminuria. *Diabetic Med.*, **14** (suppl. 1), A54.

Smits, P., Kapma, J.-A., Jacobs, M.-C., Lutterman, J. & Thien, T. (1993). Endothelium-dependent vascular relaxation in patients with type 1 diabetes. *Diabetes*, **42**, 148–53.

Ting, H.H., Timimi, F.K., Boles, K.S. et al. (1996). Vitamin C improves endothelium-dependent vasodilation in patients with non-insulin-dependent diabetes mellitus. *J. Clin. Invest.*, **97**, 22–8.

Tomlinson, D. (1999). Mitogen-activated protein kinases as glucose transducers for diabetic complications. *Diabetologia*, **42**, 1271–81.

Tooke, J.E. & Goh, K.L. (1999). Vascular function in type 2 diabetes mellitus and pre-diabetes: the case for intrinsic endotheliopathy. *Diabetic Med.*, **16**, 1–6.

Trap-Jensen, J. & Lassen, N.A. (1968). Increased capillary diffusion capacity for small ions in skeletal muscle in long-term diabetics. *Scand. J. Clin. Lab. Invest.*, **21**, 116–22.

Vehkavaara, S., Seppala-Lindroos, A., Westerbacka, J., Groop, P. & Jarvinen, H. (1999). In vivo endothelial dysfunction characterizes patients with impaired fasting glucose. *Diabetes Care*, **22**, 2055–60.

Watts, G.F., O'Brien, S.F., Silvester, W. & Millar, J.A. (1996). Impaired endothelium-dependent and independent dilatation of forearm resistance arteries in men with diet-treated non-insulin-dependent diabetes: role of dyslipidaemia. *Clin. Sci.*, **91**, 567–73.

Wautier, J.-L. & Guillausseau, P.-J. (1998). Diabetes, advanced glycation endproducts and vascular disease. *Vasc. Med.*, **3**, 131–7.

Williams, S.B., Cusco, J.A., Roddy, M.-A., Johnstone, M.T. & Creager, M.A. (1996). Impaired nitric oxide-mediated vasodilation in patients with non-insulin-dependent diabetes mellitus. *J. Am. Coll. Cardiol.*, **27**, 567–74.

Zatz, R. & Brenner, B.M. (1986). Pathogenesis of diabetic microangiopathy. The hemodynamic view. *Am. J. Med.*, **80**, 443–53.

Zenere, B.M., Arcaro, G., Saggiani, F. et al. (1995). Noninvasive detection of functional alterations of the arterial wall in IDDM patients with and without microalbuminuria. *Diabetes Care*, **18**, 975–82.

16

The vasculitides

Peter Hewins and Caroline O. S. Savage

Renal Immunobiology Group, University of Birmingham, Birmingham

Definition and introduction

Vasculitis is defined as blood vessel inflammation. The histopathological features are marked disruption of the normal vessel wall architecture, perivascular leukocyte infiltration and variable deposition of homogeneous fibrin-like material in the medial layer of the vessel wall (fibrinoid necrosis: Lie, 1990). The leukocyte infiltrate is frequently mixed, but may be predominantly neutrophilic, lymphocytic or eosinophilic. In some instances, specialized aggregates of macrophages and T cells (granulomata) are noted. Intravascular thrombosis and extravasation of blood frequently occur. Aneurysms can form through focal dilatation of the walls of muscular or elastic arteries and are at risk of rupturing. Intimal proliferation and/or fibrosis during healing can significantly narrow the vessel lumen (stenosis), leading to ischaemia or infarction. Arterial and venous vessels of any calibre, from the aorta to capillaries, can be affected. In many instances vasculitis is patchy but disseminated. Glomeruli are differentiated capillaries and, where small-vessel vasculitis involves the kidney, a segmental necrotizing glomerulonephritis (SNGN) is typically seen. The SNGN is also frequently 'crescentic', indicating the presence of inflammatory (mainly mononuclear) cells in Bowman's space surrounding the glomerular tuft. The vasculitides constitute a heterogeneous group of disorders affecting vessels of particular size and with distinct extravascular features. Pathological findings in different diseases frequently overlap.

Nonspecific early symptoms can delay diagnosis but evolving disease causes progressive organ damage which may become irreversible. Vasculitis must not be neglected in the differential diagnosis of any unexplained inflammatory response. Life-threatening manifestations mandate expedient treatment.

Traditionally, Kussmaul and Maier are accredited with the seminal description of vasculitis ('periarteritis nodosa' – now termed polyarteritis nodosa) in 1866 (Lie, 1991). All cases were initially labelled as periarteritis but subsequently distinct pathological entities were distinguished and terminology altered. Diagnostic techniques have also radically changed since the original autopsy descriptions and pathogenic mechanisms have begun to be illuminated. Serum sickness models provided the first experimental data. Animals developed arteritis and glomerulonephritis after being injected with antigens able to stimulate the production of immune complexes that deposited in vessel walls (Savage and Ng, 1986). Cellular and humoral autoimmunity (loss of self-tolerance) have since been implicated in many vasculitides. To date, however, the exact aetiology of most vasculitides remains enigmatic and their varying clinicopathological features have vexed numerous attempts to provide an encompassing classification. The utility of classification is illustrated by data indicating differing responses to treatment, mortality and relapse rates for specific vasculitides.

The most recent classification is the Chapel Hill Consensus Conference (CHCC) nomenclature (Table 16.1; Jennette et al., 1994). Vasculitides are grouped according to the size of the predominant vessel type involved: large-vessel (aorta and its main branches), medium-vessel (main visceral arteries and veins) or small-vessel (arterioles, capillaries and venules). Subclassification is based upon features such as age, the distribution of vascular involvement or associated findings. The CHCC nomenclature is not exhaustive, defining only 10 diseases and excluding vasculitis occurring secondary to either rheumatological disease or infection. The classic model of antibody-mediated small-vessel vasculitis, Goodpasture's disease (antiglomerular basement membrane (GBM) disease) is also absent from the CHCC nomenclature. Aetiology is characterized for some CHCC vasculitides, such as essential cryoglobulinaemic vasculitis, which is usually secondary to hepatitis C virus infection, and classical polyarteritis nodosa, which is associated with hepatitis B infection in some instances. Antineutrophil cytoplasmic antibodies (ANCA) may be pathogenic in certain small-vessel vasculitides. A complete classification will require determination of aetiology and pathogenesis for all vasculitides. Herein, we will consider ANCA-associated small-vessel vasculitides to illustrate important clinical features and salient pathogenic factors.

ANCA-associated systemic vasculitides (ASV)

Wegener's granulomatosis (WG), microscopic polyangiitis (MPA) and Churg–Strauss syndrome (CSS) can be distinguished from the other small-vessel vasculitides by the scarcity of immune deposits and by their frequent association with ANCA. This novel immunoglobulin G (IgG)-class autoantibody may well have a pathogenic role in ASV, although direct evidence for this has proved difficult to obtain (Hewins et al., 2000). Renal limited vasculitis (RLV or idiopathic necrotizing crescentic glomerulonephritis) is absent from the CHCC nomenclature but is

Table 16.1 Vasculitis classification according to Chapel Hill Consensus Conference nomenclature

Vessel Size	Disease name	Clinicopathological features
Large-vessel vasculitis	Giant cell (temporal) arteritis	Granulomatous arteritis of aorta and its major branches, notably temporal and other extracranial branches of the carotids. Patients aged over 50. Associated with polymyalgia rheumatica
	Takayasu arteritis	Granulomatous inflammation of aorta and major branches. Patients aged under 50
Medium-vessel vasculitis	Polyarteritis nodosa (classical)	Necrotizing medium and small arteritis without SNGN or vasculitis in smaller vessels
	Kawasaki disease	Large, medium and small arteritis plus mucocutaneous lymph node syndrome. Coronary artery involvement frequent. Mainly affects children
Small-vessel vasculitis	Wegener's granulomatosis	Granulomatous respiratory tract inflammation plus necrotizing venulitis, capillaritis, arteriolitis and arteritis. SNGN often present
	Churg–Strauss syndrome	Small- to medium-vessel necrotizing vasculitis plus granulomatous and eosinophilic respiratory tract inflammation with asthma and blood eosinophilia
	Microscopic polyangiitis	Small- to medium-vessel necrotizing vasculitis usually with SNGN ± lung capillaritis
	Henoch–Schönlein purpura	Small-vessel vasculitis (mainly in skin, glomeruli and gut) with immunoglobulin A deposits. Arthralgia /arthritis common
	Essential cryoglobulinaemic vasculitis	Small-vessel vasculitis (mainly skin and glomeruli) with cryoglobulin immune deposits plus serum cryoglobulins
	Cutaneous leukocytoclastic angiitis	Isolated skin angiitis. No systemic vasculitis or glomerulonephritis

SNGN, segmental necrotizing glomerulonephritis.

ANCA-associated and almost certainly represents a variant with no extraglomerular involvement. The ASV are not uncommon: one recent estimate of the annual incidence in Sweden was 21/million adults from 1986 to 1995 (Tidman et al., 1998). ASV also constitute the most frequent cause of rapidly progressive glomerulonephritis (RPGN).

Wegener's granulomatosis

The incidence of WG has been estimated at up to 7.9/million adults in the UK (Lane et al., 2000). There is an equal sex distribution, most patients are Caucasian and the mean age for presentation is 50–70 years. Disseminated WG is characterized by the triad of granulomatous inflammation of the respiratory tract, systemic necrotizing vasculitis and SNGN. All three features do not invariably coexist. WG limited to the respiratory tract is well described, although it usually evolves into a disseminated disease. The most dramatic manifestations of WG are RPGN and diffuse alveolar haemorrhage. The sera of most patients ($\geq 70\%$) with active disseminated WG contain ANCA directed against proteinase 3 (PR3-ANCA), a serine protease found within the neutrophil azurophilic granule. In up to 25% of WG patients, ANCA are directed against another azurophilic granule protein, myeloperoxidase (MPO) (Savige et al., 1999). A small number of patients with active disseminated WG are ANCA-negative.

Typical early symptoms, as with other vasculitides, are constitutional (fever, weight loss and malaise), rheumatological (arthralgia and myalgia) and cutaneous (purpura). Upper respiratory tract (URT) features include purulent/bloody nasal discharge, nasal pain, nasal crusting, sinusitis, otitis media, hearing loss, mastoiditis and mucosal ulcers. URT features are prominent, evident at presentation in $\sim 75\%$ of patients and occur in most ($> 90\%$) during follow-up (Anderson et al., 1992; Hoffman et al., 1992). Severe manifestations include nasal septal perforation and saddle-nose deformity, which are specific but uncommon. Nondiscriminatory ocular symptoms are common but exceptionally proptosis develops secondarily to an inflammatory retroorbital mass.

Tracheobronchial stenosis may develop as a result of granulomatous inflammation. Pulmonary granulomata cause chest X-ray nodules, which are often bilateral, multiple and cavitating. Pulmonary involvement is evident in 45–63% of patients at presentation and eventually occurs in $\sim 85\%$ (Anderson et al., 1992; Hoffman et al., 1992). Polyneuropathy and mononeuritis multiplex (reflecting vasa nervorum vasculitis) and central nervous system symptoms (due to localized granulomata or vasculitis) are well recognized. Renal involvement was diagnosed in 76% of cases in a metaanalysis of 349 patients (Bajema et al., 1997).

Open-lung biopsy offers the highest diagnostic yield for concurrent granulomata and vasculitis (Lane et al., 2000). Other granulomatous conditions such as tuberculosis must be carefully excluded. Transbronchial and upper-airways biopsy specimens are diagnostic in only $\sim 50\%$ of cases. Renal biopsy will usually provide a diagnosis where there is an active urinary sediment and/or renal impairment. Granulomata are rarely detected on the renal biopsy and the renal histology alone does not distinguish WG from MPA or RLV. None the less, renal biopsy is relatively noninvasive and the treatment of SNGN is common to all three conditions.

Microscopic polyangiitis and renal limited vasculitis

A recent UK estimate of the incidence of MPA was 7/million adults (Lane et al., 2000). MPA and RLV accounted for 77% of cases in the afore-mentioned Swedish study with a higher incidence of ASV (Tidman et al., 1998). Patient demographics closely resemble those for WG (Serra et al., 1984; Savage et al., 1985; Adu et al., 1987; Pettersson et al., 1995; Tidman et al., 1998; Westman et al., 1998; Guillevin et al., 1999a). RLV has no systemic features and presents as RPGN but many patients with MPA describe systemic symptoms preceding the development of renal disease. Constitutional, rheumatological, cutaneous and ocular features are similar in type and frequency to those in WG. URT symptoms are less prominent than in WG, although reported frequencies vary from ~ 1% to 47% (Serra et al., 1984; Savage et al., 1985; Adu et al., 1987; Pettersson et al., 1995; Tidman et al., 1998; Westman et al., 1998; Guillevin et al., 1999a). The frequency of pulmonary involvement is between 25% and 68%. Diffuse alveolar haemorrhage occurs in ~ 10–30%. Gastrointestinal symptoms are more frequent (up to 30%) and prominent than in WG, although visceral perforation is less common than in classical polyarteritis nodosa. Peripheral nervous system involvement is also frequent. A recent series of MPA patients (not recruited from a nephrology centre) recorded renal disease in 79% (Guillevin et al., 1999a). Most patients are ANCA-positive. PR3-ANCA are frequently detected ($\leq 30\%$) but a greater proportion of patients ($\geq 60\%$) with MPA and RLV have MPO-ANCA (Savige et al., 1999). Renal biopsy is the most frequently employed diagnostic technique; other affected tissues may be sampled and, when pulmonary infiltrates are present, open-lung biopsy should be considered.

Churg–Strauss syndrome (CSS)

CSS is a rare disorder, accounting for only a few per cent of younger patients with ASV. The syndrome comprises hypereosinophilia ($> 1.5 \times 10^9/l$ and $> 10\%$ of the total peripheral blood leukocyte count), asthma, eosinophilic and granulomatous inflammation, particularly affecting the respiratory tract and systemic vasculitis. Vasculitic lesions may also exhibit marked eosinophilic infiltration. The CHCC definition includes the presence of extravascular eosinophilic granulomata but some studies have suggested that extravascular granulomata may not always be detectable. Lanham et al. (1984) previously proposed the presence of asthma, hypereosinophilia and two or more extrapulmonary sites of systemic vasculitis as diagnostic.

There is typically a prior history of allergic rhinitis, sinusitis and/or nasal polyposis. Late-onset asthma follows and, after an interval, which may last some years, the second phase of hypereosinophilia and fleeting pulmonary infiltrates develops. Eventually, the third life-threatening, vasculitic phase occurs. Not all cases follow this triphasic pattern. The spectrum of systemic involvement is similar to other ASV but, in addition to pulmonary infiltrates, cardiac and gastrointestinal involvement are common and frequently severe (Guillevin, 2000). The cardiac manifestations include coronary vasculitis, cardiomyopathy and myocardial infarction. In contrast, diffuse alveolar haemorrhage and SNGN are less frequent in CSS. ANCA, with specificity for either PR3 or MPO, are detected in ~ 50% of patients with CSS (Guillevin et al., 1999b; Savige et al., 1999). Diagnosis should be based upon consistent clinical features and histopathology from biopsy of an affected organ.

Common laboratory findings in ASV

1. Elevated erythrocyte sedimentation rate and C-reactive protein
2. Neutrophilic leukocytosis (eosinophilic in CSS), anaemia, thrombocytosis and hypoalbuminaemia
3. Cytoplasmic ANCA (cANCA: PR3-ANCA) or MPO-ANCA-positivity
4. Normal complement levels and no cryoglobulins or anti-DNA antibodies (indicating essential cryoglobulinaemic vasculitis or systemic lupus erythematosus).
5. Negative anti-GBM antibodies (although ASV and anti-GBM antibody-mediated disease can coexist)
6. Negative microbiological cultures (ANCA may occur in infections such as bacterial endocarditis)

Diffuse alveolar haemorrhage in ASV

ASV are the most frequent cause of this condition, a capillaritis, although it also occurs in anti-GBM disease and very rarely in other diseases, such as systemic lupus erythematosus. The clinical features are haemoptysis, anaemia, hypoxia, diffuse chest X-ray infiltrates and an increased carbon monoxide gas transfer factor. Mechanical ventilation is often required and mortality remains high despite aggressive treatment. Frequently, diffuse alveolar haemorrhage and SNGN coexist, producing a 'pulmonary–renal syndrome'.

Renal involvement in ASV

Pauciimmune SNGN (± crescent formation) is characteristic of WG, MPA, RLV and CSS. Arteritis and/or arteriolitis is detected in 19–34% of renal biopsies. Interstitial infiltrates and tubular atrophy are also common. Eventually, the active infiltrates are replaced by fibrosis and the glomeruli become sclerosed. Characteristically in ASV, lesions of differing ages coexist in one biopsy.

Intraglomerular leukocytes were scarce in one early report of renal histopathology in WG which found mainly platelet aggregation and fibrin deposition at sites of capillary thrombosis and necrosis (Weiss and Crissman, 1984). A subsequent study of crescentic GN (of mixed aetiology) identified significantly increased numbers of intraglomerular monocytes (Hooke et al., 1987). More recently, two studies have found significantly increased numbers of intraglomerular neutrophils in ASV. The number of intraglomerular activated neutrophils correlated with the severity of renal injury in one study (Brouwer et al., 1994). In the second, neutrophils were mainly retained within capillary loops, which potentially localizes them to mediate endothelial damage (Cockwell et al., 1999). In some series monocytes/macrophages and T lymphocytes are the predominant cells detected but this does not necessarily imply their involvement in the *initiation* of inflammation (Cunningham et al., 1999). Furthermore, biopsy may not readily detect cells that are rapidly lost from sites of inflammation, either by necrosis or apoptosis (programmed cell death).

Pathogenicity of ANCA

Clinical evidence

The association of ANCA with SNGN was first described in 1982 using indirect immunofluorescence (IIF) to examine ethanol-fixed neutrophils from healthy donors incubated with sera from affected patients (Davies et al., 1982). The two typical IIF patterns seen in ASV are cANCA and perinuclear (pANCA; Savige et al., 1999). The most frequent target antigens for cANCA and pANCA in ASV are PR3 and MPO, respectively. Enzyme-linked immunosorbent assays (ELISA) are typically used to determine antigenic specificities and titres. A minority of cANCA recognize MPO and pANCA can have more diverse specificities, including lactoferrin, cathepsin G and elastase. Atypical ANCA IIF staining patterns also occur, usually in patients with nonvasculitic illnesses where the antigenic specificity is rarely PR3 or MPO. Vasculitis should not be diagnosed on the basis of a positive ANCA alone (particularly isolated IIF) due to their occurrence in other illnesses but the combination of IIF and ELISA ANCA testing is extremely valuable in patients with suspected vasculitis as an adjunct to tissue diagnosis (Hagen et al., 1998).

Circumstantial clinical evidence supports a pathogenic role for PR3-ANCA and MPO-ANCA in ASV. The majority of patients with active ASV have one or other of these antibodies in their sera. For active WG, many series report $\geq 88\%$ ANCA-positivity (Hoffman et al., 1992; Bajema et al., 1997; Tidman et al., 1998).

Results in MPA vary from ~75% to >90% (Pettersson et al., 1995; Tidman et al., 1998; Guillevin et al., 1999). A study incorporating a more sensitive technique (capture ELISA) reported 97% positivity for newly diagnosed WG and MPA (Westman et al., 1998). Furthermore, the combination of IIF and PR3/MPO ELISA testing confers a very high specificity (99%) when ASV patients are compared to disease controls (Hagen et al., 1998). Many patients become ANCA-negative when their disease remits; persistent or intermittent ANCA positivity has been reported as risk factor for relapse; a significant proportion of patients switch from ANCA-negative to -positive around the time of relapse and in some series the rise in ANCA titre precedes the clinical relapse (Cohen Tervaert et al., 1989; Gaskin et al., 1991; Jayne et al., 1995; Ara et al., 1999; Kyndt et al., 1999). Similar findings apply in WG, MPA and RLV. The favourable response to immunosuppression ($\geq$ 90% patients enter remission) also suggests an autoimmune aetiology for the ASV. Finally, ANCA are detected in the sera of ~20–40% of patients with anti-GBM disease and appear to modulate its clinical features, increasing the frequency of systemic symptoms and relapse (Jayne et al., 1990).

In vitro and ex vivo evidence

In vitro, primed neutrophils from healthy donors are activated by ANCA, causing degranulation, reactive oxygen species generation and cytokine production (Falk et al., 1990; Mulder et al., 1994; Porges et al., 1994; Radford et al., 1999). Primed and ANCA-treated neutrophils mediate cytolysis of endothelial cells in culture (Savage et al., 1992). In vivo, activated leukocytes could similarly mediate damage to nearby endothelium. Neutrophil priming, by proinflammatory cytokines such as tumour necrosis factor-α or interleukin-8, causes translocation of PR3 and MPO to the plasma membrane where they are available for interaction with autoantibodies (Falk et al., 1990; Csernok et al., 1994; Porges et al., 1994). It has recently been suggested that there are intracellular stores of PR3 in addition to the azurophilic granules and that these are mobilized by lower concentrations of priming agents (Witko-Sarsat et al., 1999a). Apoptosis also translocates PR3 and MPO to the plasma membrane (Gilligan et al., 1996). A recent report that neutrophils from an MPO-deficient donor were not activated by MPO-ANCA confirms the requirement for antigen expression (Reumaux et al., 2000). Ex vivo examination of neutrophils from patients with active ASV suggests that priming does occur and that increased PR3 membrane expression is evident (Csernok et al., 1994; Muller Kobold et al., 1998a, b). Thus, PR3 may be available in vivo to interact with ANCA. A separate report claimed that PR3 is expressed on a subset of neutrophils in all individuals and that a larger subset of PR3-positive neutrophils was a risk factor for developing ASV (Witko-Sarsat et al., 1996b). Increased plasma membrane expression of MPO has not been demonstrated in ASV.

Monocytes also surface-express ANCA antigens and in vitro ANCA induce IL-8 and MCP-1 secretion by monocytes (Casselman et al., 1995; Ralston et al., 1997). Activation of circulating monocytes in ASV has been reported (Muller Kobold et al., 1999). A major problem in interpreting such data is that some degree of leukocyte priming/activation is inevitable during their collection, isolation and study.

Although there is some debate, the balance of evidence suggests that ANCA-mediated neutrophil/monocyte activation also involves engagement of Fcγ receptors (FcγR) (Mulder et al., 1994; Porges et al., 1994; Radford et al., 1999). The physiological role of FcγR is to permit phagocytosis of IgG-coated pathogens by engaging the Fc portion of IgG. FcγR cross-linking by monoclonal antibodies induces similar, but not identical patterns of neutrophil activation to ANCA. PR3 and MPO do not have transmembrane domains and are not believed to be able directly to signal intracellularly. Thus, FcγR involvement offers an attractive mechanism to explain ANCA-mediated activation. Genetically determined polymorphisms in neutrophil-expressed FcγR correlate with the severity of renal injury in ASV (Tse et al., 2000). Other evidence indicates the need for the β_2-integrin, CD 18, in ANCA-mediated neutrophil activation (Reumaux et al., 1995).

ANCA render neutrophils temporarily adherent when superfused on to neutrophils rolling on a platelet monolayer in vitro (a surrogate endothelium; Radford et al., 2000). This mechanism is FcγR- and β_2-integrin-dependent. ANCA-induced secretion of IL-8 (a neutrophil chemoattractant) may trap neutrophils in glomerular capillary loops, preventing them from migrating into the mesangium and promoting endothelial damage (Cockwell et al., 1999). Finally, ANCA accelerate apoptosis of primed neutrophils but the process is aberrant, reducing the ability of macrophages to clear the apoptotic bodies (Harper et al., 2000). Apoptotic neutrophils may then secondarily necrose, negating the anti-inflammatory potential of apoptosis. Opsonization of already apoptotic neutrophils by ANCA may also be a proinflammatory signal to macrophages (Csernok et al., 2000; Harper et al., 2001).

Endothelial changes are also documented in ASV. Renal biopsy data indicate upregulated expression of endothelial adhesion molecules intercellular adhesion molecule 1 and vascular cell adhesion molecule 1. Furthermore, endothelial cells may produce chemokines that recruit leukocyte subsets (Cockwell et al., 1997). Neutrophil degranulation releases PR3 and MPO. In vitro, soluble PR3 and MPO bind to endothelial cells where they are available to ligate ANCA (Vargunam et al., 1992; Savage et al., 1993). In vivo, in situ immune complex formation might result, mediating tissue damage, although of course, immune deposits in ASV are scanty. We do not find evidence of native ANCA autoantigen expression by endothelial cells (King et al., 1995). ANCA have been suggested to potentiate the enzymatic activity of granule constituents, perhaps by preventing binding to inhibitors or reducing clearance. In ASV, granule constituents released in proximity to the endothelium or bound to the surface of activated neutrophils might cause direct endothelial damage. PR3 and elastase, but not MPO, have also been reported to induce endothelial cell apoptosis in vitro and in the case of PR3, this involves internalization but is not dependent upon catalytic activity (Yang et al., 1996, 2000; Pendergraft et al., 2000).

In vivo evidence

Animal models of ASV have provided limited information. Restricted interspecies homology renders it difficult to raise reactive autoantibodies by immunizing animals with human PR3. No useful models of PR3-ANCA vasculitis exist. Anti-MPO antibodies are a part of a polyclonal autoimmune response in some animal models of vasculitis but it is difficult to interpret the pathogenicity of these MPO antibodies. A more important finding is that anti-MPO autoantibodies potentiate SNGN in rats injected with subnephritogenic doses of anti-GBM antibodies (Heeringa et al., 1998). Rats not previously immunized with MPO did not develop significant SNGN in response to the same dose of anti-GBM antibodies. In a separate model, antihuman MPO antibodies were raised in rats and, although vasculitis or glomerulonephritis did not automatically develop, these lesions could be induced by infusing neutrophil products (including MPO) plus H_2O_2 (the MPO substrate) into preimmunized animals. Intriguingly, immune deposits were present in the earliest stages of disease in this model but rapidly disappeared (Heeringa et al., 1998).

In contrast to anti-GBM disease, where antibodies from affected humans induce disease when injected into animals, pathogenic transfer of ANCA has not been demonstrated. Transport of IgG across the placenta offers the opportunity to observe the transfer of pathogenic antibodies between humans. Transient neonatal myasthenia following the transfer of antiacetylcholine receptor antibodies is well recognized for example. Pregnancy is predictably unusual in ASV and transfer of ANCA has not been documented. Successful pregnancy and fetal loss during active WG have been described but the causes of fetal death were undetermined (Haber et al., 1999). Interestingly, one described a transient vasculitic rash in a neonate born to a mother who suffered a relapse of ANCA-negative MPA immediately after delivery (Morton, 1998). The neonate's symptoms indicate the acquisition of a pathogenic factor, possibly an IgG, from the maternal circulation. One final in vivo observation of note is the development of ASV in patients treated with the antithyroid drug propylthiouracil (Harper et al., 1998). Most patients develop MPO-ANCA and a propylthiouracil metabolite may act as a hapten, promoting autoantibody production.

T-lymphocyte involvement in ASV

High affinity of IgG, restricted epitope recognition and subclass switching suggest T cell help in ANCA production. Autoreactive T lymphocytes (proliferating in response to PR3 or MPO) have been identified in the peripheral blood of patients with ASV by some groups (Griffith et al., 1995; King et al., 1998). The persistence of autoreactive T cells in ASV patients in remission might explain their propensity to relapse. There is no evidence to suggest that autoreactive cytotoxic T cells initiate vascular damage in ASV, despite its pauciimmune nature. None the less, T cells are likely to be involved in sustaining and amplifying tissue damage following the initial insult, as is evident during the crescentic phase of SNGN (Cunningham et al., 1999). A common dominating T-cell receptor BV8-F/L-G-G-A/Q-G-J2S3 β-chain sequence was found in CD4 + T cells from four unrelated patients with vasculitis, all of whom were HLA-DRB1*0401 allele-positive, suggesting they had each mounted a cell-mediated immune response against a common antigen (Giscombe et al., 1998). Patients with ASV have been successfully treated with anti-T lymphocyte therapies when conventional treatments have failed (Lockwood et al., 1996).

T-lymphocyte involvement in WG

In WG, T cells almost certainly have additional roles in the pathogenesis of granulomata, and these consist predominantly of macrophages, CD4 + T cells and neutrophils. Th1 responses are important in granulomata production and maintenance. Peripheral blood from patients with active WG contain CD4 + HLA-DR + (activated) T lymphocytes that exhibit enhanced proliferative responses and selectively secrete Th1 cytokines (interferon-γ and tumour necrosis factor-α) in a interleukin-12-dependent manner (Lúdvíksson et al., 1998). A subsequent report has confirmed this Th1 profile in peripheral blood T lymphocytes and documented similar findings in T cells isolated directly from granulomata (Csernok et al., 1999). This suggests a primary role for T lymphocytes in the pathogenesis of granulomata in WG. However, the link between granulomatous disease and vasculitis is uncertain. T lymphocytes in the two studies discussed did not proliferate in response to PR3.

Infectious triggers for ASV

WG in particular most commonly develops during the winter months (Raynauld et al., 1993; Tidman et al., 1998). Chronic nasal carriage of *Staphylococcus aureus* is a risk factor for relapse in WG and co-trimoxazole therapy to eradicate *Staphylococcus* reduces relapse rates (Stegeman et al., 1994, 1996). Expanded Vβ + T cell subsets have been reported in WG and MPA suggesting superantigen involvement and relapses of WG were found to be more common in patients carrying superantigen producing *Staphylococcal* strains (Simpson et al., 1995;

Cohen Tervaeart et al., 2000). Cytokines produced in response to infection might prime leukocytes and endothelial cells, promoting ANCA mediated vascular damage. Infection may also trigger granuloma formation.

Summary of ASV pathogenesis

The majority of patients with WG, MPA and RLV, together with a significant proportion of those with CSS, have autoantibodies to MPO or PR3. These antibodies are specific for vasculitis and correlate with disease activity in many patients. In vitro, PR3-ANCA and MPO-ANCA activate primed neutrophils and monocytes and promote neutrophil-directed endothelial cell cytolysis. ANCA are likely to promote intravascular retention of neutrophils and neutrophil–endothelial adhesion in vivo. Furthermore, the products released from activated neutrophils may damage the endothelium. The ANCA response is presumed to be dependent upon T-cell help and T cells probably have additional specific roles in the pathogenesis of granulomata. While there is some evidence that the autoantigens to which T cells respond are PR3 and/or MPO, this is by no means proven. Infections may trigger ASV disease activity.

However, direct proof of ANCA pathogenicity is lacking. Identical pathology occurs in some patients who are consistently ANCA-negative and sustained rises in ANCA titres may occur without relapse. These findings suggest that, in some patients, ANCA are either unnecessary or insufficient to cause vasculitis. Some patients may not have true vasculitis: a WG-like condition due to transporter associated with the proteosome (TAP) deficiency associated with reduced leukocyte expression of MHC class I has recently been described (Moins-Teisserene et al., 1999). Autoantibodies and autoreactive T cells have not been detected in ASV lesions. Experimental models suggest only that ANCA potentiate vasculitis. It remains to be determined to what extent these negative findings reflect the limitations of our current methodologies and of our understanding of autoimmune pathogenesis.

Treatment and prognosis of ASV

The use of cyclophosphamide plus corticosteroids has transformed prognosis for ASV patients. Untreated, the 12-month mortality rate for WG was 82% (Fauci et al., 1983) but there was only 20% mortality in a large cohort followed for a median time of 8 years, 84% of whom received combined cyclophosphamide and corticosteroids (Hoffman et al., 1992). In a cohort of patients with renal vasculitis (MPA and RLV) who received combination therapy, 5-year survival was 65% but previous reports of survival without cyclophosphamide were much lower (38%) (Serra et al., 1984; Savage et al., 1985). A 74% 5-year survival was documented in the largest MPA series to include patients without renal involvement (Guillevin et al., 1999). Furthermore, combination therapy can induce complete remission (reported rates: 70–96% Hoffman et al., 1992; Jayne et al., 1995; Westman et al., 1998; Ara et al., 1999) and preserves or restores independent renal function (67–84%: Hoffman et al., 1992; Pettersson et al., 1995; Westman et al., 1998). Renal recovery can occur in patients who are dialysis-dependent at presentation. The major difficulties still to be overcome are frequent relapses (occurring in 21–54% of patients still on immunosuppression (Cohen Tervaert et al., 1989; Gaskin et al., 1991; Hoffman et al., 1992; Jayne et al., 1995; Pettersson et al., 1995; Westman et al., 1998; Guillevin et al., 1999) and the toxicity of therapy. Cyclophosphamide-related side-effects include life-threatening infections, infertility, haemorrhagic cystitis and increased rates of malignancy (particularly bladder cancer: Hoffman et al., 1992; Westman et al., 1998). The role of pulsed cyclophosphamide (using larger intermittent doses to allow a lower cumulative dose) in ASV remains to be clarified; relapses were more frequent in patients treated with pulse therapy in one controlled trial but not in another (Adu et al., 1997; Guillevin et al., 1997). Importantly, it has recently been demonstrated that azathioprine is as effective as cyclophosphamide as maintenance therapy after cyclophosphamide induced remission and azathioprine-treated patients suffered less severe side-effects (Jayne and Rasmussen, 2000). Although it is less toxic, azathioprine is not without risks, including increased malignancy rates (Westman et al., 1998).

Plasma exchange is frequently employed in patients with ASV and diffuse alveolar haemorrhage on the basis of its efficacy in anti-GBM disease. The merits of methylprednisolone and/or plasma exchange in ASV with severe renal impairment remain to be proven, but anecdotally they are often effective. Intravenous human immunoglobulin has been used in ASV and the role of anti-T cell therapy has been alluded to but these treatments currently remain second-line. In patients with nonrenal WG, methotrexate may be of benefit and the value of anti-staphylococcal therapy in preventing WG relapse is being further assessed. Finally, newer cytotoxic agents such as mycophenolate mofetil are being tested in addition to antitumour necrosis factor-α therapy which has proved effective in rheumatoid arthritis (Jayne and Rasmussen, 2000). The goal of new treatments must be to reduce further or obviate the need for cyclophosphamide or similarly toxic drugs. Our current strategy for ASV is to randomize all eligible and consenting patients to ongoing multicentre therapeutic trials. The principal treatments employed are:

1. Oral prednisolone initiated at 1 mg/kg/per day (maximum 60 mg/day), tapered to ~15 mg/day by 3 months and further reduced thereafter.
2. Cyclophosphamide, orally at 2 mg/kg/per day or by intermittent pulses at

15 mg/kg. The duration of treatment is ordinarily limited to 3–6 months according to trial protocol.

3. Azathioprine 2 mg/kg/per day after cyclophosphamide therapy.

Dose reductions are necessary in elderly patients, in renal impairment and with leukopenia ($< 4 \times 10^9$/l). The optimal duration of therapy in ASV is undetermined but it is likely to be several years at least, in contrast to the 12-month regimes often used in classical polyarteritis nodosa. Patients with endstage renal disease secondary to ASV can be successfully transplanted and maintained on normal transplant immunosuppression regimes, although vasculitis relapses still occur.

REFERENCES

Adu, D., Howie, A.J., Scott, D.G.I. et al. (1987). Polyarteritis and the kidney. *Q. J. Med.*, **62**, 221–37.

Adu, D., Pall, A., Luqmani, R.A. et al. (1997). Controlled trial of pulse versus continuous prednisolone and cyclophosphamide in the treatment of systemic vasculitis. *Q. J. Med.*, **90**, 401–9.

Anderson, G., Coles, E.T., Crane, M. et al. (1992). Wegener's granuloma. A series of 265 British cases seen between 1975 and 1985. *Q. J. Med.*, **83**, 427–38.

Ara, J., Mirapeix, E., Rodriguez, R. et al. (1999). Relationship between ANCA and disease activity in small vessel vasculitis patients with anti-MPO ANCA. *Nephrol. Dial. Transplant.*, **14**, 1667–72.

Bajema, I., Hagen, C., Van der Woude, F.J. & Bruijn, J.A. (1997). Wegener's granulomatosis: meta-analysis of 349 literary case reports. *J. Lab. Clin. Med.*, **129**, 17–22.

Brouwer, E., Huitema, M.G., Mulder, A.H.M. et al. (1994). Neutrophil activation in vitro and in vivo in WG. *Kidney Int.*, **45**, 1120–31.

Casselman, B.L., Kilgore, K.S., Miller, B.F. & Warren, J.S. (1995). Antibodies to neutrophil cytoplasmic antigens induce MCP-1 secretion from human monocytes. *J. Lab. Clin. Med.*, **126**, 495–502.

Cockwell, P., Tse, W.Y. & Savage, C.O.S. (1997). Activation of endothelial cells in thrombosis and vasculitis. *Scand. J. Rheumatol.*, **26**, 145–50.

Cockwell, P., Brooks, C.J., Adu, D. & Savage, C.O.S. (1999). IL-8: a pathogenetic role in ANCA-associated glomerulonephritis. *Kidney Int.*, **55**, 852–63.

Cohen Tervaert, J.W., van der Woude, F.J., Fauci, A.S. et al. (1989). Association between active WG and ANCA. *Arch. Intern. Med.*, **149**, 2461–5.

Cohen Tervaeart, J.W., Popa, E.R. & Brons, R.H. (2000). *Staphylococcus aureus*, superantigens and vasculitis. *Clin. Exp. Immunol.*, **120** (suppl. 1), 6–7.

Csernok, E., Ernst, M., Scmitt, W. et al. (1994). Activated neutrophils express PR3 on their plasma membranes in vitro and in vivo. *Clin. Exp. Immunol.*, **95**, 244–50.

Csernok, E., Trabandt, A., Müller, A. et al. (1999). Cytokine profiles in Wegener's granulomatosis. *Arthritis Rheum.*, **42**, 742–50.

Csernok, E., Moosig, F., Kumanovics, G. & Gross, W.L. (2000). Opsonization of apoptotic neutrophils by ANAC leads to activation of macrophages. *Clin. Exp. Immunol.*, **120** (suppl. 1), 38.

Cunningham, M.A., Huang, X.R., Dowling, J.P. et al. (1999). Prominence of cell mediated immunity effectors in pauci-immune glomerulonephritis. *J. Am. Soc. Nephrol.*, **10**, 499–506.

Davies, D.J., Morn, J.E., Niall, J.F. & Ryan, G.B. (1982). Segmental necrotising glomerulonephritis with anti-neutrophil antibodies: possible arbovirus aetiology? *Br. Med. J.*, **285**, 606.

Falk, R.J., Terrell, R.S., Charles, L.A. & Jennette, J.C. (1990). ANCA induce neutrophils to degranulate and produce oxygen radicals in vitro. *Proc. Natl Acad. Sci. U.S.A.*, **87**, 4115–19.

Fauci, A.S., Haynes, B.F., Katz, P. & Wolff, S.M. (1983). Wegener's granulomatosis: prospective clinical and therapeutic experience with 85 patients for 21 years. *Ann. Intern. Med.*, **98**, 76–85.

Gaskin, G., Savage, C.O.S., Ryan, J.J. et al. (1991). ANCA and disease activity during follow-up of 70 patients with systemic vasculitis. *Nephrol. Dial. Transplant.*, **6**, 689–94.

Gilligan, H.M., Bredy, B., Brady, H.R. et al. (1996). ANCA interact with primary granule constituents on the surface of apoptic neutrophils in the absence of neutrophil priming. *J. Exp. Med.*, **184**, 2231–41.

Giscombe, R., Nityanand, S., Lewin, N. et al. (1998). Expanded T cell populations in patients with WG: characteristics and correlates with disease activity. *J. Clin. Immunol.*, **18**, 404–13.

Griffith, M.E., Coulhart, A. & Pusey, C.D. (1995). T cell responses to MPO and PR3 in patients with systemic vasculitis. *Clin. Exp. Immunol.*, **103**, 253–8.

Guillevin, L. (2000). Polyarteritis nodosa and Churg Strauss syndrome. *Clin. Exp. Immunol.*, **120** (suppl. 1), 33–5.

Guillevin, L., Cordier, J.-F., Lhote, F. et al. (1997). A prospective, multicentre, randomized trial comparing steroids and pulse cyclophosphamide versus steroids and oral cyclophosphamide in the treatment of generalised WG. *Arthritis Rheum.*, **40**, 2187–98.

Guillevin, L., Durand-Gasselin, B., Cevallos, R. et al. (1999a). Microscopic polyangiitis. *Arthritis Rheum.*, **42**, 421–30.

Guillevin, L., Cohen, P., Gayraud, M. et al. (1999b). Churg–Strauss syndrome. Clinical study and long-term follow-up of 96 patients. *Medicine (Baltimore)*, **78**, 26–37.

Haber, M.A., Tso, A., Taheri, S. et al. (1999). Wegener's granulomatosis in pregnancy. *Nephrol. Dial. Transplant.*, **14**, 1789–91.

Hagen, E.C., Daha, M.R., Hermans, J. et al. (1998). Diagnostic value of standardized assays for ANCA in idiopathic systemic vasculitis. *Kidney Int.*, **53**, 743–53.

Harper, L., Cockwell, P. & Savage, C.O.S. (1998). Case of propylthiouracil-induced ANCA associated small vessel vasculitis. *Nephrol. Dial. Transplant.*, **13**, 455–8.

Harper, L., Radford, D.J., Adu, D. & Savage, C.O.S. (2000a). Antineutrophil cytoplasmic antibodies induce reactive oxygen-dependent disregulation of primed neutrophil apoptosis and clearance by macrophages. *Am. J. Pathol.*, **157**, 211–20.

Harper, L., Cockwell, P., Adu, D. & Savage, C.O.S. (2001). Neutrophil priming and apoptosis in anti-neutrophic cytoplasmic autoantibody-associated vasculitis. *Kidney Int.*, **59**, 1729–38.

Heeringa, P., Brouwer, E., Cohen Tervaert, J.W. et al. (1998). Animal models of ANCA-associated vasculitis. *Kidney Int.*, **53**, 253–63.

Hewins, P., Cohen Tervaert, J.W., Savage, C.O.S. & Kallenberg, C.G.M. (2000). Is Wegener's granulomatosis an autoimmune disease? *Curr. Opin. Rheumatol.*, **12**, 3–10.

Hoffman, G.S., Kerr, G.S., Leavitt, R.Y. et al. (1992). Wegener granulomatosis: analysis of 158 patients. *Ann. Intern. Med.*, **116**, 488–98.

Hooke, D.H., Gee, D.C. & Atkins, R.C. (1987). Leukocyte analysis using monoclonal antibodies in human glomerulonephritis. *Kidney Int.*, **31**, 964–72.

Jayne, D. & Rasmussen, N. (2000). European collaborative trials in vasculitis: EUVAS-update and latest results. *Clin. Exp. Immunol.*, **120** (suppl. 1), 13–14.

Jayne, D.R.W., Marshal, P.D., Jones, S.J. & Lockwood, C.M. (1990). Autoantibodies to GBM and neutrophil cytoplasm in rapidly progressive glomerulonephritis. *Kidney Int.*, **37**, 965–70.

Jayne, D.R.W., Gaskin G, Pusey, C.D. & Lockwood, C.M. (1995). ANCA and predicting relapse in systemic vasculitis. *Q. J. Med.*, **88**, 127–33.

Jennette, J.C., Falk, R.J., Andrassy, K. et al. (1994). Nomenclature of systemic vasculitides. *Arthritis Rheum.*, **37**, 187–92.

King, W.J., Adu, D., Daha, M.R. et al. (1995). Endothelial cells and renal epithelial cells do not express the Wegener's autoantigen, PR3. *Clin. Exp. Immunol.*, **102**, 98–105.

King, W.J., Brooks, C.J., Holder, R. et al. (1998). T lymphocyte responses to ANCA antigens are present in patients with ANCA-associated systemic vasculitis and persist during remission. *Clin. Exp. Immunol.*, **112**, 539–46.

Kyndt, X., Reumaux, D., Bridoux, F. et al. (1999). Serial measurements of ANCA in patients with systemic vasculitis. *Am. J. Med.*, **106**, 527–33.

Lane, S.E., Scott, D.G.I., Heaton, A. & Watts, R.A. (2000). Primary vasculitis in Norfolk-increasing incidence or increasing recognition. *Nephrol. Dial. Transplant.*, **15**, 23–7.

Lanham, J.G., Elkon, K.B., Pusey, C.D. & Hughes, G.R. (1984). Systemic vasculitis with asthma and eosinophilia: a clinical approach to CSS. *Medicine (Baltimore)*, **63**, 65–81.

Lie, J.T. (1990). Illustrated histopathologic classification criteria for selected vasculitis syndromes. *Arthritis Rheum.*, **33**, 1074–87.

Lie, J.T. (1991). Vasculitis, 1815 to 1991: classification and diagnostic specificity. *J. Rheumatol.*, **19**, 83–9.

Lockwood, C.M., Thiru, S. & Stewart, S. (1996). Treatment of refractory Wegener's granulomatosis with humanised monoclonal antibodies. *Q. J. Med.*, **89**, 903–12.

Lúdvíksson, B.J., Sneller, M.C., Chua, K.S. et al. (1998). Active WG is associated with HLA-DR and CD4 T cells exhibiting an unbalanced Th1-type T cell cytokine pattern; reversal with IL-10. *J. Immunol.*, **160**, 3602–9.

Moins-Teisserene, H., Gadola, S., Cella, M. *et al.* (1999). A syndrome resembling WG associated with low surface expression of HLA class I molecules. *Lancet*, **354**, 1598–603.

Morton, M.R. (1998). Hypersensitivity vasculitis (microscopic polyangiitis) in pregnancy with transmission to the neonate. *Br. J. Obstet. Gynaecol.*, **105**, 928–30.

Mulder, A.H.L., Heeringa, P., Brouwer, E. et al. (1994). Activation of granulocytes by ANCA; a FcγRII-dependent process. *Clin. Exp. Immunol.*, **98**, 270–8.

Muller Kobold, A.C., Kallenberg, C.G.M. & Cohen Tervaert, J.W. (1998a). Leukocyte membrane PR3 correlates with disease activity in patients with WG. *Br. J. Rheumatol.*, **37**, 901–7.

Muller Kobold, A.C., Mesander, G., Stegeman, C.A. et al. (1998b). Are circulating neutrophils intravascularly activated in patients with ANCA-associated vasculitis? *Clin. Exp. Immunol.*, **114**, 491–9.

Muller Kobold, A.C., Kallenberg, C.G.M. & Cohen Tervaert, J.W. (1999). Monocyte activation in patients with WG. *Arch. Rheum. Dis.*, **58**, 237–45.

Pendergraft, W.F., Zarella, C.S., Yang, J.J. et al. (2000). Proteolytic inactive C-terminal death domain of PR3. *Clin. Exp. Immunol.*, **120** (suppl. 1), 37.

Pettersson, E.E., Sundelin, B. & Heigl, Z. (1995). Incidence and outcome of pauci-immune necrotising and crescentic glomerulonephritis in adults. *Clin. Nephrol.*, **43**, 141–9.

Porges, A.J., Redecha, P.B., Kimberley, W.T. et al. (1994). ANCA engage and activate human neutrophils via FcγRIIa. *J. Immunol.*, **153**, 1271–80.

Radford, D.J., Lord, J.M. & Savage, C.O.S. (1999). The activation of the neutrophil respiratory burst by anti-neutrophil cytoplasm autoantibody (ANCA) from patients with systemic vasculitis requires tyrosine kinases and protein kinase C activation. *Clin. Exp. Immunol.*, **118**, 171–9.

Radford, D.J., Savage, C.O.S. & Nash, G.B. (2000). Treatment of rolling neutrophils with anti-neutrophil cytoplasm autoantibodies causes conversion to firm integrin-mediated adhesion. *Arthritis Rheum.*, **43**, 1337–44.

Ralston, D.R., Marsh, C.B., Lowe, M.P. & Wewers, M.D. (1997). ANCA induce monocyte IL-8 release. Role of surface PR3, α1-antitrypsin and Fcγ receptors. *J. Clin. Invest.*, **100**, 1416–24.

Raynauld, J.P., Bloch, D.A. & Fries, J.F. (1993). Seasonal variation in onset of WG, PAN and giant cell arteritis. *J. Rheumatol.*, **20**, 1524–6.

Reumaux, D., Vossebeld, P.J.M., Roos, D. & Verhoeven, A.J. (1995). Effect of TNF-induced integrin activation on FcγRII-mediated signal transduction: relevance for activation of neutrophils by anti-PR3 or anti-MPO antibodies. *Blood*, **86**, 3189–95.

Reumaux, D., de Boer, M,. Duthilleul, P. et al. (2000). Neutrophils from a completely MPO deficient donor are not activated by anti-MPO antibodies. *Clin. Exp. Immunol.*, **120** (suppl. 1), 40.

Savage, C.O.S. & Ng, Y.C. (1986). The aetiology and pathogenesis of major systemic vasculitides. *Postgrad. Med. J.*, **62**, 627–36.

Savage, C.O.S., Winearls, C.G., Evans, D.J. et al. (1985). Microscopic polyarteritis: presentation, pathology and prognosis. *Q. J. Med.*, **56**, 467–83.

Savage, C.O.S., Pottinger, B.E., Gaskin, G. et al. (1992). Autoantibodies developing to MPO and PR3 in systemic vasculitis stimulate neutrophil cytotoxicity towards cultured endothelial cells. *Am. J. Pathol.*, **141**, 335–42.

Savage, C.O.S., Gaskin, G., Pusey, C.D. & Pearson, J.D. (1993). ANCA can recognise vascular endothelial cell-bound ANCA-associated autoantigens. *Exp. Nephrol.*, **1**, 190–5.

Savige, J., Gillis, D., Benson, E. et al. (1999). International consensus statement on testing and reporting of ANCA. *Am. J. Clin. Pathol.*, **111**, 507–13.

Serra, A., Cameron, J.S., Turner, D.R. et al. (1984). Vasculitis affecting the kidney. *Q. J. Med.*, **53**, 181–207.

Simpson, I.J., Skinner, M.A., Geursen, A. et al. (1995). Peripheral blood T lymphocytes in systemic vasculitis: increased TCR Vβ_2 gene usage in microscopic polyarteritis. *Clin. Exp. Immunol.*, **101**, 220–6.

Stegeman, C.A., Cohen Tervaert, J.W., Sluiter, W.J. et al. (1994). Association of chronic nasal carriage of *Staphylococcus aureus* and higher relapse rates in WG. *Ann. Intern. Med.*, **120**, 12–17.

Stegeman, C.A., Cohen Tervaert, J.W., de Jong P.E. et al. (1996). Trimethoprim-sulfa-methoxazole (co-trimoxazole) for the prevention of relapses of Wegener's granulomatosis. *N. Engl. J. Med.*, **335**, 16–20.

Tidman, M., Olander, R., Svalander, C. & Danielsson, D. (1998). Patients hospitalized because of small vessel vasculitis with renal involvement in the period 1975–1995. *J. Intern. Med.*, **244**, 133–41.

Tse, W., Abadeh, S., Jefferis, R. et al. (2000). Fcγ receptor polymorphisms are predictors of renal outcome in ASV. *Clin. Exp. Immunol.*, **120** (suppl. 1), 60.

Vargunam, M., Adu, D., Taylor, C.M. et al. (1992). Endothelial MPO-anti-MPO interaction in vasculitis. *Nephrol. Dial. Transplant.*, **7**, 1077–81.

Weiss, M.A. & Crissman, J.D. (1984). Renal biopsy findings in Wegener's granulomatosis. *Hum. Pathol.*, **15**, 943–56.

Westman, K.W., Bygren, P.G., Olsson, H. et al. (1998). Relapse rate, renal survival and cancer morbidity in patients with WG or MPA with renal involvement. *J. Am. Soc. Nephrol.*, **9**, 842–52.

Witko-Sarsat, V., Cramer, E.M., Hieblot, C. et al. (1999a). Presence of PR3 in secretory vesicles: evidence of a novel, highly mobilizable intracellular pool distinct from azurophil granules. *Blood*, **94**, 2487–96.

Witko-Sarsat, V., Lesavre, P., Lopez, S. et al. (1999b). A large subset of neutrophils expressing membrane PR3 is a risk factor for vasculitis and rheumatoid arthritis. *J. Am. Soc. Nephrol.*, **10**, 1224–33.

Yang, J.J., Kettriz, R., Falk, R.J., Jennette, J.C. & Gaido, M.L. (1996). Apoptosis of endothelial cells induced by the neutrophil serine proteases PR3 and elastase. *Am. J. Pathol.*, **149**, 1617–26.

Yang, J.J., Preston, G.A., Pendergraft, W.F. et al. (2000). Internalization of PR3 and MPO is concomitant with endothelial cell damage. *Clin. Exp. Immunol.*, **120** (suppl. 1), 37.

17

Pulmonary hypertension

Tim Higenbottam[1] and Helen Marriott[2]

[1]Clinical Sciences, AstraZeneca R&D Charnwood, Loughborough, Leicestershire
[2]Section of Medicine and Pharmacology, Division of Clinical Sciences, Medical School,
University of Sheffield, Sheffield

Introduction

Pulmonary hypertension was first recognized as a distinct illness in the nineteenth century (Romberg, 1891). It required the detailed clinical descriptions of primary pulmonary hypertension (PPH) from Dresdale et al. (1951) and Wood (1952) to facilitate the modern diagnosis. In 1973, as a result of the widespread use of cardiac catheterization and detailed histopathology, a World Health Organization (WHO)-sponsored meeting was held to classify the many different forms of pulmonary hypertension. The meeting classified pulmonary hypertension into primary or unexplained pulmonary hypertension and those forms that are secondary to other disease (Hantano and Strasser, 1975). Also, the concept of pulmonary vasodilatation was introduced to encourage specific therapies for the illness. The establishment of the National Institute of Health (NIH)-sponsored register of PPH patients in the 1980s led to further changes in clinical practice, as well as basic understanding of the disease. The place of right heart catheterization was established as the essential step in diagnosis and quantification of the severity of the disease (Rich et al., 1987). Evidence of right heart failure proved valuable in predicting survival (D'Alonzo et al., 1991). In only a relatively small proportion of patients is it possible to vasodilate the pulmonary circulation.

Interest in pulmonary hypertension was increased by successful heart–lung and lung transplant surgery (Reitz et al., 1982). Limited numbers of suitable donors, however, preclude this form of treatment for the majority of patients. For example, in the UK, over the last decade, an average of 10 lung and heart–lung transplant surgery for PPH have been performed, with at least 120 adult patients each year being diagnosed. In the 1980s long-term intravenous prostacyclin proved effective therapy to increase survival and quality of life (Higenbottam et al., 1984; Jones et al., 1987). Initially proposed as a bridge to transplantation, it has since been used as a substitute treatment instead of surgery. From these developments have followed the testing of new analogues of prostacyclin with simpler delivery systems. Interesting alternatives to prostaglandins offer potentially simpler and more effective means to improve survival for these unfortunate patients.

In the NIH registry, 6% of patients were identified as exhibiting a familial disposition (Rich et al., 1987). The chromosome 2q 31–32 was identified as associated with familial PPH (Nichols et al., 1997). Recently those mutations causing the familial disease were identified as responsible for the gene for bone morphogenetic protein receptor-2 (BMPR-2) (Deng et al., 2000; Thomson et al., 2000). Of particular interest is that this is a subunit of the receptor complex for transforming growth factor-β, an important cytokine and mitogen in vascular control (Blobe et al., 2000).

It is against the background of these rapid advances in medical science that this chapter has been designed to draw together the basic and clinical themes to illustrate this exciting story that has begun to improve the life of many patients.

The new classification of pulmonary hypertension (1998 WHO)

The advances in treatment and understanding during the last two decades prompted the second world conference on pulmonary hypertension in 1998 in Evian. The WHO again sponsored the meeting (Rich, 1998), which led to a new classification of pulmonary hypertension.

It had become evident that prostacyclin was effective both in improving quality of life and survival of PPH patients (Higenbottam et al., 1993; Barst et al., 1996). Not all forms of pulmonary hypertension however benefit from prostaglandin therapy. Furthermore, the characteristic pathological abnormalities of the different forms of pulmonary hypertension had become clearly defined from study of explant tissue of lung transplant recipients (Chazova et al., 1995).

This led to a classification of five types of pulmonary hypertension:
1. Pulmonary arterial hypertension
2. Pulmonary venous hypertension
3. Pulmonary hypertension from hypoxia and hypoxaemia
4. Chronic thromboembolic pulmonary hypertension
5. Miscellaneous types of pulmonary hypertension

Pulmonary arterial hypertension

In this form of pulmonary hypertension the characteristic morphological change is extensive intimal thickening of the precapillary arteries (Figure 17.1). This is a result of proliferation of fibroblast and vascular smooth muscle cells. There is narrowing of the lumen of the vessels that can become obliterated (Hislop and

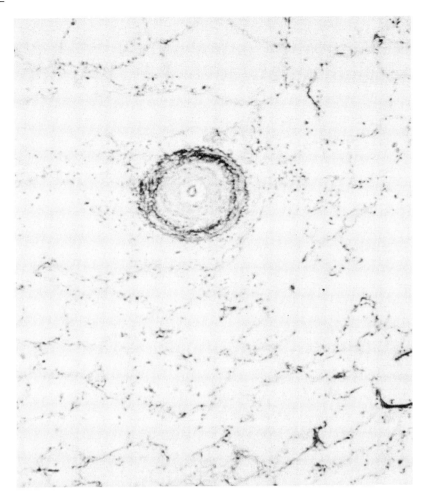

Figure 17.1   Intimal thickening of a pulmonary artery in pulmonary hypertension. From Chazova et al. (1995) with permission.

Reid, 1976). Indeed, it has been estimated that at the time of diagnosis over 80% of the precapillary arteries have been lost (Reeves and Noonan, 1973).

There are a number of types of pulmonary artery hypertension:

1. PPH, which can be either sporadic or familial
2. Pulmonary arterial hypertension associated with diseases, such as human immunodeficiency virus (HIV) infection, congenital heart and lung disease, scleroderma, portal hypertension, and systemic lupus erythematosus, or use of appetite-suppressant drugs such as fenfluramine and dexfenfluramine

All these forms of pulmonary artery hypertension appear to benefit from long-term prostacyclin therapy (Kuo et al., 1997; Rosenzweig et al., 1999; Badesch et al., 2000).

Pulmonary venous hypertension

Postcapillary veins are affected by this vascular disease, with again intimal proliferation representing the principal change in morphology and causing narrowing of the lumen.

There are two unexplained forms:
1. Pulmonary venoocclusive disease
2. Pulmonary capillary haemangiomatosis

The most common causes of this form of pulmonary hypertension are left ventricular failure and left-sided valvular disease, both of which cause chronic elevation of pulmonary venous pressure. Treatment of the heart disease resolves the pulmonary hypertension.

Prostacyclin therapy does not improve patients with pulmonary venous hypertension (Nicod et al., 1989; Humbert et al., 1998). It is speculated that the increased pulmonary blood flow from the treatment leads to pulmonary oedema in the face of an inability to reduce the pulmonary venous pressure.

Pulmonary hypertension from hypoxia and hypoxaemia

Alveolar hypoxia, from chronic lung disease and central hypoventilation, together with obstructive sleep apnoea, causes pulmonary hypertension in a significant number of afflicted patients. In chronic obstructive pulmonary disease (COPD) patients in respiratory failure, the pulmonary hypertension can be reversed or progression delayed by long-term oxygen therapy (LTOT: Weitzenblum et al., 1985). Indeed, this form of treatment significantly increases survival (Anon, 1980, 1981).

Chronic thromboembolic pulmonary hypertension

Here the pulmonary hypertension results from obstruction of the pulmonary arteries with either chronic pulmonary emboli and/or intravascular thrombosis. This illness is divided into two forms according to the principal site of obstruction. It is important to separate the proximal obstruction (Figure 17.2) from the peripheral (Figure 17.3), as the former can, in selected patients, be treated surgically (Jamieson, 1998).

Miscellaneous types of pulmonary hypertension

A number of diseases result in physical obstruction of the pulmonary arteries. These include tumours, such as leiomyosarcomas, fibrosing mediastinitis, filariasis and schistosomiasis.

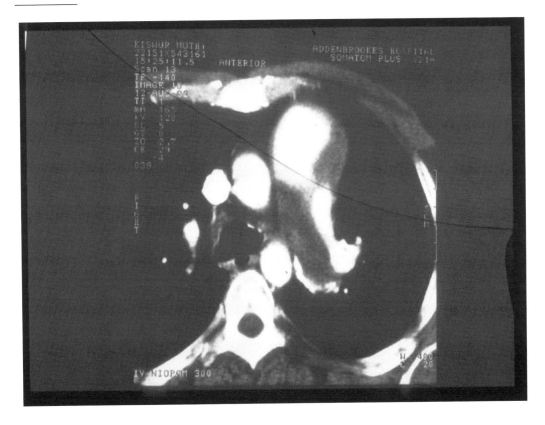

Figure 17.2 Proximal obstruction.

Pathobiology of pulmonary hypertension

Heart–lung and lung transplant surgery has not only advanced the therapy of pulmonary hypertension, it has also improved understanding of the pathobiology through the use of 'live' tissue for physiological studies and histopathology. Similarly the genetic studies that have followed precision in diagnosis have identified further mechanisms involved in the disease. Together, these advances will surely expand the range of treatments that may influence the disease.

Familial primary pulmonary hypertension

Identification of the gene mutations responsible for familial PPH illustrates the remarkable advances that have occurred in medical science in the last few years. Detailed family studies developed the idea of an autosomal-domininant inherited condition with reduced penetrance (Loyd et al., 1984). There was evidence of anticipation, with a falling age of occurrence in successive generations (Loyd et al., 1995).

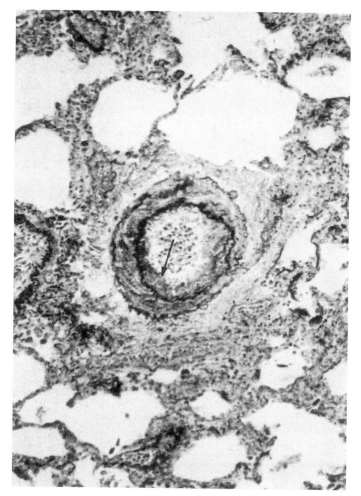

Figure 17.3 Peripheral obstruction.

In 1997 the gene for familial PPH was mapped to chromosome 2q 31–32 (Morse et al., 1997; Nichols et al., 1997). All affected families studied linked to this locus, which was termed PPH1. Screening for candidate genes within this interval revealed mutations in the gene *BMPR-2* (Thomson et al., 2000). BMPR-2 is a receptor member of the transforming growth factor-β (TGF-β) family (Blobe et al., 2000: Figure 17.4). These cytokines are potent regulators of other growth factors that are overexpressed in lung tissue in a variety of forms of pulmonary hypertension (Botney et al., 1994). The TGF-β family is important in the regulation of vascular development and integrity. In the disease hereditary haemorrhagic pulmonary telangiectasia (Rendu–Osler–Weber syndrome) there are mutations of the gene for endoglin and activin receptor like kinase-1 (ALK-1: Shovlin and

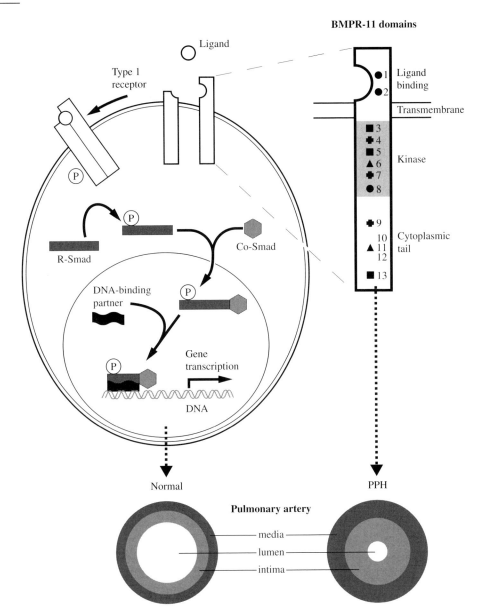

Figure 17.4 Bone morphogenetic protein receptor-1 (BMPR-II) signalling pathway. PPH, primary pulmonary hypertension. From Thomson et al. (2000) with permission.

Letarte, 1999), which are members of TGF-β receptor complexes (Massague and Chen, 2000).

The importance of the mutations of *BMPR-2* in the development of pulmonary vascular disease has been highlighted by the finding that up to 26% of sporadic cases of PPH exhibit the mutations (Thomson et al., 2000).

Endothelial dysfunction

The role of endothelial dysfunction in vascular disease is now well established. There is evidence of widespread changes in the phenotype of pulmonary endothelium in the various forms of pulmonary hypertension.

Reduction in endothelial production of prostacyclin

In PPH patients there is evidence that the rate of production of prostacyclin is reduced (Tuder et al., 1999). The expression of the endothelial enzyme prostacyclin synthase is also reduced (Christman et al., 1992). These findings underlined the logic of long-term infusion of prostacyclin as a treatment of PPH.

Reduction of nitric oxide production

In all forms of pulmonary hypertension there is evidence that nitric oxide (NO) release is reduced, especially in hypoxia-associated pulmonary hypertension (Dinhxuan et al., 1991; Cremona et al., 1994, 1999). In the endothelium of pulmonary arteries, NO synthase is underexpressed (Giaid and Saleh, 1995). In PPH patients there is localized overexpression of NO synthase in plexiform lesions, a proliferative angiogenic lesion associated with severe pulmonary hypertension.

Again, this provides support for the use of NO therapies, particularly in hypoxic pulmonary hypertension.

Endothelin-1 overexpression

Endothelin-1 (ET-1), a powerful vasoconstrictor and mitogen, is overexpressed in lung tissue of all forms of pulmonary hypertension (Giaid et al., 1993). These findings are common for PPH, pulmonary arterial hypertension associated with congenital heart–lung disease, chronic thromboembolic pulmonary hypertension, and hypoxia-induced pulmonary hypertension (Giaid et al., 1993; Kim et al., 1999). Evidence is not so consistent with circulating levels of ET-1 but differing rates of metabolism may account for these varying results (Stewart et al., 1991).

On the strength of these observations, antagonists for the ET-1 receptors A and/or B are now entering clinical trials for PPH (Williamson et al., 2000).

Endothelial cell proliferation

Isolation of endothelial cells from the plexiform lesions of the lungs of PPH patients and those with pulmonary arterial hypertension from anorectic use has added a further specific abnormality of the endothelium. These cells show a monoclonal expansion (Lee et al., 1998), not unlike the changes associated with certain tumours. Whether this represents a selective expansion within an area of angiogenesis remains unknown, but it further emphasizes the striking and widespread changes of behaviour of vascular cells of the pulmonary circulation.

Phenotypic changes in other vascular cells

In experimental models of pulmonary hypertension most vascular cells have been shown to undergo phenotypic changes. In cultured vascular smooth muscle cells from PPH patients' pulmonary arteries there is evidence of underexpression of a subunit of the voltage-dependent potassium channel. This Kv 1.5 subunit is reduced in these cells from PPH arteries (Yuan et al., 1998).

A diagnostic algorithm for pulmonary hypertension

The patient's presenting signs and symptoms

The most common symptoms of all forms of pulmonary hypertension are non-specific. They are breathlessness, angina and syncope. The latter two symptoms are only seen in advanced disease and are often associated with peripheral oedema and ascites, suggesting right ventricular failure.

The most important clue for the clinician is the inappropriate severity of breathlessness, which is out of proportion to the signs from lung or heart disease. Physical signs are absent in the lungs unless there is COPD or interstitial pulmonary fibrosis (IPF). The cardiac signs are of a loud second heart sound in the pulmonary area and, later, a right ventricular heave. There may also be central cyanosis and peripheral oedema.

Screening tests

Echocardiography with Doppler provides evidence of dilatation of the right atrium and ventricle. It also provides a measure of systolic pulmonary artery pressure (Eysmann et al., 1989). The exclusion of left ventricular failure and left-sided valvulopathy are the other valuable attributes of this investigation.

Lung functions tests are used to determine evidence of COPD or IPF and measurement of arterial blood gas tensions allows diagnosis of respiratory failure. Screening for liver dysfunction and HIV infections aids diagnosis of these forms of pulmonary arterial hypertension.

Systemic diseases are usually diagnosed by a combination of serological tests and a detailed clinical examination for signs of lupus erythematosus and sclero-derma.

All patients should undergo ventilation and perfusion lung scintigraphy to look for evidence of pulmonary embolism.

Currently all patients undergo an exercise test. The most popular are the shuttle (Singh et al., 1992) or 6-min walking (Miyamoto et al., 2000) tests. The distance covered in each test correlates with cardiac output and allows patients to be graded according to severity of disease.

In all patients, diagnosis of pulmonary hypertension is made at right heart cardiac catheterization. This should only be undertaken in those medical centres with specialized expertise.

Right heart cardiac catheterization

Patients receive premedication with a sedative. Intravenous access is through the internal jugular vein in either the neck or the femoral vein. Each site has its devotees. Measurements of mean right atrial pressure, mean pulmonary artery pressure and pulmonary wedge pressure can be obtained with a Swan–Ganz floatation catheter. This device also provides a measurement of cardiac output using the thermodilution method. Arterial blood pressure is obtained indirectly with a Doppler device and arterial oxygen saturation is obtained with a pulse oximeter.

It is ideal to record stable measurements: many investigators record six or eight measurements as baseline.

Vasodilator trials are performed, with intravenous prostacyclin (Raffy et al., 1996), adenosine (Morgan et al., 1991) or inhaled NO (Sitbon et al., 1998) being the most commonly used drugs. The vasodilator tests should only be performed in a specialist hospital as they carry a mortality risk.

Medical and surgical treatments for pulmonary hypertension

Pulmonary arterial hypertension

This includes PPH, both sporadic and familial, pulmonary arterial hypertension with HIV, congenital heart–lung disease, portal pulmonary hypertension, anorectic pulmonary hypertension and pulmonary hypertension with systemic disease.

Treatment is decided according to the severity of the haemodynamics, as follows.

Mild-to-moderate disease

This is gauged by New York Heart Association (NYHA) grade I–II, or a shuttle walking test distance of more than 200 m. Such patients do not have angina or syncope.

At right heart catheter the mean right atrial pressure is less than 10 mmHg, mean pulmonary artery pressure is below 50 mmHg, and cardiac output is greater than 2.5 l/min.

These patients are treated with anticoagulants which improve survival chances (Fuster et al., 1984). If, in the acute vasodilator trial during right heart catheterization, there had been a fall in mean pulmonary artery pressure of 20% or an improvement of cardiac output of 20% was observed, then oral vasodilators can

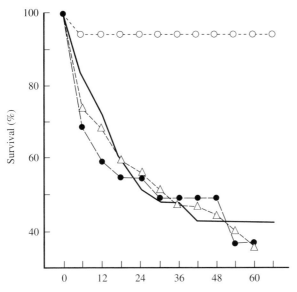

Figure 17.5 The effect of calcium channel blockers on survival in primary pulmonary hypertension. From Rich et al. (1992) with permission.

be tried. Diltiazem and amlodopine are the most popular vasodilators in use. These should be started in hospital whilst monitoring systemic blood pressure to avoid dangerous falls in systemic blood pressure (Packer, 1985). Again, for a selected number of patients this improves survival (Figure 17.5; Rich et al., 1992).

The efficacy of treatment is gauged with a walking test, which should increase if the treatment is to be continued. Failure to demonstrate an improvement would be an indication for a further right heart catheter study.

Moderate-to-severe disease

Here the patient may complain of breathlessness as well as angina and syncope. The shuttle walk test will be below 200 m. The NYHA grade would be III or IV.

The right atrial pressure will be above 10 mmHg., the mean pulmonary artery pressure may be up to 70 mmHg and the cardiac output may be low (less than 2.5 l/min). It is very unlikely that there will be any vasodilation.

Currently these patients should receive continuously infused prostacyclin (Higenbottam et al., 1993, 1998; Barst et al., 1996). This treatment is technically challenging and should only be attempted in units with expertise. Common problems are underdosing and cannulae infection, both of which can be fatal.

With successful therapy, patients survive and enjoy a good quality of life (Figures 17.6 and 17.7). Again, progress is monitored with shuttle walk tests. The dose of prostacyclin may need to be increased or alternative treatments such as lung transplant surgery may be required.

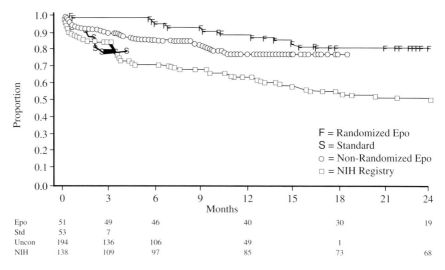

Epo	51	49	46	40	30	19
Std	53	7				
Uncon	194	136	106	49	1	
NIH	138	109	97	85	73	68

Figure 17.6   Long-term continuous infusions of prostacyclin improves survival. NIH, National Institute of Health; NYHA, New York Heart Association.

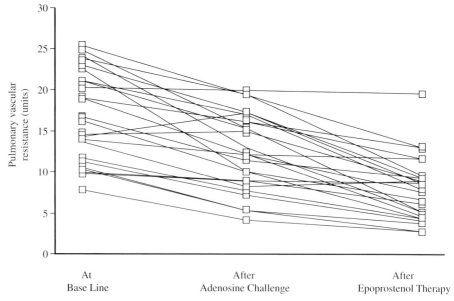

Figure 17.7   Long-term prostacyclin may reverse pulmonary hypertension. From McLaughlin et al. (1998) with permission.

Pulmonary venous hypertension

There is no medical treatment for this condition and prostacyclin worsens the patients with pulmonary venous hypertension (Figure 17.8). It is easily diagnosed where there is left ventricular failure or left valvulopathy. At echocardiography left

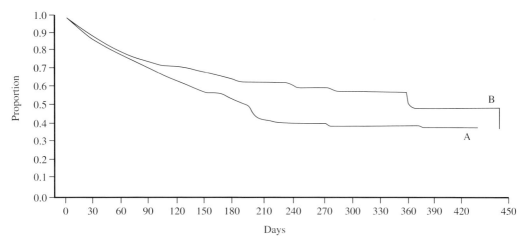

Figure 17.8 Prostacyclin worsens venous pulmonary hypertension.

ventricular and valve abnormalities are found in this condition. When the disease is a result of either venoocclusive disease or pulmonary capillary haemangiomatosis, the only abnormality is an elevated pulmonary wedge pressure. In such cases a high-resolution computed tomography scan may detect distinctive features of a reticular appearance (Dufour et al., 1998).

Pulmonary hypertension from hypoxia and hypoxaemia

For these patients the current therapy is the use of LTOT for COPD patients in respiratory failure. These patients need to have arterial oxygen tensions below 7.3 kPa and forced expiratory volume in 1 s less than 1.5 l. The use of 2 l/min flow rate of oxygen overnight for 14 h (Anon, 1987) or 24 h (Anon, 1980) improves survival and quality of life. There remains some uncertainty in the use of ambulatory oxygen. Presently it is advised for those patients who show significant arterial oxygen desaturation during exercise (Wedzicha, 1999).

In IPF, oxygen is advised for patients with pulmonary hypertension, although evidence of benefit is difficult to find.

In patients with obstructive sleep apnoea, continuous positive airway pressure overnight restores sleep and improves pulmonary hypertension. Alveolar hypoventilation may need home-assisted ventilation, but this is used palliatively as clear effects on pulmonary hypertension have not been demonstrated.

Alternatives to oxygen that affect the pulmonary vasculature, such as calcium channel blockers or inhaled NO, can cause worsening of gas exchange in chronic lung disease. They overcome hypoxic vasoconstriction leading to increased mismatch between the distribution of ventilation and perfusion (Bratel et al., 1985; Barbera et al., 1996). Selective distribution of such agents to those regions of high ventilation would be required if this problem of worsening gas exchange is to be overcome.

Chronic thromboembolic pulmonary hypertension

Proximal obstructions of the pulmonary arteries

Careful selection of patients is critical for success of thromboendarterectomy surgery (Jamieson, 1998). The ideal is to locate obstructions, complete and incomplete, distributed from the main left and right pulmonary arteries to level of the subsegmental arteries. Conventionally this is undertaken using pulmonary angiography.

Patients should have right atrial pressure measures below 10 mmHg and cardiac output measurements above 2.5 l/min (Moser et al., 1992). They should have no evidence of coronary heart disease and should be under 65 years old.

The success of this form of surgery depends on a highly trained surgeon and postoperative care team. There are only a few recognized centres with satisfactory results.

Distal obstruction of the pulmonary arteries

In those patients with unsuitable haemodynamic measurements, and those with distal postsegmental pulmonary artery obstructions, then management is as for pulmonary arterial hypertension. For example, if cardiac output is below 2.5 l/min and there is elevated right atrial pressure, then long-term intravenous prostacyclin enhances survival (Sitbon et al., 1999).

Miscellaneous causes of pulmonary hypertension

There are no guidelines for care of these forms of pulmonary hypertension.

Atrial septostomy

In selected patients the provision of an atrial septal defect can improve exercise tolerance and survival (Figure 17.9). The procedure in adults makes use of balloon dilators at the time of right heart catheterization, progressively enlarging the defect until the cardiac output increases (Kerstein et al., 1995; Sandoval et al., 1998).

This is again a procedure for specialized centres, as the procedure carries a mortality risk. It cannot be used in patients with advanced disease.

Transplantation surgery

For all forms of pulmonary hypertension, transplant surgery offers a treatment. Currently, medical treatment is used where appropriate and the patient is followed by exercise testing. Deterioration in functional status is an indication for further right heart catheterization; if the condition has worsened then transplant surgery is considered (Anon, 1998).

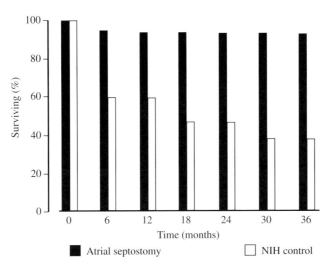

Figure 17.9 Atrial septostomy improves survival in pulmonary hypertension. From Higenbottam et al. (1999) with permission.

The options are single-lung transplantation, sequential double-lung and heart–lung transplantation. Most centres offer either sequential double or heart–lung transplantation. These probably provide a better outcome (Pasque et al., 1990). The long-term survival after transplant surgery is a median of 2.8 years (Keck et al., 1998): obliterative bronchiolitis is the main cause of fatalities.

Use of prostacyclin before surgery and introduction of newer immunosuppressant therapy has enhanced survival in the last 5 years. Pretransplant treatment of portal pulmonary hypertension patients with prostacyclin enhances the survival after liver transplantation (Conte et al., 1998).

In those types of pulmonary hypertension where there is no effective medical treatment, e.g. pulmonary venous hypertension and miscellaneous causes, then transplant surgery may be offered to selected patients.

It is not indicated for any untreated tumours, e.g. leiomyosarcomas or in HIV-associated pulmonary hypertension (Anon, 1998).

The future for pulmonary hypertension

The main challenges facing the care of patients with pulmonary hypertension is the requirement to demonstrate that the newer analogues of prostacyclin perform adequately with fewer complications. Alternatives to prostacyclin, such as the ET-1 antagonists, need to be shown to be safer than prostacyclin and as effective, if not better.

For the common forms of pulmonary hypertension such as pulmonary venous hypertension with left ventricular failure and hypoxic pulmonary hypertension, new therapies are needed. In each disorder it is necessary to avoid complications associated with relief of the pulmonary hypertension.

In left ventricular failure, relief of pulmonary venous hypertension with prostacyclin leads to pulmonary oedema. The speculation is that the development of pulmonary venous hypertension protects the lungs from pulmonary hypertension. Lessening the pulmonary hypertension in hypoxic pulmonary hypertension worsens gas exchange in chronic lung disease. In both conditions selective therapeutic effects are needed.

Finally, evidence from prostacyclin therapy in PPH indicates that long-term treatment may 'reverse' in part the structural changes characteristic of the illness (McLaughlin et al., 1998). In experimental models of pulmonary hypertension it has proved possible to reverse the disease with serine protease inhibitors (Cowan et al., 2000) and ET-1 antagonists (Chen et al., 1995). The hope is that these approaches will translate into real treatments for all forms of pulmonary hypertension.

REFERENCES

Badesch, D.B., Tapson, V.F., McGoon, M.D. et al. (2000). Continuous intravenous epoprostenol for pulmonary hypertension due to the scleroderma spectrum of disease. A randomized, controlled trial (see comments). *Ann. Intern. Med.*, **132**, 425–34.

Barbera, J.A., Roger, N., Roca, J. et al. (1996). Worsening of pulmonary gas exchange with nitric oxide inhalation in chronic obstructive pulmonary disease. *Lancet*, **347**, 436–40.

Barst, R.J., Rubin, L.J., Long, W.A. et al. (1996). A comparison of continuous intravenous epoprostenol (prostacyclin) with conventional therapy for primary pulmonary hypertension. The Primary Pulmonary Hypertension Study Group (see comments). *N. Engl. J. Med.*, **334**, 296–302.

Blobe, G.C., Schiemann, W.P. & Lodish, H.F. (2000). Role of transforming growth factor beta in human disease. *N. Engl. J. Med.*, **342**, 1350–8.

Botney, M.D., Bahadori, L. & Gold, L.I. (1994). Vascular remodeling in primary pulmonary hypertension. Potential role for transforming growth factor-beta. *Am. J. Pathol.*, **144**, 286–95.

Bratel, T., Hedenstierna, G., Nyquist, O. & Ripe, E. (1985). The effect of a new calcium antagonist, felodipine, on pulmonary hypertension and gas exchange in chronic obstructive lung disease. *Eur. J. Respir. Dis.*, **67**, 244–53.

Chazova, I., Loyd, J.E., Zhdanov, V.S. et al. (1995). Pulmonary artery adventitial changes and venous involvement in primary pulmonary hypertension. *Am. J. Pathol.*, **146**, 389–97.

Chen, S.J., Chen, Y.F., Meng, Q.C. et al. (1995). Endothelin-receptor antagonist bosentan prevents and reverses hypoxic pulmonary hypertension in rats. *J. Appl. Physiol.*, **79**, 2122–31.

Christman, B.W., McPherson, C.D., Newman, J.H. et al. (1992). An imbalance between the excretion of thromboxane and prostacyclin metabolites in pulmonary-hypertension. *N. Engl. J. Med.*, **327**, 70–5.

Conte, J.V., Gaine, S.P., Orens, J.B., Harris, T. & Rubin, L.J. (1998). The influence of continuous intravenous prostacyclin therapy for primary pulmonary hypertension on the timing and outcome of transplantation. *J. Heart Lung Transplant.*, **17**, 679–85.

Cowan, K.N., Heilbut, A., Humpl, T. et al. (2000). Complete reversal of fatal pulmonary hypertension in rats by a serine elastase inhibitor. *Nat. Med.*, **6**, 698–702.

Cremona, G., Higenbottam, T., Borland, C. & Mist, B. (1994). Mixed expired nitric-oxide in primary pulmonary-hypertension in relation to lung diffusion capacity. *Q. J. Med.*, **87**, 547–51.

Cremona, G., Higenbottam, T.W., Bower, E.A., Wood, A.M. & Stewart, S. (1999). Hemodynamic effects of basal and stimulated release of endogenous nitric oxide in isolated human lungs. *Circulation*, **100**, 1316–21.

D'Alonzo, G.E., Barst, R.J., Ayres, S.M. et al. (1991). Survival in patients with primary pulmonary hypertension. Results from a national prospective registry. *Ann. Intern. Med.*, **115**, 343–9.

Deng, Z., Morse, J.H., Slager, S.L. et al. (2000). Familial primary pulmonary hypertension (gene PPH1) is caused by mutations in the bone morphogenetic protein receptor-II gene. *Am. J. Hum. Genet.*, **67**, 737–44.

Dinhxuan, A.T., Higenbottam, T.W., Clelland, C.A. et al. (1991). Impairment of endothelium-dependent pulmonary-artery relaxation in chronic obstructive lung-disease. *N. Engl. J. Med.*, **324**, 1539–47.

Dresdale, D.T., Schutz, M. & Michtom, R.J. (1951). Primary pulmonary hypertension I. Clinical and hemodynamic study. *Am. J. Med.*, **11**, 686–70.

Dufour, B., Maitre, S., Humbert, M. et al. (1998). High-resolution CT of the chest in four patients with pulmonary capillary hemangiomatosis or pulmonary venoocclusive disease. *Am. J. Roentgenol.*, **171**, 1321–4.

Eysmann, S.B., Palevsky, H.I., Reichek, N., Hackney, K. & Douglas, P.S. (1989). Two-dimensional and Doppler-echocardiographic and cardiac catheterization correlates of survival in primary pulmonary hypertension. *Circulation*, **80**, 353–60.

Fuster, V., Steele, P.M., Edwards, W.D. et al. (1984). Primary pulmonary hypertension: natural history and the importance of thrombosis. *Circulation*, **70**, 580–7.

Giaid, A. & Saleh, D. (1995). Reduced expression of endothelial nitric oxide synthase in the lungs of patients with pulmonary hypertension. *N. Engl. J. Med.*, **333**, 214–21.

Giaid, A., Yanagisawa M, Langleben, D. et al. (1993). Expression of endothelin-1 in the lungs of patients with pulmonary hypertension. *N. Engl. J. Med.*, **328**, 1732–9.

Hantano, S. & Strasser, T. (eds) (1975). *Primary Pulmonary Hypertension. Report on the WHO Meeting.* Geneva: World Health Organization.

Higenbottam, T., Wells, F., Wheeldon, D. & Wallwork, J. (1984). Long-term treatment of primary pulmonary-hypertension with continuous intravenous epoprostenol (prostacyclin). *Lancet*, **1**, 1046–7.

Higenbottam, T.W., Spiegelhalter, D., Scott, J.P. et al. (1993). Prostacyclin (epoprostenol) and heart–lung transplantation as treatments for severe pulmonary-hypertension. *Br. Heart J.*, **70**, 366–70.

Higenbottam, T.W., Butt, A.Y., DinhXaun, A.T. et al. (1998). Treatment of pulmonary hypertension with the continuous infusion of a prostacyclin analogue, iloprost. *Heart*, **79**, 175–9.

Higenbottam, T., Stenmark, K. & Simonneau, G. (1999). Treatments for severe pulmonary hypertension. *Lancet*, **353**, 338–40.

Hislop, A. & Reid, L. (1976). New findings in pulmonary arteries of rats with hypoxia-induced pulmonary hypertension. *Br. J. Exp. Pathol.*, **57**, 542–54.

Humbert, M., Maitre, S., Capron, F. et al. (1998). Pulmonary edema complicating continuous intravenous prostacyclin in pulmonary capillary hemangiomatosis. *Am. J. Respir. Crit. Care Med.*, **157**, 1681–5.

Jamieson, S.W. (1998). Pulmonary thromboendarterectomy. *Heart*, **79**, 118–20.

Jones, D.K., Higenbottam, T.W. & Wallwork, J. (1987). Treatment of primary pulmonary-hypertension with intravenous epoprostenol (prostacyclin). *Br. Heart J.*, **57**, 270–8.

Keck, B.M., Bennett, L.E., Fiol, B.S. et al. (1998). Worldwide thoracic organ transplantation: a report from the UNOS/ISHLT International Registry for Thoracic Organ Transplantation. *Clin. Transplant.*, **12**, 39–52.

Kerstein, D., Levy, P.S., Hsu, D.T. et al. (1995). Blade balloon atrial septostomy in patients with severe primary pulmonary hypertension. *Circulation*, **91**, 2028–35.

Kim, H., Yung, G.L., Morris, T.A., Marsh, J.J. et al. (1999). Endothelin antagonism inhibits pulmonary vascular remodeling in canine chronic pulmonary embolism. *Am. J. Respir. Crit. Care Med.*, **159**, A566.

Kuo, P.C., Johnson, L.B., Plotkin, J.S. et al. (1997). Continuous intravenous infusion of epoprostenol for the treatment of portopulmonary hypertension. *Transplantation*, **63**, 604–6.

Lee, S.D., Shroyer, K.R., Markham, N.E. et al. (1998). Monoclonal endothelial cell proliferation is present in primary but not secondary pulmonary hypertension. *J. Clin. Invest.*, **101**, 927–34.

Loyd, J.E., Primm, R.K. & Newman, J.H. (1984). Familial primary pulmonary hypertension: clinical patterns. *Am. Rev. Respir. Dis.*, **129**, 194–7.

Loyd, J.E., Butler, M.G., Foroud, T.M. et al. (1995). Genetic anticipation and abnormal gender ratio at birth in familial primary pulmonary hypertension. *Am. J. Respir. Crit. Care Med.*, **152**, 93–7.

Massague, J. & Chen, Y.G. (2000). Controlling TGF-beta signaling. *Genes Dev.*, **14**, 627–44.

Maurer, J.R., Frost, A.E., Glanville, A.R., Estenne, M. & Higenbottam, T.W. (1998). International guidelines for the selection of lung transplant candidates. The American Society for Transplant Physicians (ASTP)/American Thoracic Society (ATS)/European Respiratory Society (ERS)/International Society for Heart and Lung Transplantation (ISHLT). *Am. J. Respir. Crit. Care Med.*, **158**, 335–9.

McLaughlin, V.V., Genthner, D.E., Panella, M.M. & Rich, S. (1998). Reduction in pulmonary vascular resistance with long-term epoprostenol (prostacyclin) therapy in primary pulmonary hypertension (see comments). *N. Engl. J. Med.*, **338**, 273–7.

Medical Research Council Working Party (1981). Long term domiciliary oxygen therapy in chronic hypoxic cor pulmonale complicating chronic bronchitis and emphysema. Report of the Medical Research Council working party. *Lancet*, **1**, 681–6.

Miyamoto, S., Nagaya, N., Satoh, T. et al. (2000). Clinical correlates and prognostic significance of six-minute walk test in patients with primary pulmonary hypertension. Comparison with cardiopulmonary exercise testing. *Am. J. Respir. Crit. Care Med.*, **161**, 487–92.

Morgan, J.M., McCormack, D.G., Griffiths, M.J. et al. (1991). Adenosine as a vasodilator in primary pulmonary hypertension (see comments). *Circulation*, **84**, 1145–9.

Morse, J.H., Jones, A.C., Barst, R.J. et al. (1997). Mapping of familial primary pulmonary hypertension locus (PPH1) to chromosome 2q31–q32. *Circulation*, **95**, 2603–6.

Moser, K.M., Auger, W.R., Fedullo, P.F. & Jamieson, S.W. (1992). Chronic thromboembolic pulmonary hypertension: clinical picture and surgical treatment. *Eur. Respir. J.*, **5**, 334–42.

Nichols, W.C., Koller, D.L., Slovis, B. et al. (1997). Localization of the gene for familial primary pulmonary hypertension to chromosome 2q31–32. *Nat. Genet.*, **15**, 277–80.

Nicod, P. & Moser, K.M. (1989). Primary pulmonary hypertension. The risk and benefit of lung biopsy (see comments). *Circulation*, **80**, 1486–8.

Nocturnal Oxygen Therapy Trial Group (1980). Continuous or nocturnal oxygen therapy in hypoxemic chronic obstructive lung disease: a clinical trial. Nocturnal oxygen therapy trial group. *Ann. Intern. Med.*, **93**, 391–8.

Packer, M. (1985). Vasodilator therapy for primary pulmonary hypertension. Limitations and hazards. *Ann. Intern. Med.*, **103**, 258–70.

Pasque, M.K., Cooper, J.D., Kaiser, L.R. et al. (1990). Improved technique for bilateral lung transplantation: rationale and initial clinical experience. *Ann. Thorac. Surg.*, **49**, 785–91.

Raffy, O., Azarian, R., Brenot, F. et al. (1996). Clinical significance of the pulmonary vasodilator response during short-term infusion of prostacyclin in primary pulmonary hypertension. *Circulation*, **93**, 484–8.

Reeves, J.T. & Noonan, J.A. (1973). Microarteriographic studies of primary pulmonary hypertension. A quantitative approach in two patients. *Arch. Pathol.*, **95**, 50–5.

Reitz, B.A., Wallwork, J.L., Hunt, S.A. et al. (1982). Heart–lung transplantation: successful therapy for patients with pulmonary vascular disease. *N. Engl. J. Med.*, **306**, 557–64.

Rich, S.E. (1998). Primary pulmonary hypertension: executive summary from the world symposium – primary pulmonary hypertension. Available from the World Health Organization via the internet: http://www.who.int/ncd/cvd/pph.thml 1998.

Rich, S., Dantzker, D.R., Ayres, S.M. et al. (1987). Primary pulmonary hypertension. A national prospective study. *Ann. Intern. Med.*, **107**, 216–23.

Rich, S., Kaufmann, E. & Levy, P.S. (1992). The effect of high doses of calcium-channel blockers on survival in primary pulmonary hypertension (see comments). *N. Engl. J. Med.*, **327**, 76–81.

Romberg, E. (1891). Über Skelerose der Lungen Arterie. *Dtsch. Arch. Kun. Med.*, **48**, 197–206.

Rosenzweig, E.B., Kerstein, D. & Barst, R.J. (1999). Long-term prostacyclin for pulmonary hypertension with associated congenital heart defects. *Circulation*, **99**, 1858–65.

Sandoval, J., Gaspar, J., Pulido, T. et al. (1998). Graded balloon dilation atrial septostomy in severe primary pulmonary hypertension. A therapeutic alternative for patients nonresponsive to vasodilator treatment. *J. Am. Coll. Cardiol.*, **32**, 297–304.

Shovlin, C.L. & Letarte, M. (1999). Hereditary haemorrhagic telangiectasia and pulmonary arteriovenous malformations: issues in clinical management and review of pathogenic mechanisms. *Thorax*, **54**, 714–29.

Singh, S.J., Morgan, M.D., Scott, S., Walters, D. & Hardman, A.E. (1992). Development of a shuttle walking test of disability in patients with chronic airways obstruction. *Thorax*, **47**,

1019–24.

Sitbon, O., Humbert, M., Jagot, J.L. et al. (1998). Inhaled nitric oxide as a screening agent for safely identifying responders to oral calcium-channel blockers in primary pulmonary hypertension (see comments). *Eur. Respir. J.*, **12**, 265–70.

Sitbon, O., Humbert, N., Nunes, H. et al. (1999). Long term Epopprostenol (PGI₂) therapy in pulmonary hypertension (PH) associated with HIV infection, portal hypertension, Eisenmenger syndrome and distal chronic thromboembolic disease (CTSD): comparison with primary PH and PH associated with connective tissue diseases (PH-CTD). *Eur. Respir. J.*, **14** (s30), 426s.

Stewart, D.J., Levy, R.D., Cernacek, P. & Langleben, D. (1991). Increased plasma endothelin-1 in pulmonary hypertension – marker or mediator of disease. *Ann. Intern. Med.*, **114**, 464–9.

Thomson, J.R., Machado, R.D., Pauciulo, M.W. et al. (2000). Sporadic primary pulmonary hypertension is associated with germline mutations of the gene encoding BMPR-II, a receptor member of the TGF-beta family. *J. Med. Genet.*, **37**, 741–5.

Tuder, R.M., Cool, C.D., Geraci, M.W. et al. (1999). Prostacyclin synthase expression is decreased in lungs from patients with severe pulmonary hypertension. *Am. J. Respir. Crit. Care Med.*, **159**, 1925–32.

Wedzicha, J.A. (1999). Domiciliary oxygen therapy services: clinical guidelines and advice for prescribers. Summary of a report of the Royal College of Physicians. *J. R. Coll. Physicians Lond.*, **33**, 445–7.

Weitzenblum, E., Sautegeau, A., Ehrhart, M., Mammosser, M. & Pelletier, A. (1985). Long-term oxygen therapy can reverse the progression of pulmonary hypertension in patients with chronic obstructive pulmonary disease. *Am. Rev. Respir. Dis.*, **131**, 493–8.

Williamson, D.J., Wallman, L.L., Jones, R. et al. (2000). Hemodynamic effects of Bosentan, an endothelin receptor antagonist, in patients with pulmonary hypertension. *Circulation*, **102**, 411–18.

Wood, P. (1952). Pulmonary hypertension. *Br. Med. Bull.*, **8**, 348–53.

Yuan, X.J., Wang, J., Juhaszova, M., Gaine, S.P. & Rubin, L.J. (1998). Attenuated K⁺ channel gene transcription in primary pulmonary hypertension (letter). *Lancet*, **351**, 726–7.

18

Role of endothelial cells in transplant rejection

Marlene L. Rose

Division of Cardiothoracic Surgery, Imperial College School of Medicine, Harefield, Middlesex

Introduction

Approximately 36 000 transplants are performed throughout the world each year, of which the majority are kidney transplants. About 5000 hearts, 6500 livers and 1200 lung transplants are performed. Rejection remains the most common complication following transplantation and is the major cause of morbidity and mortality. Endothelial cells form the interface between donor tissue and recipient blood and so are the first donor cells to be recognized by the host's immune system. This fact, and the observation that they express numerous molecules able to stimulate lymphocytes, has led to much research into their precise role in transplant rejection. It is our view that endothelial cells are pivotal both in controlling the egress of inflammatory cells into the allografted organ and also as specific antigen-presenting cells (APCs), by presenting foreign molecules to the immune system (Figure 18.1).

Rejection is mediated by both cell-mediated and humoral mechanisms but the relative importance of these pathways differs in acute and chronic rejection. This chapter briefly describes the features of acute and chronic rejection and then outlines the role of endothelial cells in this process.

Basic mechanism of rejection

The major stimulus for rejection of allografted organs is recognition that the donor cells are foreign, by recognition of antigens that are coded by the major histocompatibility complex (MHC). There are two classes of MHC: class I (human leukocyte antigen, HLA) ABC) and class II (HLA-DR, DP, DQ). Both sets of antigens are highly polymorphic glycoproteins encoded by the MHC locus found

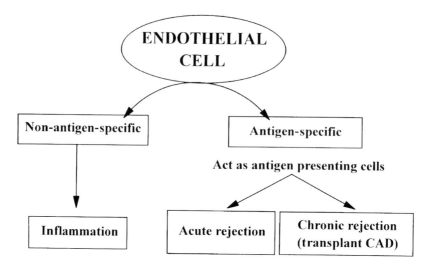

Figure 18.1   Diagram to illustrate the role of endothelial cells in transplant rejection.

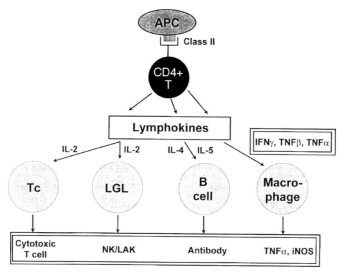

Figure 18.2   Diagrammatic representation of T-cell (Tc) activation, illustrating the pivotal role of major histocompatibility complex class II antigens (presented by antigen-presenting cells (APC) within the graft) in initiating rejection. Activation of CD4 + T cells results in a cascade of lymphokines causing the maturation of a number of possible effector mechanisms (in double-lined boxes). Note that the cytokines interferon-γ (IFN-γ), tumour necrosis factor-β (TNF-β) and TNF-α may be directly damaging to tissue. Il-1, interleukin-2; LGL, large granular lymphocyte; NK, natural killer; LAK, lymphokine-activated killer cell; iNOS, inducible nitric oxide synthase.

on chromosome 6 in humans. The number of T cells which are able to recognize foreign MHC molecules is very large (estimated at an astounding 0.1–1% of circulating T cells) – a fact which almost certainly accounts for the vigour of the rejection response.

Rejection is initiated by the CD4 + T-cell subset recognizing MHC class II antigens on APC within the graft (Figure 18.2). This recognition results in activation of recipient CD4 + T cells and the release of cytokines (interleukin-2 IL-2), IL-4, IL-5, IL-6, interferon-γ (IFN-γ), tumour necrosis factor-β(TNF-α), TNF-β) by these cells. This produces the effector mechanisms of rejection, namely maturation of CD8 + cytotoxic T cells, infiltration of macrophages, maturation of natural killer (NK) cells and lymphokine-activated killer cells (LAK) and antibody formation (Figure 18.2). These effector mechanisms have been listed for the sake of completeness, but there is little evidence that NK or LAK cells are important in allograft rejection. Indeed, the precise mediators which cause graft dysfunction are unknown; for although CD8 + cytotoxic T cells can cause graft destruction, they are not essential for rejection; it is quite possible that a direct effect of cytokines, in particular TNF-α and IFN-γ, is toxic to the allografted cells. For example, TNF-α has a negative inotropic effect on cardiac myocytes. Similarly, induction of inducible nitric oxide synthase (iNOS) by activated macrophages and endothelial cells may be an important effector mechanism.

Activation of CD4 + T cells is thus a pivotal event in initiating acute rejection (Figure 18.2). Foreign MHC class II molecules initiate activation of CD4 + T cells, so understanding the distribution and density of these molecules on the allografted organ is important. Advances in immunocytochemical techniques, including the use of monoclonal antibodies and frozen sections, have revolutionzed knowledge about the normal distribution of MHC molecules in different tissues. Class II (HLA-DR and DP) antigens, which were originally thought to be restricted to macrophages, dendritic cells, monocytes and activated T cells, have now been described on human endothelial cells and epithelial cells (for a review, see Rose, 1992). The expression of class II antigens on human endothelial cells has been described in every organ (Rose, 1992) and it is particularly striking on the microvessels, i.e. capillaries, arterioles and venules. The large-vessel endothelium (such as aorta, pulmonary artery, saphenous vein), however, does not express MHC class II.

The expression of MHC antigens is not a constant feature of a cell; they can be upregulated or induced by cytokines (Halloran et al., 1986). Thus, the distribution of MHC class I and class II antigens changes during acute rejection of the graft. After cardiac transplantation there is massive upregulation of MHC class I antigens (normally only on the interstitial cells) so that cardiac myocytes become MHC class I-positive (Rose, 1992). Upregulation of MHC class I antigens has also been described after renal, liver and pancreatic transplantation. There is upregulation of MHC class II antigens on renal tubular epithelial cells (Fuggle et al., 1986) after renal transplantation. There is also upregulation of adhesion molecules on endothelial cells during acute rejection (Briscoe et al., 1991: Taylor et al., 1992, and see below). The upregulation of these molecules is almost certainly mediated by local production of cytokines by infiltrating cells; thus, some cytokines (such as TNF-α and IFN-γ) have been directly visualized in graft biopsies using immunocytochemical methods (Arbustini et al., 1991); others (IL-2, IL-1, IL-4, IL-6, IL-10) have been detected using polymerase chain reaction to amplify cytokine mRNA (Cunningham et al., 1994).

The consequences of T-cell activation described above lead to infiltration of the graft with inflammatory cells (T cells and monocytes) – this process is termed acute rejection. The majority of heart transplant recipients have one or two acute rejection episodes in the first 6 months following transplantation. Acute rejection may be suspected clinically but it is always confirmed by histological assessment of endomyocardial biopsy tissue; this is an essential part of the management of patients following cardiac transplantation.

Chronic rejection

Chronic rejection in heart transplant recipients produces a rapidly progressing obliterative vascular disease in the transplanted heart. It is the major cause of late death and repeat transplantation after cardiac transplantation. This disease is variously termed cardiac allograft vasculopathy or transplant-associated coronary artery disease. This same phenomenon is also present in renal, lung and liver allografts and has been designated chronic rejection, obliterative bronchiolitis and vanishing bile duct syndrome, respectively. The reported incidence of transplant coronary artery disease, as detected by routine coronary artery angiography, varies greatly between cardiac transplant centres. A recent multicentre study of 3,837 patients reported a 5-year incidence of angiographically detectable disease of 42% at 5 years (Costanzo et al., 1998). Higher incidences of diseases are reported using intravascular ultrasound (Yeung et al., 1995). There are a number of reviews which describe the histological differences between transplant-associated coronary artery disease and naturally occurring coronary artery disease and the various risk factors, both immunological and nonimmunological, have been described (Gao et al., 1989; Hosenpud et al., 1992). Transplant coronary artery disease is a more diffuse disease, affecting the entire length of all coronary vessels, compared with spontaneous coronary artery disease. There is concentric intimal proliferation down the length of the coronary arteries in transplant coronary artery disease, as opposed to the eccentric plaques found in spontaneous coronary artery disease. These differences suggest the whole endothelium is the target of damage in transplant coronary artery disease. As the epicardial branches, including the intramyocardial branches, are affected by transplant-associated coronary artery disease, coronary artery bypass surgery for revascularization is usually precluded.

This vasculopathy of allografted organs is almost certainly of multifactorial aetiology. It is highly likely that the obstructive vascular lesions progress through repetitive endothelial injury followed by repair, smooth muscle cell (SMC) proliferation and hypertrophy, all of which gradually produce luminal obliteration. It is useful to think of the disease in terms of the Ross hypothesis (Ross, 1993) – namely, an initial damage to the endothelium resulting in release of growth factors and intimal proliferation. The latter process will be assisted by risk factors (circulating cholesterol, insulin resistance) common to both spontaneous and transplant-associated coronary artery disease. Most investigators would acknowledge that the initial damage to the endothelium is mediated by the alloimmune response, although it can also be argued that nonimmunological damage such as ischaemia, surgical manipulation and perfusion/reperfusion injury could also initially damage the endothelial cells (Tullius and Tilney, 1995). Precisely which pathways of antigen presentation are involved, which endothelial antigens are recognized and the relative importance of cell-mediated and humoral immunity in this process are unknown (see below for discussion of these topics).

Properties of endothelial cells

The phenotypic properties of endothelial cells and their response to cytokines give them a pivotal role in controlling rejection in three distinct ways:
1. They allow extravasation of inflammatory cells into the graft
2. They act as APCs
3. They are the target of the alloimmune response

Adhesion molecules and lymphocyte migration

There is currently extensive research on the role of endothelial adhesion molecules in controlling lymphocyte recirculation and extravasation of inflammatory cells. These processes are controlled by sequential interactions between different families of molecules on the endothelial cells (the selectins, β_1-and β_2-integrins and members of the immunoglobulin family) and their respective ligands on leukocytes. There are excellent reviews of this subject (Springer, 1994). Our own studies have investigated the expression of adhesion molecules (platelet endothelial cell adhesion molecule-1 (PECAM-1), intercellular (ICAM-1) and vascular adhesion molecules cell (VCAM-1) and E-selectin) and other markers of endothelial cells (such as von Willebrand factor) on endothelial cells within the cardiovascular system and have explored how these change during rejection (Page et al., 1992; Taylor et al., 1992). Immunocytochemistry of frozen sections of human heart, coronary artery, aorta, pulmonary artery and endocardium have revealed differences with regard to basal expression of these molecules (Table 18.1). PECAM or CD31, generally acknowledged to be a marker of endothelial cells, was strongly expressed on all endothelium. In contrast, von Willebrand factor, also used as a marker of endothelial cells, was strongly expressed on the larger vessels but was very weakly expressed on capillaries. ICAM-1 was constitutively expressed on endothelial cells from all vessels but was particularly strong on capillaries and endothelial cells lining the coronary artery. The coronary arteries were rather surprising, as they were found basally to express VCAM-1 as well as ICAM-1. VCAM-1 was not found to be expressed on any of the other large vessels. All coronary arteries investigated at this centre have expressed an 'activated phenotype'; possible explanations are discussed below. Immunocytochemistry of frozen sections of normal endomyocardial biopsies show weak expression of E-selectin and VCAM-1: the capillaries are negative for these markers and venules show patchy expression of E-selectin and VCAM-1. During acute (cell-mediated) rejection, there is upregulation of VCAM-1 on capillary endothelial cells in close apposition to infiltrating T cells. This is not surprising, as interaction between endothelial VCAM-1 with the T-cell β_1-integrins ($\alpha_4\beta_1$) is a requirement for T-cell migration across endothelial cells.

Endothelial expression of MHC molecules

As MHC antigens initiate allograft rejection, it is of interest to describe the distribution of these molecules on endothelial cells of different origins (Table 18.1). All endothelial cells constitutively express MHC class I molecules and many endothelial cells constitutively express MHC class II molecules; however, there is an interesting heterogeneity with regard to constitutive expression of class II antigens; the large vessels (aorta, pulmonary artery, endocardium, umbilical vein, umbilical artery) are negative but the capillaries within all organs examined are strongly positive (Table 18.1; Pober and Cotran, 1990; Page et al., 1992). Arterioles and venules within the heart show weak or patchy basal expression of MHC class II antigens. It was surprising to find that all pieces of coronary artery we examined expressed MHC class II molecules, as well as VCAM-1. The coronaries were either obtained from heart donors deemed unsuitable for transplantation, or they were removed from the explanted heart of patients requiring transplantation (for diseases not involving the coronary artery). These molecules may therefore have been upregulated during procedures prior to harvest. The most common endothelial cells used in cell culture are those derived from umbilical vein endothelial cells. These cells do not express MHC class II antigens in situ and it is

Table 18.1 Distribution of adhesion molecules, major histocompatibility complex molecules and von Willebrand factor in endothelial cells derived from microvessels and large vessels of the human cardiovascular system

	Myocardial biopsies			Large vessels		
	Capillaries	Arterioles	Venules	Coronary	Pulmonary artery	Aorta
CD31	+ +	+ +	+ +	+ +	+ +	+ +
ICAM-1	+ +	+	+	+ +	+	+
VCAM-1	−	±	±	+	−	−
E-selectin	−	−	±	+	±	±
von Willebrand factor	±	+ +	+ +	+ +	+ +	+ +
Class I	+ +	+	+	+ +	+	+
Class II	+ +	±	±	+ +	−	−

ICAM-1, intercellular adhesion molecule-1; VCAM-1, vascular cell adhesion molecule-1.
+ +, strong, even expression; +, strong but patchy expression; ±, weak and patchy expression;
−, negative.
Source: summarized from Page et al. (1992) and Taylor et al. (1992).

therefore not surprising that they are also negative in vitro. Interestingly, cardiac microvascular endothelial cells, which are positive in situ, lose their class II after 2 weeks in culture (McDougall et al., 1996). This observation raises the intriguing possibility that factors in normal serum act to maintain class II expression in vivo. In vitro, cytokines are used extensively to upregulate MHC and adhesion molecules in a variety of cell types, but endothelial cells are unique in the sense that only IFN-γ upregulates MHC class II expression in vitro (Pober and Cotran, 1990).

Pathways of antigen presentation and antigen-presenting cells

The term 'antigen-presenting cell' has a specific meaning to immunologists: it means the cell is able to present antigen to resting T cells, i.e. is able to cause activation of resting T cells. Only specialized cells (traditionally recognized as B cells, dendritic cells and monocytes) can perform this task. T cells recognize nominal antigen as processed peptides presented by self MHC molecules. An important step in the understanding of alloreactivity came with the discovery that T cells can engage and respond to allogenic MHC molecules directly (Figure 18.3). This form of antigen recognition, termed direct presentation or the direct

Direct Presentation   **Indirect Presentation**

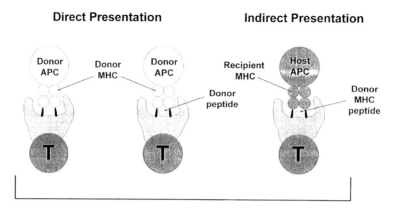

Recipient T cells

Figure 18.3 Diagrammatic representation of mechanisms whereby recipient T cells recognize allo-class II determinants. Recipient T cells recognize donor major histocompatibility complex (MHC) determinants on donor antigen-presenting cells (APC: direct presentation) or they recognize donor MHC peptides which have been released from donor cells and processed and presented by host APC within self MHC molecules (indirect presentation). Adapted from Shoskes and Wood (1994) with permission.

pathway, is responsible for the strong proliferative response to alloantigens seen in vitro and quite possibly the early acute rejection seen in nonimmunosuppressed animals after transplantation of MHC mismatched organs. T cells can also recognize allogeneic peptides that have been processed and presented within self MHC molecules by recipient APC in the same manner than T cells recognize nominal antigen (Figure 18.3). This pathway is termed the indirect route or indirect pathway of T-cell activation (Shoskes and Wood, 1994). Alloantigens shed from the graft are likely to be treated as exogenous antigen by recipient APC and will therefore be presented within MHC class II molecules to activate recipient CD4 + T cells.

Any graft cell expressing class II antigens will be able to activate the indirect pathway – it is likely that damaged endothelial cells are an important source of graft-derived MHC class II antigens – as these are the only parenchymal cells expressing class II in the heart. The contribution indirect recognition of endothelial MHC class II makes to cellular rejection is currently not known. The question which has received much attention from a number of groups in recent years is whether endothelial cells can cause direct allostimulation of resting T lymphocytes (for a review, see Pober et al., 1996). The reason for this is that direct recognition of allo-MHC molecules results in a 'strong' response; the number of T cells recognizing MHC molecules directly is 10–100 higher than those recognizing nominal antigen, resulting in a strong in vitro proliferative response.

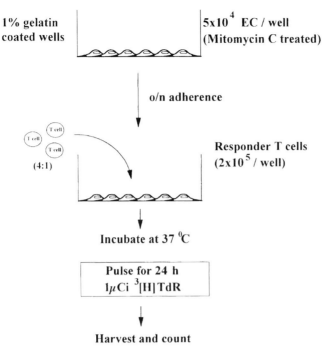

Figure 18.4 Method of measuring the proliferative response of purified CD4 + T cells to human
endothelial cells (EC). Addition of mitomycin C (or irradiated) human EC to gelatin-coated
tissue culture wells results in a monolayer of EC to which can be added appropriate
numbers of responder T cells. The EC and T cells are cocultured for 6 days, in the presence
of ^{3}[H]thymidine (^{3}[H]TdR) for the last 24 h. The cultures are harvested and counted on a
β-counter – the counts (cpm) represent the proliferative response of T cells.

In order to discover whether endothelial cells directly cause allostimulation of
resting T cells, we and others (Savage et al., 1993; Page et al., 1994a) have cultured
stringently purified CD4 + T cells with pure passaged endothelial cells and looked
for T-cell proliferation (measured by uptake of [^{3}H]thymidine) at day 6. The
endothelial cells are treated with mitomycin C to stop them proliferating; any cell
proliferation which is detected is thus due to responding T cells (Figure 18.4). The
results in Figure 18.5 show the response of CD4 + T cell to human endothelial cells
(Eahy.926), porcine aortic endothelial cells (PAEC) and fetal lung fibroblasts. It
can be seen that, provided IFN-γ is used to upregulate MHC class II, there is a
strong proliferative response to human endothelial cells, but not to fibroblasts.
There is also a strong response to PAEC, which is independent of IFN-γ treatment.
The reason for this is that PAEC class II expression persists in culture. That the
response was direct and not indirect was proven by the findings that responder T
cells were free of contaminating APC (Page et al., 1994a).

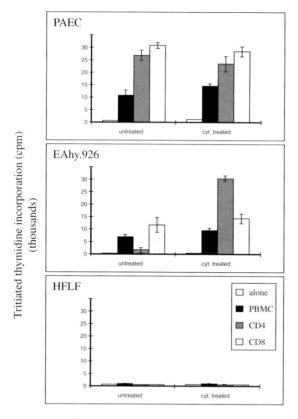

Figure 18.5 Response at day 6 of purified peripheral blood mononuclear cells (PBMC) CD4 + and CD8 + T cells to untreated and interferon-γ (IFN-γ)-treated porcine aortic endothelial cells (PAEC), human endothelial cells (Eahy.926) and human fetal lung fibroblasts (HFLF). CD4+ and CD8+ T cells respond strongly to PAEC, regardless of cytokine treatment. CD4+ T cells respond well to human endothelial cells, providing they have been pretreated with IFN-γ to upregulate major histocompatibility complex class II antigens. CD8+ T cells respond to human endothelial cells in the absence of cytokine treatment. There is no proliferative response of human lymphocytes to the fibroblasts.

It must be concluded, therefore, that donor endothelial cells can present alloantigen to recipient T cells. It is interesting to note that there is a species difference between rodents and humans, as rodents do not constitutively express MHC class II antigens on their endothelial cells. This difference may explain why it is easier to suppress transplant rejection in rodents than it is in humans. It follows, therefore, that understanding the signals that allow human endothelial cells to stimulate T cells may lead to new strategies of preventing rejection. One of the important concepts to emerge in recent years is the knowledge that T cells require two signals to become activated (Janeway and Bottomly, 1994): one is occupancy of the T-cell receptor and the second is activation of one of the many accessory

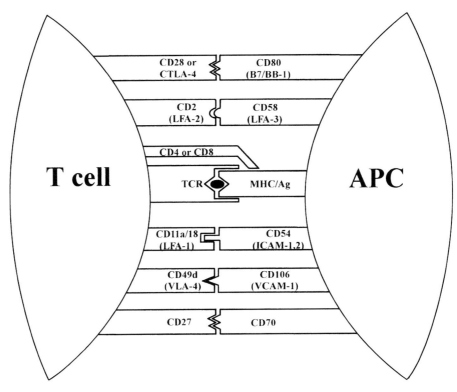

Figure 18.6 Diagrammatic representation of possible interactions between receptors on T cells and their appropriate ligands on antigen-presenting cells (APC). CTLA-4, cytotoxic T late antigen-4; LFA, leukocyte function antigen; TCR, T-cell receptor; MHC, major histocompatibility complex; Ag, antigen; ICAM, intercellular adhesion molecule; VCAM-1, vascular cell adhesion molecule 1.

molecules' present on T cells (Figure 18.6). Much attention has focused on the B7 family of receptors, known to be essential as second signals on APC of bone marrow origin (e.g. monocytes, B cells and dendritic cells); blockade of this pathway inhibits dendritic cell-stimulated mixed lymphocyte responses in vitro and also inhibits allograft and indeed xenograft rejection in rodents (Pearson et al., 1994). We have questioned whether endothelial cells utilize the B7 pathway to stimulate T cells, and our results (Page et al., 1994b)) and those of others (Pober et al., 1996) demonstrate that human endothelial cells do not express B7 receptors and stimulate T cells via another accessory molecule leukocyte function antigen-3 (LFA)-3).

Role of endothelial cells in chronic rejection

It is paradoxical that, despite the heavy immunosuppression received by patients after solid organ transplantation, the majority make a vigorous antibody response against the allografted organ (for a review, see Rose, 1993). The most common way of detecting these antibodies is a complement-dependent cytotoxicity test against a panel of HLA-typed leukocytes (termed panel-reactive antibodies or PRA test) or donor cells (termed a donor-specific response). Many clinical studies have reported an association between antibody producers and development of chronic rejection (Rose, 1993). Thus Suciu-Foca et al. (1991) reported a 90% 4-year actuarial survival in patients who had not made antibody following cardiac transplantation versus a 38% 4-year survival in the antibody-producers. These authors looked for anti-HLA antibodies, but our own studies have shown a correlation between antiendothelial antibodies and chronic rejection (Dunn et al., 1992). Using gel electrophoresis to separate endothelial peptides according to molecular weight followed by probing blots with patients' sera, we found that the majority of patients who had transplant-associated coronary artery disease (TxCAD) had antibodies against endothelial peptides of 56–58 kDa. Other groups have also reported that antiendothelial antibodies are associated with chronic rejection and poor patient survival after cardiac (Faulk et al., 1999; Frederich et al., 1999) or renal transplantation (Ferry et al., 1997). As this test (Dunn et al., 1992) detected antibodies against unrelated human umbilical vein endothelial cells, it is clear that donor-specific HLA antigens could not be involved. Use of sodium dodecyl sulphate gel electrophoresis and amino acid sequencing revealed that the most immunogeneic endothelial peptide (at 56–58 kDa) was the intermediate filament vimentin and other immunoreactive peptides were identified as triose phosphate isomerase and glucose-regulating protein. In all, 40 different proteins were identified, which reacted with patients immunoglobulin M (Wheeler et al., 1995). Vimentin is the intermediate filament characteristic of, but not restricted to, endothelial cells and fibroblasts. Whereas SMCs predominantly express desmin as their intermediate filament, they coexpress desmin and vimentin when migrating or proliferating. Vimentin is diffusely expressed in the intima and media of normal and diseased coronary arteries. We have developed a simple enzyme-linked immunoassay to measure antivimentin antibodies (Jurcevic et al., 1998), which has been shown to be an independent risk factor for TxCAD (Jurcevic et al., 2001). Our working hypothesis is that antibodies to vimentin reflect disease activity in the coronary arteries – but the outstanding questions are how vimentin, a cytosolic protein, is exposed to the immune system and whether and how the antibodies are damaging.

It is highly likely that endothelial cells are damaged early after transplantation (possibly by nonimmunological factors such as ischaemia–reperfusion injury) and vimentin is released into the circulation. There it binds to host B cells. Our hypothesis to explain the presence of antivimentin antibodies after transplantation is that host T cells recognize vimentin fragments, presented indirectly by host

B cells. A database of MHC-binding peptides has revealed sequence homology between epitopes of vimentin and class II presented peptides, these being an HLA-DRα peptide and a heat shock protein peptide (hsp65), suggesting that the T cells 'see' vimentin as a foreign class II peptide. Such cross-reactions between DRα and infectious agents/normal components of tissues have been suggested as a mechanism for a number of autoimmune diseases (Baum et al., 1996). It is likely that damaged endothelial cells are a source of many other peptides which will be presented indirectly to recipient T cells.

One of the major drawbacks to ascribing a role for antibodies in the pathogenesis of rejection is lack of understanding about the way antibodies interact with their cellular targets. Serum derived from our transplant patients does not exhibit complement-dependent or antibody-dependent cellular cytotoxicity against endothelial cells derived from HUVEC or aorta. Complement-mediated lysis is a severe and acute form of damage, usually associated with hyperacute rejection. It is more important to investigate whether antiendothelial antibodies can cause more subtle forms of change, such as endothelial cell activation. Recently, a number of reports have demonstrated that antibodies from patients with autoimmune disease (Carvalho et al., 1996) or transplant patients (Pidwell et al., 1995) can upregulate adhesion molecules on endothelial cells. Importantly, it has been shown that monoclonal antibodies against MHC class I antigens and alloantisera from patients cause signal transduction in human endothelial cells (Bian and Reed, 1999), including activation of nuclear factor κB (NF-κB) and endothelial cell proliferation (Smith et al., 2000). For example, patients' immunoglobulin G containing anti-HLA-A2 antibodies were found to activate (NF-κB) in A_2-positive human umbilical vein or cardiac microvascular endothelial cells in an antigen-specific manner (Figure 18.7). We believe the information that antibodies can activate endothelial cells is very promising and should be explored as a mechanism whereby antibodies could damage endothelial cells in both autoimmune disease and chronic rejection after solid organ transplantation.

In conclusion, the immunological properties of endothelial cells suggest they perform a pivotal role in rejection following solid organ transplantation. Expression of MHC class II molecules allows them to activate recipient T cells by the direct and indirect route. Release of non-HLA antigens as a result of immunological or nonimmunological damage provides a stimulus for antibody formation which may further damage or activate donor endothelial cells. The costimulatory molecules used by endothelial cells appear to differ from those used by traditional APC, such as B cells and dendritic cells. Further understanding of the molecules involved is warranted, as development of specific strategies to block endothelial cell recognition may provide better ways of preventing rejection than methods currently used.

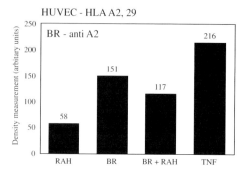

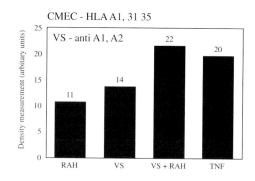

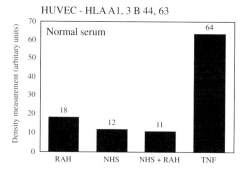

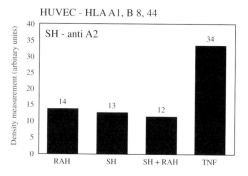

Figure 18.7   Effect of patients' immunoglobulin G (IgG) on nuclear factor (NF-κB) activation. Human umbilical vein endothelial cells (HUVEC) bearing specific human leukocyte antigen (HLA-A2) antigens were incubated with patients' IgG anti-A2 antibodies ((a) patients BR) HUVEC, or cardiac microvascular endothelial cells (CMEC) bearing HLA-A1 antigen was incubated with patients' sera containing anti-A1 antibodies ((b) patient VS), (c) normal serum or patients' IgG containing anti-A2 antibodies ((d) patient SH) for 30 min. Cells were also incubated with media alone (not shown), media plus rabbit antihuman IgG, human IgG plus rabbit antihuman IgG and tumour necrosis factor-α (TNF-α). The amount of binding of nuclear extracts to [α-^{32}P]dCTP-labelled oligodeoxynucleotides complementary to the consensus sequence of the NF-κB DNA binding sites is shown on the y-axis as density measurements in arbitrary units. It can be seen that, in two instances human IgG anti-HLA significantly enhanced binding of NF-κB compared to rabbit antihuman serum (RAH) controls (a and b), and this was not increased by addition of cross-linking antibody. Normal serum (c) or anti-A2 added to irrelevant cells (d) had no effect on NF-κB binding to HUVEC. These are the results from individual experiments. From Smith et al. (2000), with permission.

REFERENCES

Arbustini, E., Grasso, M., Diegoli, M. et al. (1991). Expression of tumour necrosis factor in human acute cardiac rejection. An immunohistochemical and immunoblotting study. *Am. J. Pathol.*, **139**, 709–15.

Baum, H., Davies, H. & Peakman, M. (1996). Molecular mimicry in the MHC: hidden clues to autoimmunity? *Immunol. Today*, **17**, 64–70.

Bian, H. & Reed, E.F. (1999). Alloantibody mediated class I signal transduction in endothelial cells and smooth muscle cells: enhancement by IFN-γ and TNF-α. *J. Immunol.*, **163**, 1010–15.

Briscoe, D.M., Schoen, F.J., Rice, G.E. et al. (1991). Induced expression of endothelial-leukocyte adhesion molecules in human cardiac allografts. *Transplantation*, **51**, 537–9.

Carvalho, D., Savage, C.O.S., Black, C.M. & Pearson, J.D. (1996). IgG antiendothelial cell autoantibodies from scleroderma patients induce leukocyte adhesion to human vascular endothelial cells in vitro. *J. Clin. Invest.*, **97**, 1–97.

Costanzo, M.R. Naftel, D.C., Pritzker, M.R. et al. (1998). Heart transplant coronary artery disease detected by coronary angiography: a multiinstitutional study of preoperative donor and receipient factors. *J. Heart Lung Transplant.*, **17**, 744–53.

Cunningham, D.A., Dunn, M.J., Yacoub, M.J. & Rose, M.L. (1994). Local production of cytokines in the human cardiac allograft. *Transplantation*, **57**, 1333–7.

Dunn, M.J., Crisp, S.J., Rose, M.L., Taylor, P.M. & Yacoub, M.H. (1992). Antiendothelial antibodies coronary artery disease after cardiac transplantation. *Lancet*, **339**, 1566–70.

Faulk, W.P., Rose, M.L., Meroni, P.L. et al. (1999). Antibodies to endothelial cells identify myocardial damage and predict development of coronary artery disease in patients with transplanted hearts. *Hum. Immunol.*, **60**, 826–32.

Ferry, B.L., Welsh, K.I., Dunn, M.J. et al. (1997). Anti-cell surface endothelial antibodies in sera from cardiac and kidney transplant recipients; association with chronic rejection. *Transplant. Immunol.*, **5**, 17–24.

Frederich, R., Toyoda, M., Czer, L.S. et al. (1999). The clinical significance of antibodies to human vascular endothelial cells after cardiac transplantation. *Transplantation*, **67**, 383–91.

Fuggle, S.V., McWhinnie, D.L., Chapman, J.R., Taylor, H.M. & Morris, P.J. (1986). Sequential analysis of HLA-class II antigen expression in human renal allografts. *Transplantation*, **42**, 144–9.

Gao, S.J., Schroeder, J.S., Alderman, E.L. et al. (1989). Prevalence of accelerated coronary artery disease in heart transplant survivors. Comparison of cyclosporine and axathiprine regimens. *Circulation*, **8**, 100–5.

Halloran, P.F., Wadgymar, A. & Autenreid, P. (1986). The regulation of the expression of major histocompatibility complex products. *Transplantation*, **4**, 413–20.

Hosenpud, J.D., Shipley, G.D. & Wagner, C.R. (1992). Cardiac allograft vasculopathy; current concepts, recent developments, and future directions. *J. Heart Lung Transplant.*, **11**, 9–23.

Janeway, C.A. & Bottomly, K. (1994). Signals and signs for lymphocyte responses. *Cell*, **76**, 275–85.

Jurcevic, S., Dunn, M.J., Crisp, S. et al. (1998). A new enzyme linked immunosorbent assay to measure anti-endothelial antibodies after cardiac transplantation demonstrates greater inhibition of antibody formation by tacrolimus compared to cyclosporine. *Transplantation*, **15**, 1197–1202.

Jurcevic, S., Ainsworth, M.E., Pomernace, A. et al. (2001). Antivimentin antibodies are an independent predictor of transplant-associated coronary artery disease after cardiac transplantation. *Transplantation*, **71**, 886–982.

Leung, D.Y., Collins, M.T., Lapierre, L.A., Geha, R.S. & Pober, J.S. (1986). Immunoglobulin M antibodies present in the acute phase of Kawasaki syndrome lyse cultured vascular endothelial cells stimulated by gamma interferon. *J. Clin. Invest.*, **77**, 1428–35.

McDougall, R.M., Yacoub, M.H. & Rose, M.L. (1996). Isolation, culture and characterisation of MHC class II positive microvascular endothelial cells from the human heart. *Microvasc.*, **51**, 137–52.

Page, C.S., Holloway, N., Smith, H., Yacoub, M.H. & Rose, M.L. (1994a). Alloproliferative responses of purified CD4$^+$ and CD8$^+$ T cell subsets to human vascular endothelial cells in the absence of contaminating accessory cells. *Transplantation*, **57**, 1628–37.

Page, C., Rose, M.L., Yacoub, M.H. & Pigott, R. (1992). Antigenic heterogeneity of vascular endothelium. *Am. J. Pathol.*, **141**, 673–83.

Page, C.S., Thompson, C., Yacoub, M.H. & Rose, M.L. (1994b). Human endothelial cell stimulation of allogeneic T cells via a CTLA-4 independent pathway. *Transplant Immunol.*, **2**, 342–7.

Pearson, T.C., Alexander, D.Z., Winn, K.J. et al. (1994). Transplantation tolerance induced by CTLA4-Ig. *Transplantation*, **57**, 1701–6.

Pidwell, D.W., Heller, M.J., Gabler, D. & Orosz, C. (1995). In vitro stimulation of human endothelial cells by sera from a subpopulation of high percentage panel reactive antibody patients. *Transplantation*, **60**, 563–9.

Pober, J.S. & Cotran, R.S. (1990). The role of endothelial cells in inflammation. *Transplantation*, **50**, 537–44.

Pober, J.S., Orosz, C.G., Rose, M.L. & Savage, C.O.S. (1996). Can graft endothelial cells initiate a host anti-graft immune response? *Transplantation*, **61**, 343–9.

Rose, M.L. (1992). HLA antigens in tissues. In: *Methods in Clinical Histocompatibility Testing*, ed. Dyer, P. & Middleton, D., pp. 192–210. Oxford: IRL Oxford University Press.

Rose, M.L. (1993). Antibody mediated rejection following cardiac transplantation. *Transplant. Rev.*, **7**, 140–52.

Ross, R. (1993). The pathogenesis of atherosclerosis: a perspective for the 1990s. *Nature*, **362**, 801–9.

Savage, C.O.S., Hughes, C.C.W., McIntyre, B.W., Picard, J.K. & Pober, J.S. (1993). Human CD4$^+$ T cells proliferate to HLA-DR$^+$ allogeneic vascular endothelium: identification of accessory interactions. *Transplantation*, **56**, 34.

Shoskes, D.A. & Wood, K.J. (1994). Indirect presentation of MHC antigens in transplantation. *Immunol. Today*, **15**, 32–8.

Smith, J.S., Lawson, C., Yacoub, M.H. & Rose, M.L. (2000). Activation of NF-κB in human endothelial cells induced by monoclonal and allospecific HLA antibodies. *Int. Immunol.*, **12**, 563–71.

Springer, T.A. (1994). Traffic signals for lymphocyte recirculation and leukocyte emigration.

The multistep paradigm. *Cell*, **76**, 301–14.

Suciu-Foca, N., Reed, E., Marboe, C. et al. (1991). The role of anti-HLA antibodies in heart transplantation. *Transplantation*, **51**, 716–24.

Taylor, P.M., Rose, M.L., Yacoub, M.H. & Piggott, R. (1992). Induction of vascular adhesion molecules during rejection of human cardiac allografts. *Transplantation*, **54**, 451–7.

Tullius, S.G. & Tilney, N.J. (1995). Both alloantigen-dependent and independent factors influence chronic allograft rejection. *Transplantation*, **59**, 313–18.

Wheeler, C.H., Collins, A., Dunn, M.J. et al. (1995). Characterisation of endothelial antigens associated with transplant associated coronary artery disease. *J. Heart Lung Transplant.*, **14**, S188–97.

Yeung, C.A., Davis, S.F., Hauptman, P.J. et al. (1995). Incidence and progression of transplant coronary artery disease over one year: results of a multicenter trial with use of intravascular ultrasound. Multicenter Intravascular Ultrasound Transplant Study Group. *J. Heart Lung Transplant.*, **14**, S215–20.

19

Vascular function in normal pregnancy and preeclampsia

Lucilla Poston[1] and David Williams[2]

[1]Department of Obstetrics and Gynaecology, Guy's, King's and St Thomas' School of Medicine, King's College, London
[2]Department of Obstetrics and Gynaecology, Imperial College School of Medicine, London

The maternal cardiovascular system undergoes remarkable adaptive physiological changes in pregnancy in order to provide the growing conceptus with an adequate blood supply, while simultaneously ensuring that the mother's own blood pressure remains within normal limits. The complex processes involved remain incompletely understood but are essential to our understanding of the common cardiovascular disorders in pregnancy, particularly gestational hypertension and preeclampsia. In this review an attempt will be made to summarize the mechanisms known to influence vascular function in the mother in normal pregnancy and to extend this to a discussion of preeclampsia.

Normotensive pregnancy

Cardiovascular haemodynamics

One of the earliest manifestations of the response to pregnancy is a fall in peripheral vascular resistance (Robson et al., 1989). Longitudinal studies using Doppler ultrasound and echocardiography indicate that the decline in systemic peripheral vascular resistance occurs by 5 weeks of gestation and is 85% complete by 16 weeks (Robson et al., 1989; Clapp and Capeless, 1997). As a result, blood flow to several maternal organs increases dramatically; perfusion of the kidneys is raised by 80%, flow to the skin of the hands and feet increases by over 200% and uterine artery flow is elevated by 1000%. Data from the pregnant baboon (Phippard et al., 1986) and pregnant women (Chapman et al., 1998) suggest that the fall in peripheral resistance provides the stimulus for early activation of the renin–angiotensin–aldosterone axis and the resultant rise in plasma volume and cardiac output which is characteristic of normal pregnancy. The cardiac output rises as a result of an increase in both stroke volume and heart rate (Easterling et al., 1987; Robson et al., 1989); both changes are detectable as early as 5 weeks after conception. Stroke volume reaches a plateau by 16 weeks and heart rate continues upwards, albeit modestly, until 32 weeks. Although the cardiac output is elevated, the fall in peripheral resistance is sufficient to prevent maternal blood pressure from increasing; indeed, the blood pressure actually falls, reaching its nadir in the second trimester.

The temporal relationship between stroke volume, heart rate, peripheral resistance and the concentrations of the hormones which contribute to sodium and volume homeostasis is well described and has provided valuable insight into the origin of the raised cardiac output. However, the cause of the primary event – the fall in vascular resistance – remains controversial. Resistance to flow, i.e. a reduction in the resistance to steady flow, is determined in part by parameters contributing to the pulsatile arterial load, including arterial compliance, arterial impedance and physical indices of pulse wave propagation. In turn these depend on the physical structure of the vessels and on vascular tone. The important role of increased systemic vascular compliance through remodelling of the maternal vasculature is reviewed in Chapter 2 and will therefore not be considered in detail here. The emphasis on recent research has focused on an explanation for reduced vascular tone in pregnancy which by reducing the pulsatile arterial load and peripheral vascular resistance will make a substantial contribution to cardiovascular homeostasis. Over the years, a range of hypotheses has been proposed, including altered sympathetic activity (Heesch and Rogers, 1995), reduced vascular smooth muscle constrictor responsiveness (Gant et al., 1973) and enhanced synthesis of vasodilators (Poston et al., 1995). These will now be considered in detail.

The autonomic nervous system in normal pregnancy

Basal sympathetic tone does not seem to be affected by pregnancy. Ganglionic or selective α-adrenoreceptor blockade produces an equivalent fall in blood pressure in pregnant and nonpregnant rats (Pan et al., 1990) and renal sympathetic nerve activity is not influenced by pregnancy in late gestation in the pregnant rabbit (O'Hagan and Casey, 1998). In pregnant women, skeletal muscle sympathetic activity is also unchanged compared with the nonpregnant state (Schobel et al., 1996). A decrease in basal sympathetic activity would therefore seem unlikely to contribute to tonic vasodilatation. Studies of the baroreceptor response produce a confusing picture, but suggest that pregnancy is associated with an exaggerated lowering of heart rate when blood pressure is elevated (Heesch and Rogers, 1995). The systemic vasoconstrictor response to hypotension seems diminished, although cardiac response – tachycardia – is maintained. This might have physiological benefit as it would maintain blood flow to peripheral circulations, including the uterine vascular bed, in the face of a hypotensive challenge. The alternative approach to investigation of sympathetic control of the vasculature is to evaluate responsiveness to infusion of adrenergic agonists. Nisell et al. (1985) found that the absolute blood pressure response to noradrenaline (norepinephrine) infusion was no different between pregnant and nonpregnant women. However, the pressor response in pregnancy was found to be the result of an increase in cardiac output, whereas the rise in blood pressure in the nonpregnant women was because of an increase in systemic vasoconstriction. The conclusion was that the arteries from the pregnant women were less responsive to noradrenaline.

Reduced sensitivity to vasoconstrictor stimuli in normal pregnancy

The reduced sensitivity to noradrenaline described by Nisell et al. (1985) is unlikely to be due to altered characteristics or density of α-adrenoceptors since reduced responsiveness to other vasoconstrictors has long been recognized in normal pregnancy. The increased plasma renin activity in pregnancy generates an elevation in plasma angiotensin II (AII), but this is paradoxically associated with a reduced pressor response to exogenous AII (Gant et al., 1973). Reduced constriction to vasopressin and noradrenaline has also been recorded (Chesley, 1978; Williams et al., 1997).

The vascular endothelium in normotensive pregnancy

The discovery that the vascular endothelium, through the synthesis of vasodilators, could blunt responses to vasoconstictor stimuli led to the hypothesis that reduced vasoconstriction in pregnancy might be reinterpreted as a state of enhanced endothelium-dependent vasodilatation.

The role of endothelial nitric oxide

Studies in the rat (Chu and Beilin, 1993; Conrad et al., 1993; Yallampalli and Garfield, 1993; Xu et al., 1996, Cockell and Poston, 1997a) and guinea pig (Weiner et al., 1994) have generally suggested that the L-arginine–nitric oxide (NO) pathway makes a major contribution to vasodilatation in pregnancy (for review, see Sladek et al., 1997). However, animal studies have also indicated there may be some species/vascular bed heterogeneity in NO synthesis; one laboratory (Conrad and Vernier, 1989; Danielson and Conrad, 1995) has proposed that NO plays a particularly important role in renal vasodilatation in the rat, and studies in the pregnant sheep highlight an increase in NO synthase (NOS) which is specific to the uterine artery (Magness et al., 1997).

In human pregnancy, different methodologies and conflicting results present a rather confused picture of the role of NO. Urinary concentrations of cyclic guanosine 3,5-monophosphate (cGMP), the second messenger for NO and a surrogate but nonspecific marker for NOS activity, increase early in pregnancy and remain elevated until term (Chapman et al., 1998). An increase in plasma cGMP has also been reported during normal pregnancy (Boccardo et al., 1996). Several laboratories have measured the serum concentration of nitrite (NO_2^-) and nitrate (NO_3^-), or their product, NOx, during healthy pregnancy but most have ignored the influence of dietary nitrate and consequently these studies have variously concluded that NO is increased (Seligman et al., 1994; Shaamash et al., 2000), decreased (Hata et al., 1999) or unchanged (Curtis et al., 1995; Smarason et al., 1997). Two groups have restricted the dietary nitrate intake in pregnant women and one has found that NOx measured after a 12–15-h fast is significantly elevated (Nobunaga et al., 1996). The other (Conrad et al., 1999) measured NOx in plasma and urine as well as plasma cGMP in pregnant women subjected to a reduced NOx intake. A marked rise in plasma cGMP was observed, especially in the first trimester but, in contrast to the findings of Nobunaga et al., this occurred without any alteration in plasma or urinary NOx.

In vivo studies have provided much more convincing and direct evidence for NOS upregulation in the maternal circulation during normal pregnancy. Infusion of the NO synthase inhibitor, N^G-monomethyl-L-arginine (L-NMMA), into the brachial artery in early pregnancy caused a greater reduction in hand blood flow of pregnant compared with nonpregnant women (Williams et al., 1997). In late pregnancy (36–41 weeks), L-NMMA returned the elevated hand blood flow back to nongravid levels, implicating a major role for NO in peripheral vasodilatation. A similar study, investigating blood flow to the forearm rather than the hand, and which eliminated the potential influence of increased blood flow during pregnancy, has confirmed these findings (Anumba et al., 1999a). The same group has also shown that responses to endothelium-dependent dilators and the endothelium-independent NO donor (glyceryl trinitrate) were similar in pregnant and nonpregnant women, indicating that sensitivity to NO was unaffected by pregnancy (Anumba et al., 1999b).

An alternative approach to investigation of the endothelium is the study of isolated arteries, usually obtained during caesarean section. Small arteries from subcutaneous fat, omentum and myometrium have been studied using the technique of small-vessel wire myography (Mulvany and Halpern, 1977) or small-vessel perfusion myography (Halpern et al., 1984), enabling the measurement of tension, pressure and vessel diameter in small arterioles. The classical method of evaluating endothelium-dependent dilatation is to carry out concentration responses to known endothelium-dependent vasodilators, e.g. acteycholine (ACh) or bradykinin (BK) in arteries preconstricted with a vasoconstrictor, usually noradrenaline. Using this method, we investigated responses to the endothelium-dependent vasodilator, ACh, in small arteries (250–300 μm internal diameter) from subcutaneous fat and found similar responses in arteries from pregnant women and those from nonpregnant women (obtained during routine abdominal surgery; McCarthy et al., 1994). Interestingly, neither the NOS inhibitor, L-NMMA, nor the cyclooxygenase inhibitor, indometacin, completely inhibits relaxation to ACh. In the presence of both inhibitors, the residual relaxation was greater in arteries from the pregnant women, suggesting increased synthesis of an endothelium-dependent dilator other than NO or prostacyclin (PGI_2), possibly an endothelium-derived hyperpolarizing factor (see below). In contrast, we later found that pregnancy was associated with increased relaxation to BK, in small subcutaneous arteries (Knock and Poston, 1996). To complicate the issue further, and using arteries from the omental circulation, Pascoal and Umans (1996) concluded that ACh- and BK-mediated relaxation was similar in arteries from term pregnant women and nonpregnant women. However, these authors proposed that pregnancy was associated with an increase in a novel component of BK-mediated relaxation, identified using specific pharmacological inhibitors of the different pathways involved, and concluded that this was possibly attributable to a hyperpolarizing factor. Another study showed no difference in relaxation to BK in small myometrial arteries from pregnant women and from nonpregnant women obtained during hysterectomy (Ashworth et al., 1997), although an investigation of isolated uterine arteries has shown enhanced relaxation to ACh in vessels from pregnant women (Nelson et al., 1998).

These comparisons of the uterine circulation in arteries from pregnant and nonpregnant women must be interpreted with some caution since the substantial alteration of structure of the uterine vasculature in pregnancy is likely to influence constrictor and dilator tone. In summary, consideration of all the investigations of isolated arteries has shown little consensus regarding the role of agonist-stimulated NO synthesis in the vasodilatation of pregnancy.

Flow-mediated endothelium-dependent vasodilatation

The endothelium also releases NO in response to shear force (shear stress) created as blood flows through the artery (Chapter 3). Shear is arguably a far more physiologically relevant dilator stimulus than either ACh or BK. We have shown that small subcutaneous arteries from pregnant women demonstrate a remarkably increased dilatory response to flow compared to those from nonpregnant women, and that this is totally inhibited by nitro-L-arginine (L-NAME: Cockell and Poston, 1997a). This substantiated our earlier investigations in arteries from pregnant rats (Cockell and Poston, 1996; Learmont et al., 1996), confirmed by Ahokas et al. (1997). Using the same technique, substantial NO-mediated responses to flow have been observed in small myometrial arteries from pregnant women at term (Kublickiene et al., 1997, 2000a) although, perhaps wisely, these were not compared to arteries from nonpregnant women.

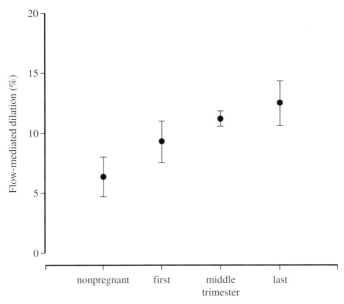

Figure 19.1   Flow-mediated dilation in 8 women studied in the first, middle and last trimesters of pregnancy. Five of the women also had a vascular scan 1–5 months (median 1.5 month) before pregnancy. Values are means ± SE. There was a significant difference between flow-mediated dilatation before pregnancy and in the last trimester. From Dorup et al. (1999) with permission.

Flow-mediated relaxation may also be investigated in vivo using a noninvasive method (Chapter 3). Fluid shear stress may be induced in the human arm by application of a distal cuff around the lower arm or wrist. Release of the cuff leads to hyperaemic dilatation and an increase in flow (and shear stress) in the brachial artery. This leads to vasodilatation, predominantly mediated by NO, which may be monitored with high-resolution Doppler ultrasound. Using this method two groups have recently shown that pregnant women demonstrate an increased response to flow (Veille et al., 1998; Dorup et al., 1999: Figure 19.1) when compared to nonpregnant subjects. These studies all concur that an enhanced response to shear stress is an important stimulus to vasodilatation in pregnancy.

Prostacyclin

Although previously considered to be a systemic vasodilator in pregnancy, PGI_2 is now thought more likely to play a role as a local autocoid. Urinary excretion of 2,3-dinor-6-keto-$PGF_{1\alpha}$, the major systemic enzymic metabolite of PGI_2, is raised early during human pregnancy and increases with each trimester (Goodman et al., 1982; Fitzgerald et al., 1987a). However, Barrow et al. (1983) reported that concentrations of the nonenzymic circulating PGI_2 metabolite, 6-oxo-$PGF_{1\alpha}$, were too low for PGI_2 to function as a circulating hormone – a conclusion upheld by data from pregnant animals and women showing that infusion of indometacin did not affect blood pressure or peripheral resistance (Conrad and Colpoys, 1986; Sorensen et al., 1992). In the sheep, PGI_2 biosynthesis seems to be increased preferentially in the uterine circulation during pregnancy, possibly in response to the elevatation of AII (Magness et al., 1992). Pregnancy in the ewe is also associated with a dramatic rise in the expression of cyclooxygenase-1 (COX-1) mRNA and protein in the uterine artery endothelium (Janowiak et al., 1998), but not COX-2 (Habermehl et al., 2000). Neither COX-1 nor COX-2 was found to be increased in a systemic (omental) artery (Habermehl et al., 2000).

Human pregnancy is associated with increased synthesis of the constrictor prostanoid thromboxane (TxA_2) as assessed by measurement of its stable systemic metabolite 2,3-dinor-TxB_2. TxA_2, which in pregnancy seems to be mainly derived from platelets (Fitzgerald et al., 1987b) increases three- to fivefold during gestation and remains elevated throughout (Fitzgerald et al., 1987a).

Endothelium-derived hyperpolarizing factor

Several reports suggest that PGI_2 and NO-independent, but endothelium-dependent mechanisms of relaxation are enhanced in human pregnancy (McCarthy et al., 1994; Pascoal and Umans, 1996), an observation supported in arteries from pregnant rats (Bobadilla et al., 1997; Gerber et al., 1998; Dalle Lucca et al., 2000). Vasodilation induced by ACh induced relaxation that is insensitive to cyclooxygenase blockade and inhibition of NO synthase is greater in pregnant rats compared with virgin animals. In both groups elevation of the potassium concentration in the organ bath totally abolished any remaining relaxation. This is strongly indicative of a role for enhanced synthesis of the putative endothelium-derived hyperpolarizing factor (EDHF). The chemical nature of EDHF is hotly disputed; the various candidates include a cytochrome P450-derived metabolite of arachidonic acid, one of the epoxyeicosatrienoic acids (EETs) and a cannabinoid (Feletou and Vanhoutte, 1999).

Role of oestrogens in endothelial adaptation to pregnancy

The oestrogens undoubtedly play an important role in cardiovascular homeostasis in pregnancy. Oestrogens are involved in stimulation of the renin–angiotensin system, in the upregulation of NO and PGI_2 synthesis and also may contribute to remodelling of the heart and vasculature. A detailed description of the subject lies beyond the scope of this review, but possibly the most convincing evidence in relation to oestrogen-mediated peripheral vasodilatation lies in the now well-established observation that oestrogens stimulate vasodilatation, achieved at least in part through NO. Thus, the increase in uterine blood flow following 17β-

estradiol infusion in nonpregnant sheep (Magness and Rosenfeld, 1989) is blunted by simultaneous local infusion of L-NAME (Van Buren et al., 1992) and is related to greater NOS activity (Veille et al., 1996). 17β-estradiol pretreatment of isolated arteries from nonpregnant rats (Cockell and Poston, 1997b) and from nonpregnant women (Kublickiene et al., 2000b) also induces an increase in endothelium-dependent NO-mediated flow-induced dilatation equivalent to that observed in arteries in pregnancy. These data are corroborated by numerous reports in nonpregnant subjects, e.g. those describing improvement of agonist- and flow-mediated vasodilatation in postmenopausal women receiving hormone replacement therapy (for review, see Mendelsohn and Karas, 1999).

The mechanism by which oestrogen modulates NO production has not been fully elucidated, but there are 11 copies of an incomplete (half palindromic motif) oestrogen response element (ERE) on the NOS III gene 5' flanking 'promoter' region (Robinson et al., 1994). In other genes these 'half motifs' interact to form a complete ERE and the occupied oestrogen receptor may similarly activate NOS-III by binding to these regions. Recent evidence also strongly supports the presence of an oestrogen receptor on the plasma membrane (Russell et al., 2000a) which is likely to mediate the prompt 'nongenomic' responses to estradiol. The immediate release of NO was inhibited by a specific oestrogen receptor anatgonist (ICI 182,780) suggesting structural similarity with the nuclear receptor. The observation that oestrogens stimulate the acute expression of endothelial cell heat shock protein 90 (hsp90), calcium-independent activation of NOS (Russell et al., 2000b) and mitogen-activated protein (MAP) kinase (Russell et al., 2000a) may have direct relevance to the enhanced flow-mediated relaxation observed in pregnancy. As described in Chapter 3, activation of hsp90, calcium-independent NOS activation and MAP kinase activation are also features of the 'nongenomic' response of endothelial cells exposed to shear stress. Oestrogens, by 'priming' these pivotal pathways of the endothelial response to respond to shear stress, may thus contribute to stimulation of flow-mediated vasodilatation.

Other functions of the endothelium in pregnancy

Despite an increase in synthesis of endothelium-dependent vasodilators which are also potent 'antiplatelet' agents, and the associated haemodilution that accompanies volume expansion, normal pregnancy is characterized by low-grade intravascular coagulation (Letsky, 1995). Indeed, the risk of thromboembolism increases sixfold during pregnancy and is the most common direct cause of maternal death in the UK. Plasma fibrinogen (Bonnar, 1987) and endothelium-derived von Willebrand factor (Sorensen et al., 1995) are raised in pregnancy. There is also a gestational increase in endothelium production of plasminogen activator inhibitor (PAI-1) and tissue plasminogen activator (tPA), with the effect of both inhibition and promotion of fibrinolysis, respectively (Sorensen et al., 1995). Thrombin generation is also increased, as are circulating levels of fibrin degradation products (FDP; de Boer et al., 1989; Sorensen et al., 1995), although the ratio of thrombin to FDP remains unchanged. The procoagulant state of the endothelium therefore does not appear to be compensated by upregulation of the fibrinolytic system (Bremme et al., 1992; Sorensen et al., 1995). In late pregnancy, the procoagulant state is further aggravated as the gravid uterus partially obstructs the inferior vena cava, causing venous stasis in the lower limbs.

Maternal vascular function in preeclampsia

Preeclampsia or the threat of this syndrome is the commonest cause of antenatal admissions and affects approximately 4% of all pregnancies. As delivery is at present the only cure, preeclampsia is also responsible for many premature deliveries. The diagnosis of the preeclampsia is determined by a pregnancy-induced increase in blood pressure accompanied by proteinuria, oedema or both. Hypertension and proteinuria are simply measurable endpoints of the disease; they give no indication of the underlying complexity of the problem. Preeclampsia occurs as a spectrum of disorders which may include eclampsia (fitting), dysfunction of the liver, kidneys and lungs and profound abnormalities of the cardiovascular system and haemostasis.

The last decade has seen considerable strides towards an understanding of the origin of this extraordinary syndrome. There is an undoubted hereditary element to preeclampsia and intensive effort is currently underway to discover the associated gene or genes. None the less, preeclampsia does not follow a simple pattern of inheritance. There is also good evidence that paternal genes may play a role, which complicates the search. The observation that preeclampsia often occurs in pregnancies of women with other disorders, such as diabetes or systemic lupus erythematosus, all characterized by microvascular dysfunction, has led many to suggest that it is highly unlikely that a single associated gene will be found, and that it will emerge that there are several 'preeclampsia-susceptibility' genes. Indeed, it is wise to consider preeclampsia as a polygenic disease (for review, see Ward and Lindheimer, 1999). Immunogenetic factors have also been implicated, with the suggestion that the mother mounts an immunological response to paternal antigens in the placenta. The normal recognition of the foreign placental antigens as 'self' is likely to involve a complex interaction between the expression of human leukocyte antigens (HLAs: possibly HLA-G) on the invading trophoblast and its abillity to prevent attack by large uterine granular leukocytes, the natural killer (NK) cells (Chumbley et al., 1994). This process may fail in preeclampsia. Failure of maternal immune tolerance might explain the higher incidence of preeclampsia in first pregnancies than in subsequent pregnancies, when antigenic 'tolerance' may have developed, and the higher incidence of preeclampsia if a woman changes partners and is challenged with 'new' paternal antigens (Ward and Lindheimer, 1999).

Cardiovascular function in preeclampsia

Central haemodynamics

Established preeclampsia is a 'low-cardiac-output, high-resistance' syndrome (Visser and Wallenburg, 1991) associated with a low plasma volume and reduced aldosterone concentrations. Easterling et al. (1987) conducted a longitudinal study in which cardiac output was measured serially by Doppler echocardiography. Patients destined to develop preeclampsia had a raised cardiac output throughout. Bosio et al. (1999) confirmed the early elevation of cardiac output in women who later developed preeclampsia, but during the clinical phase noted there was a 'cross-over' to a state of low cardiac output, high resistance. This carefully conducted longitudinal study explains the previous disagreement between those who consider preeclampsia is a high-cardiac-output state and those who recognize it as a low-cardiac-output, high-peripheral-resistance state.

The sympathetic nervous system

A well-designed investigation has shown that women with preeclampsia have increased sympathetic nerve activity in skeletal muscle (Schobel et al., 1996). Further evidence for an influence of sympathetic tone on the hypertensive state is provided by a report of raised plasma noradrenaline levels (Manyonda et al., 1998), in which the authors propose that excessive noradrenaline leads to breakdown of triglycerides to free fatty acids, increasing the pool available for lipid peroxidation (see the section on the role of oxidative stress, below). Facilitation of the sympathetic regulation of heart rate has been reported in cases of preeclampsia, with associated diminution of parasympathetic influence (Yang et al., 2000). Involvement of the sympathetic system in elevation of the blood pressure in preeclampsia is also suggested by the relative lack of functional vasodilatory β_2-adrenoreceptors compared with normal pregnancy (Aune et al., 2000).

The uteroplacental circulation

The pivotal role of the placenta in preeclampsia is unchallenged. Moreover, it is now clear that a well-defined histological abnormality is present in the uteroplacental circulation of most women who develop preeclampsia. In normal pregnancies, perfusion of the placenta is ensured by the development of a massively reduced resistance in the uterine vasculature. In part this is achieved by dilatation and remodelling of the uterine artery and its major branches (Chapter 2), but also by extensive remodelling of the smaller spiral arteries in the decidua and myometrium, at the site of attachment of the placenta (the placental bed). This is achieved by invasion of the walls of the maternal uterine spiral arteries by endovascular trophoblast cells from the placenta. The spiral arteries thus invaded show a marked increase in luminal diameter with intramural fibrinoid deposition surrounding embedded trophoblasts and an absence of musculoelastic tissue (Brosens et al., 1967; de Wolf et al., 1980). This process begins at approximately 10 weeks of gestation and is complete by 18–22 weeks. The mechanism by which trophoblast invasion effects such dramatic alteration in the vasculature has been, and is still, subject to intensive investigation. It is suggested that the trophoblasts express a range of 'stage-specific' genes as the cells progress through mitosis to an invasive phenotype. Altered expression of cytokines, integrin cell adhesion molecules, matrix metalloproteinases, HLA-G and human placental lactogen have all been implicated in trophoblast invasion (for review, see Fisher and Roberts, 1999). Recent postulates include an inhibitory role for transforming growth factor (TGF-β_3), the expression of which is 'switched off' during invasion (Caniggia et al., 1999) and the local synthesis of NO, although this has recently been disputed (Lyall et al., 1999). Others suggest that cytokine release by decidual NK cells (Loke and King, 2000) and local macrophages (Reister et al., 1999) may modulate trophoblast invasion.

In preeclampsia, failure of trophoblast invasion often occurs (Brosens et al., 1972; Robertson et al., 1986; Pijnenborg et al., 1991), leading to persistence of small arterioles with muscular coats and maintained high resistance, which in turn results in reduced placental perfusion. Preeclamptic spiral and basal arteries are also found to be more tortuous or densely distributed than normal placental bed arteries, with smaller-calibre lumens and wall thickening due to medial hyperplasia (Starzyk et al., 1997). Acute atherosis with fibrinoid necrosis may also be present (Robertson et al., 1976). Since the process of placentation occurs early in pregnancy and usually many weeks before the symptoms of the preeclampsia, it is widely held that the observed failure of placentation is a pivotal event. It may also represent the abnormal maternal immune response to male placental antigens. However, failed placentation is not confined to preeclampsia alone, as it may occur in the placental bed of pregnancies associated with a variety of abnormal outcomes, particularly intrauterine growth restriction (IUGR; Khong et al., 1986; Brosens et al., 1997). Failed placentation can therefore only be considered as an important facilitatory factor in preeclampsia. Impaired trophoblast invasion, together with maternal vulnerability, is now generally considered to be the combination of factors required to precipitate preeclampsia (Roberts and Hubel, 1999).

Flow velocity waveforms

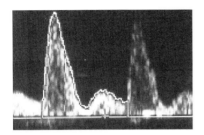   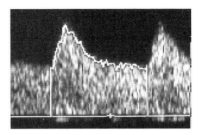

Abnormal FVW: Normal FVW:

RI ≥ 95th centile for   low RI, no notch
gestation ± early diastolic
notch

Figure 19.2 Doppler ultrasound scan of the uterine artery of (left) a woman with an abnormal flow
velocity waveform (FVW 23 weeks' gestation) and (right) a normal flow profile (23 weeks'
gestation). A high resistance index (RI) and the appearance of a diastolic notch are
indicative of high resistance and poor placentation.

Women may be vulnerable to preeclampsia for many reasons. These include
preexisting maternal vascular disease, obesity (hyperlipidaemia), thrombophilia
and undoubtedly other as yet unidentified factors. Many theories for the shallow
trophoblast invasion are proposed, including abnormal expression of several of
the 'stage-specific genes', including the integrin cell adhesion molecules (Zhou et
al., 1997) and TGF-β_3 (Caniggia et al., 1999). Clinically, these histological data are
consistent with the finding of increased impedance to blood flow in women with
IUGR and preeclampsia, as assessed indirectly by uterine artery Doppler waveform analysis (Campbell et al., 1983; Figure 19.2). The Doppler waveform characteristically has a high resistance index, often associated with a diastolic notch – a
pattern typical of the normal high-resistance uterine circulation in nonpregnant
women. Many studies have investigated the possibility that the abnormal waveform could be a useful predictive indicator of preeclampsia (Chappell and Bewley,
1998) in the clinic, but analysis is confounded by lack of conformity in the

definition of the disease and in the absence of any agreed standard protocol. Whilst of inadequate specificity for use in a low-risk population, uterine artery Doppler waveform analysis is undoubtedly useful in the research setting where it has been used successfully for identification of women at risk of the disease for intervention studies (for review, see Chien et al., 2000).

The vascular endothelium in preeclampsia

A name still often given to preeclampsia is 'toxaemia' of pregnancy, stemming from the hypothesis that the maternal disease is caused by a toxin or toxic factors originating from the placenta. This theory is little changed; indeed, it is now stronger than ever. The present 'version' includes a fundamental role for the maternal vascular endothelium; it is now hypothesized that poor perfusion of the placenta resulting from failed invasion provides the stimulus for leakage into the maternal circulation of factors which lead to endothelial cell dysfunction. Endothelial cell activation will promote platelet and neutrophil activation, and failure of the normal dilatory mechanisms will lead to vasospasm. Intense vasoconstriction will give rise to cerebral ischaemia and to eclamptic convulsions, and also to hepatic and lung dysfunction. In the kidney, damage to the glomerular capillary endothelium will cause proteinuria.

The defects described in the maternal vascular endothelium in preeclampsia are legion. Glomerular endotheliosis, swelling of the capillary endothelium, a lesion peculiar to preeclampsia, was first correctly described in 1950 (for review, see Sheehan, 1950). In the last decade endothelial dysfunction in preeclampsia has become widely accepted. Our laboratory showed that small arteries obtained from women with preeclampsia demonstrate impaired endothelium-dependent dilation (McCarthy et al., 1993; Knock and Poston, 1996), subsequently confirmed by others (Ashworth et al., 1997; Pascoal et al., 1998). This was followed by the demonstration of failure of the small arteries to dilate to flow (Cockell and Poston, 1997a; Kublickiene et al., 2000c). Many tens of publications itemize the variety of markers of endothelial cell activation which appear in the plasma of women with the disease, including endothelin-1, cellular fibronectin, thrombomodulin, plasminogen activator inhibitor type 1 and von Willebrand factor (for review, see Dekker and Sibai, 1998; Taylor and Roberts, 1999). The concentrations of some endothelial cell adhesion molecules, including vascular cell adhesion molecule, intravascular cell adhesion molecule and P-selectin, are also elevated in preeclampsia. The procoagulant state of healthy pregnancy is exacerbated by women who inherit low levels of anticoagulants, including antithrombin III, protein C and protein S (Dekker et al., 1995). Resistance to activated protein C, an inherited trait associated with mutation of the factor V Leiden gene, has also been implicated as some cohorts of preeclamptic patients have a higher incidence of this mutation (Dizon-Towson et al., 1996). However, other more recent studies have not reported such a high prevalence in other populations.

Assessment of nitric oxide in preeclampsia

The L-arginine–NO pathway is an expected casualty of endothelial cell damage in preeclampsia, and all studies in isolated arteries strongly suggest failure of NO-mediated dilatation (see above). In contrast, and probably because of methodological limitations, there is no consensus whether systemic NO synthesis is altered. Most studies have either shown no change (Cameron et al., 1993; Curtis et al., 1995; Silver et al., 1996) or an increase (Nobunaga et al., 1996; Smarason et al., 1997) in circulating or urinary NOx, probably reflecting variable nitrate intake, although Conrad et al. (1999) have found no evidence for NO depletion in women on restricted nitrate intake. Only Seligman et al. (1994) documented lower plasma NOx concentrations in women with preeclampsia. Paradoxically, two groups (Cameron et al., 1993; Nobunaga et al., 1996) have reported a correlation between systolic blood pressure and *increasing* urinary and plasma concentrations of NOx, respectively. In the latter study, volunteers were starved for 12–15 h in an attempt to control for dietary nitrogen. The periods of starvation or dietary nitrogen deprivation are necessarily short in pregnant women and are very likely to be insufficient for adequate 'washout'. Moreover, plasma and urine concentrations of NOx, as well as being influenced by the diet, are also not entirely derived from the endothelium, being reflective of synthesis by activated leukocytes. Granulocyte and monocyte activation are well described as part of the 'inflammatory' characteristics of the disease (Redman et al., 1999), and may provide a substantive source of NO.

NOS is competitively inhibited by an endogenous guanidino-substituted arginine analogue, N^GN^G-dimethylarginine (asymmetric dimethylarginine, ADMA). In normal pregnancy, the plasma concentration of ADMA is lower than in nonpregnant women (Fickling et al., 1993). Interestingly, plasma ADMA levels are significantly higher in women with preeclampsia than gestational-matched, normotensive controls (Holden et al., 1998). Consequently, endogenous inhibition of NOS by a specific inhibitor is a possible mechanism whereby NO production could be reduced in preeclampsia.

Potential origins of endothelial cell dysfunction

Other than the controversial NOx data, the evidence for endothelial cell dysfunction in preeclampsia is undisputed and it is hardly unexpected that the search for the possible cause or causes has been intense. Few are of the opinion that a single molecular species is responsible, and few would argue with the fact that the placenta is involved in some way. One attractive hypothesis is that preeclampsia is an exaggeration of the normal 'inflammatory' response to pregnancy (Redman et al., 1999), triggered by placental factors arising from poor perfusion. According to this hypothesis, endothelial cell activation is but one component of the excessive inflammatory response. In support, there is good evidence for endothelial and leukocyte activation in normal pregnancy. As described above, the endothelium expresses procoagulant markers in normal pregnancy. Redman's group (Sacks et al., 1998) have shown increased expression of surface markers of peripheral blood leukocyte activation, CD11b and CD64, on granulocytes and monocytes together with an increase in synthesis of reactive oxygen species (ROS). Leukocyte activation leads to synthesis and release of certain proinflammatory cytokines, particularly tumour necrosis factor alpha-α (TNF-α). Elevation of plasma TNF-α is well described in preeclampsia, but it may also originate from the placenta as TNF-α is a major secretory product of trophoblast, and secretion increases in response to hypoxia. Whatever the source, TNF-α and other products of leukocyte activation are likely to contribute to endothelial cell damage. Additionally, a feedforward system may come into play since endothelial cell activation and subsequent cell adhesion molecule expression will attract leukocytes and lead to further activation. A vicious cycle of endothelial cell damage could ensue.

A number of complementary theories of endothelial activation have received justified and increasing attention. Redman's group have evidence that leukocyte/endothelial activation may arise from excessive deportation of shed particles of placental trophoblast. Trophoblasts are deported from the placenta to the maternal circulation in normal pregnancy, and in increased numbers in preeclampsia (Chua et al., 1991). However, due to their size, few are likely to reach the arterial circulation, whereas the much smaller microvilli are much more likely to gain access. Knight et al. (1998) have detected syncytiotrophoblast microvilli in the plasma of pregnant women by the method of flow cytometry and with a fluoro-immunoassay using antiplacental alkaline phosphatase antibodies. Significantly higher levels were found in women with preeclampsia and concentrations were higher in uterine venous plasma than in concurrently sampled peripheral venous plasma, suggestive of placental origin. Studies from the same group have also shown that normal placental microvilli drastically reduce proliferation of cultured human umbilical venous endothelial cells (Smarason et al., 1993). More recently, von Dadelszen et al. (1999) have reported that supernatants from a coculture of endothelial cells and syncytiotrophoblast microvilli led to activation of granulocytes and monocytes, indicating that the microvilli may cause leukocyte activation as a result of endothelial cell activation.

Whilst focus has been placed on the role of the endothelium, some studies have also suggested that vascular smooth muscle may be abnormal in preeclampsia. The contractile response to TxA$_2$ has been shown to be upregulated in human omental resistance arteries from women with preeclampsia (Suzuki et al., 2000), and to be unafffected by endothelial removal, suggesting a smooth muscle defect. This study also demonstrated a reduced response to endothelium-derived NO which appeared, at least in part, to be due to a reduced GMP-mediated response in the vascular smooth muscle. Human omental resistance arteries have also been shown to undergo remodelling in women with preeclampsia (Aalkjaer et al., 1985), although it is not clear if this remodelling is an adaptation to hypertension of a cause of reduced perfusion.

A role for oxidative stress and dyslipidaemia?

The theory which one of us (LP) has recently focused upon is the postulate that endothelial dysfunction may arise from oxidative stress. Directly, and particularly through synthesis of lipid peroxides, ROS can cause endothelial dysfunction. The evidence for oxidative stress in preeclampsia is substantial and growing. Plasma nonenzymatic antioxidants, particularly ascorbic acid, are the primary line of defence against oxidative damage. Decreased plasma ascorbate concentrations in preeclampsia were first reported in 1964 (Clemetson and Andersen, 1964), an observation repeated many times (for review, see Hubel, 1999). We have shown recently that plasma vitamin C concentrations are reduced many weeks prior to the development of the disease (Chappell et al., 2000a) and Hubel et al. (1997) have reported that the plasma from women with preeclampsia leads to an escalated oxidative depletion of ascorbic acid in vitro. In contrast, vitamin E is usually raised in the plasma in preeclampsia (Uotila et al., 1993; Schiff et al., 1996). This is probably explicable on the basis of the hyperlipoproteinaemia associated with preeclampsia, since vitamin E is transported in plasma lipoproteins. Reduced activity of glutathione peroxidase and of superoxide dismutase (Poranen et al., 1996; Wang and Walsh, 1996) has also been reported, and both enzymes are important antioxidant defences. Additionally, plasma concentrations of the antioxidant glutathione are reduced (Raijmakers et al., 2000). Finally, there are scores of reports that lipid peroxidation products are increased in the plasma in preeclampsia (for review, see Hubel, 1999). These have been evaluated by estimation of antibodies to oxidized low-density lipoprotein (LDL; Branch, 1994) and in many instances by measurement of plasma concentrations of malondialdehyde (e.g. Hubel et al., 1996). Malondialydehyde concentrations are approximately 50% higher in sera from women with preeclampsia and decrease within 48 h postpartum. There is also evidence of raised plasma concentrations of the isoprostane, 8-epi-PGF$_{2\alpha}$ (Barden et al., 1996). Isoprostanes are formed by free radical-induced oxidation of arachidonic acid and are increasingly recognized as stable lipid peroxidation products which may accurately reflect oxidative damage in vivo. There are also reports of lipid peroxidation products in platelets and erythrocytes. Roggensack et al. (1999) have shown that small arteries from subcutaneous fat of women with preeclampsia demonstrate increased immunostaining for peroxynitrite. This occurred together with reduced intensity of staining for superoxide dismutase and increased staining for NOS. An increase in superoxide and NO production is the likely cause of the peroxynitrite deposition as these two radicals react to form peroxynitrite. Peroxynitrite will evoke endothelial dysfunction and at the same time reduce NO availability; these data accord therefore with the blunted endothelium-dependent relaxation observed in isolated arteries from the same circulation (McCarthy et al., 1993).

The peripheral blood leukocytes, and probably the maternal endothelium, are likely contributors to ROS synthesis but the placenta undoubtedly plays a major role. Placental ischaemia accelerates trophoblast cell turnover, thereby increasing the concentration of purines, which are substrates for xanthine dehydrogenase/oxidase (Many et al., 1996). Under hypoxic conditions, xanthine oxidase predominates over xanthine dehydrogenase to produce urate and ROS. This process could explain why hyperuricaemia often precedes clinically recognizable preeclampsia and occurs prior to any fall in glomerular filtration rate. In support of the suggestion that the placenta is the source of ROS synthesis, numerous studies have reported evidence of oxidative stress in the placenta of women with preeclampsia. These include decreased superoxide dismutase activity (Poranen et al., 1996), decreased glutathione peroxidase activity (Wang and Walsh, 1996) and increased xanthine oxidase activity (Many et al., 2000). There is also evidence for nitrotyrosine staining (indicating protein nitration by peroxynitrite; Myatt et al., 1996; Many et al., 2000) and for formation and secretion of 8-epi-PGF$_{2\alpha}$ (Walsh et al., 2000) in the placenta. The content of free 8-epi-PGF$_{2\alpha}$ is also increased in the decidua (Staff et al., 1999) and a recent study has shown that free 8-epi-PGF$_{2\alpha}$ reduces invasion of a cultured trophoblast cell line (JAR cells) through Transwell filters, an in vitro model of the placentation process (Staff et al., 2000).

The abnormal plasma lipid profile in preeclampsia is also likely to contribute to the generation of lipid oxidation products. Towards the end of normal pregnancy, maternal plasma levels of cholesterol and triglyceride increase by 50% and 300%, respectively (Potter and Nestel, 1979). Women with preeclampsia have even higher circulating levels of triglyceride, free fatty acid and total cholesterol (Sattar et al., 1996), with a relative increase in LDL cholesterol, and these disturbances are evident as early as 10 weeks of gestation in women destined to develop the disease. Free fatty acids themselves may stimulate ROS generation. Under conditions of oxidant stress and hypertriglyceridaemia, increased amounts of unsaturated fatty acids will be oxidized to lipid peroxides (Chirico et al., 1993; Sattar et al., 1996). There is also a qualitative change in LDLs in established preeclampsia, with a shift towards small dense particles (Hubel et al., 1998), a characteristic which

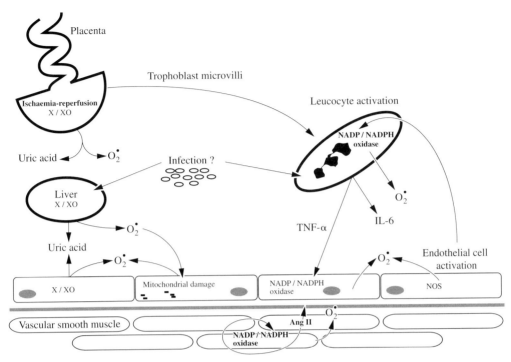

Figure 19.3   Oxidative stress in preeclampsia: possible origins of reactive oxygen species ($O_2^{\bullet}$). X/XO, xanthine/xanthine oxidase. TNF-α, tumour necrosis factor-α; NOS, nitric oxide synthase; NADPH, nicotinamide-adenine dinucleotide phosphate; Ang II, angiotensin II.

predisposes the LDL particle to oxidation.

Another possible contributory influence on synthesis of ROS is hyperhomocysteinaemia, frequently reported in women with preeclampsia (Ray and Laskin, 1999). Hyperhomocysteinaemia is known to induce endothelial dysfunction through ROS synthesis, an effect which has now been found to be reversible by antioxidant supplementation in normal nonpregnant volunteers subjected to acute experimental hyperhomocysteinaemia (Nappo et al., 1999; Figure 19.3).

The overwhelming evidence in favour of oxidative stress in preeclampsia has prompted the suggestion that antioxidant supplementation may be beneficial in the prevention or amelioration of the disease. Two studies of vitamin supplementation, both in women with *established* severe early-onset preeclampsia, have reported no substantial clinical benefit. Stratta et al. (1994) using 100–300 mg/day vitamin E in a nonrandomized trial and Gulmezoglu et al. (1997) in a randomized controlled trial of 1000 mg/day vitamin C, 800 IU/day vitamin E and 200 mg/day allopurinol, reported no significant improvement in clinical outcome. However, the second of these reported a trend towards later delivery in the treated group, and as late intervention may have precluded maximum benefit, both reports

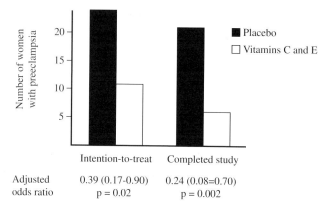

Figure 19.4 Reduced incidence of preeclampsia in intention-to-treat and completed study groups in a randomized trial of vitamin C and E supplementation; see Chappell et al. (1999).

proposed earlier initiation of therapy. We have recently reported a study in which we identified women at risk of preeclampsia on the basis of a previous history of the disease, or because they demonstrated an abnormal uterine artery Doppler waveform (see above; Chappell et al., 1999). A total of 283 women identified to be at risk were randomized to vitamin C (1000 mg/day) and vitamin E (400 IU/day) or to placebo at 16–22 weeks' gestation. Plasma markers of endothelial activation (PAI-1) and placental dysfunction (PAI-2) and plasma vitamin C and E concentrations were evaluated longitudinally until delivery. Supplementation with vitamins C and E was associated with a 61% reduction in the odds of developing preeclampsia on an intention-to-treat basis and a 76% reduction in the odds of developing the disease in the group who received the vitamins compared with those on placebo (Figure 19.4). Recently we reported (Chappell et al., 2000b) that the vitamin-treated group had a lower concentration of plasma 8-epi-PGF$_{2\alpha}$ than the placebo group, which returned to values similar to those of a pregnant low-risk control group, suggesting prevention/reversal of lipid peroxidation. This encouraging result in high-risk women has now paved the way for multicentre trials which will determine the potential benefit in lower-risk women, and establish that these supplements bring no harm to the fetus.

Conclusion

This short review has attempted to cover areas of topical interest relating to maternal vascular function in normal pregnancy and in preeclampsia. Many interesting areas of research have only been touched upon as they fall outside the focus of discussion. Neither has there been any attempt to cover fetal circulation, which alone could be the subject of an entire chapter. The convergence of interest in the endothelium in normal pregnancy and preeclampsia provides an excellent example of successful interaction between the physiological and clinical sciences.

REFERENCES

Aalkjaer, C., Danielsen, H., Johannesen, P. et al. (1985). Abnormal vascular function and morphology in pre-eclampsia: a study of isolated resistance vessels. *Clin. Sci.*, **69**, 477–82.

Ahokas, R.A., Friedman, S.A. & Sibai, B.M. (1997). Effect of indomethacin and N omega-nitro-L-arginine methyl ester on the pressure/flow relation in isolated perfused hindlimbs from pregnant and nonpregnant rats. *J. Soc. Gynecol. Invest.*, **4**, 229–35.

Anumba, D.O., Robson, S.C., Boys, R.J. & Ford, G.A. (1999a). Nitric oxide activity in the peripheral vasculature during normotensive and preeclamptic pregnancy. *Am. J. Physiol.*, **277**, H848–54.

Anumba, D.O., Ford, G.A., Boys, R.J. & Robson, S.C. (1999b). Stimulated nitric oxide release and nitric oxide sensitivity in forearm arterial vasculature during normotensive and preeclamptic pregnancy. *Am. J. Obstet. Gynecol.*, **181**, 1479–84.

Ashworth, J.R., Warren, A.Y., Baker, P.N. & Johnson IR. (1997). Loss of endothelium-dependent relaxation in myometrial resistance arteries in pre-eclampsia. *Br. J. Obstet. Gynaecol.*, **104**, 1152–8.

Aune, B., Vartun, A., Oian, P. & Sager, G. (2000). Evidence of dysfunctional beta-2 adrenoreceptor signal system in pre-eclampsia. *Br. J. Obstet. Gynaecol.*, **107**, 116–21.

Barden, A., Beilin, L.J., Ritchie, J. et al. (1996). Plasma and urinary 8-iso prostane as an indicator of lipid peroxidation in preeclampsia and normal pregnancy. *Clin. Sci.*, **91**, 711–18.

Barrow, S.E., Blair, I.A., Waddell, K.A. et al. (1983). Prostacyclin in late pregnancy: analysis of 6-oxo-prostaglandin F$_1$ in maternal plasma. In: *Prostacyclin in Pregnancy*, ed. Lewis, P.J., Moncada, S. & O'Grady, J., pp. 79–85. New York: Raven Press.

Bobadilla, R.A., Henkel, C.C., Henkel, E.C., Escalante, B. & Hong, E. (1997). Possible involvement of endothelium-derived hyperpolarizing factor in vascular responses of abdominal aorta from pregnant rats. *Hypertension*, **30**, 596–602.

Boccardo, P., Soregaroli, M., Aiello, S. et al. (1996). Systemic and fetal–maternal nitric oxide synthesis in normal pregnancy and pre-eclampsia. *Br. J. Obstet. Gynaecol.*, **103**, 879–86.

Bonnar, J. (1987). Haemostasis and coagulation disorders in pregnancy. In *Haemostasis and Thrombosis*, ed. Bloom, A.L. & Thomas, D.P., pp. 570–84. Edinburgh: Churchill Livingstone.

Bosio, P.M., McKenna, P.J., Conroy, R. & O'Herlihy, C. (1999). Maternal central hemodynamics in hypertensive disorders of pregnancy. *Obstet. Gynecol.*, **94**, 978–84.

Branch, D.W. (1994). Pre-eclampsia and serum antibodies to oxidized low-density lipoprotein. *Lancet*, **343**, 645–6.

Bremme, K., Ostlund, E., Almquist, I., Heinonen, K. & Blomback, M. (1992). Enhanced thrombin generation and fibrinolytic activity in normal pregnancy and the puerperium. *Obstet. Gynecol.*, **80**, 132–7.

Brosens, I., Robertson, W.B. & Dixon, H.G. (1967). The physiological response of the vessels of the placental bed to normal pregnancy. *J. Pathol. Bacteriol.*, **93**, 569–79.

Brosens, I., Robertson, W.B. & Dixon, H.G. (1972). The role of the spiral arteries in the pathogenesis of pre-eclampsia. *Obstet. Gynecol. Annu.*, **1**, 177–91.

Brosens, I., Dixon, H.G. & Robertson, W.B. (1997). Fetal growth retardation and the arteries of the placental bed. *Br. J. Obstet. Gynaecol.*, **84**, 656–63.

Cameron, I.T., van Papendorp, C.L., Palmer, R.M.J., Smith, S.K. & Moncada, S. (1993). Relationship between nitric oxide synthesis and increase in systolic blood pressure in women with hypertension in pregnancy. *Hypertens. Pregnancy*, **12**, 85–92.

Campbell, S., Diaz-Recasens J., Griffin, D.R. et al. (1983). New Doppler technique for assessing uteroplacental blood inflow. *Lancet*, **8326**, 675–7.

Caniggia, I., Grisaru-Gravnosky, S., Kuliszewsky, M., Post, M. & Lye, S.J. (1999). Inhibition of TGF-beta 3 restores the invasive capability of extravillous trophoblasts in preeclamptic pregnancies. *J. Clin. Invest.*, **103**, 1641–50.

Chapman, A.B., Abraham, W.T., Zamudio, S. et al. (1998). Temporal relationships between hormonal and hemodynamic changes in early human pregnancy. *Kidney Int.*, **54**, 2056–63.

Chappell, L.C. & Bewley, S. (1998). Pre-eclamptic toxaemia: the role of uterine artery Doppler. *Br. J. Obstet. Gynaecol.*, **105**, 379–82.

Chappell, L.C., Seed, P.T., Briley, A.L. et al. (1999). Effect of antioxidants on the occurrence of pre-eclampsia in women at increased risk: a randomized trial. *Lancet*, **354**, 810–16.

Chappell, L.C., Lee, R., Kelly, F.J. et al. (2000a). Plasma ascorbic acid concentrations are reduced in women with abnormal uterine artery doppler waveform and are independent of pregnancy outcome. *Hypertens. Pregnancy*, **19**, 54.

Chappell, L.C., O'Brien Coker, I., Mallet, A, Briley, A.L. & Poston, L. (2000b). Reduction in occurrence of pre-eclampsia with antioxidants is associated with decreased concentrations of plasma 8-epi-prostaglandin-F2α. *J. Soc. Gynecol. Invest.*, **7**, 182A.

Chesley, L.C. (1978). *Hypertensive Disorders in Pregnancy*, pp. 126–31. New York: Appleton-Century-Crofts.

Chien, P.R.W., Anrott, N., Gordon, A. & Khan, K.S. (2000). How useful is uterine artery Doppler flow velocimetry in the prediction of pre-eclampsia, intrauterine growth retardation and perinatal death? An overview. *Br. J. Obstet. Gynecol.*, **107**, 196–208.

Chirico, S., Smith, C., Merchant, C., Mitchinson, M.J. & Halliwell, B. (1993). Lipid peroxidation in hyperlipidaemic patients: a study of plasma using an HPLC-based thiobarbituric acid test. *Free Radical Res. Commun.*, **19**, 51–7.

Chu, Z.M. & Beilin, L.J. (1993). Mechanisms of vasodilatation in pregnancy: studies of the role of prostaglandins and nitric oxide in changes of vascular reactivity in the in situ blood perfused mesentry of pregnant rats. *Br. J. Pharmacol.*, **109**, 322–9.

Chua, W.S., Wilkins, T., Sargent, I. & Redman, C. (1991). Trophoblast deportation in pre-eclamptic pregnancy. *Br. J. Obstet. Gynaecol.*, **98**, 973–9.

Chumbley, G., King, A., Robertson, K., Holmes, N. & Loke, Y.W. (1994). Resistance of HLA-G and HLA-A$_2$ transfectants to lysis by decidual NK cells. *Cell Immunol.*, **155**, 312–22.

Clapp, J.F. & Capeless. E. (1997). Cardiovascular function before, during, and after the first and subsequent pregnancies. *Am. J. Cardiol.*, **80**, 1469–73.

Clemetson, C.A.B. & Andersen, L. (1964). Ascorbic acid metabolism in pre-eclampsia. *Obstet. Gynecol.*, **24**, 774–82.

Cockell, A.P. & Poston, L. (1996). Isolated small mesenteric arteries from pregnant rats show enhanced flow mediated relaxation but normal myogenic tone. *J. Physiol.*, **495**, 545–51.

Cockell, A.P. & Poston, L. (1997a). Flow mediated vasodilatation is enhanced in normal pregnancy but reduced in preeclampsia. *Hypertension*, **30**, 247–51.

Cockell, A.P. & Poston, L. (1997b). 17β estradiol stimulates flow-induced vasodilatation in isolated small mesenteric arteries from prepubertal female rats. *Am. J. Obstet. Gynecol.*, **177**, 1432–8.

Conrad, K.P. & Colpoys, M.C. (1986). Evidence against the hypothesis that prostaglandins are the vasodepressor agents of pregnancy. *J. Clin. Invest.*, **77**, 230–45.

Conrad, K.P. & Vernier, V.A. (1989). Plasma levels, urinary excretion and metabolic production of cGMP during gestation in rats. *Am. J. Physiol.*, **257**, R847–53.

Conrad, K.P., Joffe, G.M., Kruszyna, H. et al. (1993). Identification of increased nitric oxide biosynthesis during pregnancy in rats. *FASEB J.*, **7**, 566–71.

Conrad, K.P., Krechner, L.J. & Mosher, M.D. (1999). Plasma and 24-h NO(x) and cGMP during normal pregnancy and preeclampsia in women on a reduced NO(x) diet. *Am. J. Physiol.*, **277**, F48–57.

Curtis, N.E., Gude, N.M., King, R.G. et al. (1995). Nitric oxide metabolites in normal human pregnancy and preeclampsia. *Hypertens. Pregnancy*, **23**, 1096–105.

Dalle Lucca, J.J., Adeagbo, A.S.O. & Alsip, N.L. (2000). Influence of oestrous cycle and pregnancy on the reactivity of the rat mesenteric vascular bed. *Hum. Reprod.*, **15**, 961–8.

Danielson, L.A. & Conrad, K.P. (1995). Acute blockade of nitric oxide synthase inhibits renal vasodilation and hyperfiltration during pregnancy in chronically instrumented conscious rats. *J. Clin. Invest.*, **96**, 482–90.

de Boer, K., ten-Cate, J.W., Sturk, A., Borm, J.J. & Treffers, P.E. (1989). Enhanced thrombin generation in normal and hypertensive pregnancy. *Am. J. Obstet. Gynecol.*, **160**, 95–100.

Dekker, G.A. & Sibai, B.M. (1998). Etiology and pathogenesis of preeclampsia. *Am. J. Obstet. Gynecol.*, **179**, 1359–75.

Dekker, G.A., de Vries, J.I.P., Doelitzsch, P.M. et al. (1995). Underlying disorders associated with severe early onset preeclampsia. *Am. J. Obstet. Gynecol.*, **173**, 1042–8.

de Wolf, F., De Wolf-Peeters, C., Brosens, I. & Robertson, W.D. (1980). The human placental bed: electron microscope study of trophoblastic invasion of spiral arteries. *Am. J. Obstet. Gynecol.*, **137**, 58–70.

Dizon-Towson, D.S., Nelson, L.M., Easton, K. & Ward, K. (1996). The factor V Leiden mutation may predispose women to severe preeclampsia. *Am. J. Obstet. Gynecol.*, **175**, 902–5.

Dorup, I., Skajaa, K. & Sorensen, K.E. (1999). Normal pregnancy is associated with enhanced endothelium-dependent flow-mediated vasodilation. *Am. J. Physiol.*, **276**, H821–5.

Easterling, T.R., Watts, H., Schumucker, B.C. & Benedetti, T.J. (1987). Measurement of cardiac output during pregnancy: validation of Dopper technique and clinical observations in pre-eclampsia. *Obstet. Gynecol.*, **69**, 845–50.

Feletou, M. & Vanhoutte, P.M. (1999). The third pathway: endothelium dependent hyperpolarization. *J. Physiol. Pharmacol.*, **50**, 525–34.

Fickling, S.A., Williams, D., Vallance, P., Nussey, S.S. & Whitley, G.S. (1993). Plasma concentrations of endogenous inhibitor of nitric oxide synthesis in normal pregnancy and preeclampsia. *Lancet*, **342**, 242–3.

Fisher, S.J. & Roberts, J.M. (1999). Defects in placentation and perfusion in *Chesley's Hypertensive Disorders in Pregnancy*, ed. Lindheimer, M.D., Roberts, J.M. & Cunningham, G., Connecticut: Appleton & Lang.

Fitzgerald, D.J., Entman, S.S., Mulloy, K. & FitzGerald, G.A. (1987a). Decreased prostacyclin biosynthesis precedes the clinical manifestation of pregnancy induced hypertension. *Circulation*, **75**, 956–63.

Fitzgerald, D.J., Mayo, G., Catella, F., Entman, S.S. & FitzGerald, G.A. (1987b). Increased thromboxane biosynthesis in normal pregnancy is mainly derived from platelets. *Am. J. Obstet. Gynecol.*, **157**, 325–30.

Gant, N.F., Daley, G.L., Chand, S., Whalley, P.J. & MacDonald, P.C. (1973). A study of angiotensin II pressor response throughout primigravid pregnancy. *J. Clin. Invest.*, **52**, 2682–9.

Gerber, R.T., Anwar, M.A. & Poston, L.(1998). Enhanced acetylcholine induced relaxation in small mesenteric arteries from pregnant rats: an important role for endothelium-derived hyperpolarizing factor (EDHF). *Br. J. Pharmacol.*, **125**, 455–532.

Goodman, R.P., Killam, A.P., Brash, A.R. & Branch, R.A. (1982). Prostacyclin production during pregnancy and pregnancy complicated by hypertension. *Am. J. Obstet. Gynecol.*, **142**, 817–22.

Gulmezoglu, A.M., Hofmeyr, G.J. & Oosthuizen, M.M. (1997). Antioxidants in the treatment of severe pre-eclampsia: an explanatory randomised controlled trial. *Br. J. Obstet. Gynaecol.*, **104**, 689–96.

Habermehl, D.A., Janowiak, M.A., Vagnoni, K.E., Bird, I.M. & Magness R.R. (2000). Endothelial vasodilator production by uterine artery and systemic arteries IV. Cyclooxygenase isoform expression during the ovarian cycle and pregnancy in sheep. *Biol. Reprod.*, **62**, 781–8.

Halpern, W., Osol, G. & Coy, G.S. (1984). Mechanical behaviour of pressurized in vitro prearteriolar vessels determined with a video system. *Ann. Biomed. Eng.*, **12**, 4673–79.

Hata, T., Hashimoto, M., Kanenishi, K. et al. (1999). Maternal circulating nitrite levels are decreased in both normotensive pregnancies and pregnancies with pre-eclampsia. *Gynecol. Obstet. Invest.*, **48**, 93–7.

Heesch, C.M. & Rogers, R.C. (1995). Effects of pregnancy and progesterone metabolites on regulation of sympathetic outflow. *Clin. Exp. Pharmacol. Physiol.*, **22**, 136–42.

Holden, D.P., Fickling, S.A., Whitley, G.S. & Nussey, S.S. (1998). Plasma concentrations of asymmetric dimethylarginine, a natural inhibitor of nitric oxide synthase, in normal pregnancy and pre-eclampsia. *Am. J. Obstet. Gynecol.*, **178**, 551–6.

Hubel, C.A. (1999). Oxidative stress in the pathogenesis of preeclampsia. *Proc. Soc. Exp. Biol. Med.*, **222**, 222–35.

Hubel, C.A., McLaughlin, M.K., Evans, R.W. et al. (1996). Fasting serum triglycerides, free fatty acids and malondialdehyde are increased in preeclampsia, are positively correlated, and decrease within 48 hours post partum. *Am. J. Obstet. Gynaecol.*, **174**, 975–82.

Hubel, C.A., Kagan, V.E., Kisin, E.R., McLaughlin, M.K. & Roberts, J.M. (1997). Increased ascorbic acid radical formation and ascorbate depletion in plasma from women with pre-eclampsia: implications for oxidative stress. *Free Radical Biol. Med.*, **23**, 597–609.

Hubel, C.A., Lyall, F., Gandley, R.E. & Roberts, J.M. (1998). Small low-density lipoproteins and vascular cell adhesion molecule (VCAM-1) are increased in association with hyperlipidaemia in preeclampsia. *Metabolism*, **47**, 1281–8.

Janowiak, M.A., Magness, R.R., Habermehl, D.A. & Bird, I.M. (1998). Pregnancy increases ovine uterine artery endothelial cyclooxygenase expression. *Endocrinology*, **139**, 765–71.

Khong, T.Y., De Wolf, F., Robertson, W.B. & Brosens, I. (1986). Inadequate maternal vascular response to placentation in pregnancies complicated by pre-eclampsia and by small-for-gestational age infants. *Br. J. Obstet. Gynaecol.*, **93**, 1049–59.

Knight, M., Redman, C.W.G., Linton, E.A. & Sargent, I.L. (1998). Shedding of syncytiotrophoblast microvilli into the maternal circulation in pre-eclamptic pregnancies. *Br. J. Obstet. Gynaecol.*, **105**, 632–40.

Knock, G.A. & Poston, L. (1996). Bradykinin-mediated relaxation of isolated maternal resistance arteries in normal pregnancy and preeclampsia. *Am. J. Obstet. Gynecol.*, **175**, 1668–74.

Kublickiene, K.R., Cockell, A.P., Nisell, H. & Poston, L. (1997). Role of nitric oxide in the regulation of vascular tone in pressurised and perfused resistance myometrial arteries from term pregnant women. *Am. J. Obstet. Gynecol.*, **177**, 1263–9.

Kublickiene, K.R., Nisell, H., Poston, L., Kruger, K. & Lindblom, B. (2000a). Modulation of vascular tone by nitric oxide and endothelin 1 in myometrial resistance arteries from pregnant women at term. *Am. J. Obstet. Gynecol.*, **182**, 87–93.

Kublickiene, K.R., Nisell, H. & Poston, L. (2000b). 17β-estradiol upregulates flow-mediated relaxation in small sub-cutaneous arteries from postmenopausal women. *J. Soc. Gynecol. Invest.*, **7**, 186A.

Kublickiene, K.R., Lindblom, B., Kruger, K. & Nisell, H. (2000c). Preeclampsia: evidence for impaired shear stress-mediated nitric oxide release in uterine circulation. *Am. J. Obstet. Gynecol.*, **183**, 160–6.

Learmont, J.G., Cockell, A.P., Knock, G.A. & Poston, L. (1996). Myogenic and flow mediated responses in isolated mesenteric small arteries from pregnant and non-pregnant rats. *Am. J. Obstet. Gynecol.*, **174**, 1631–6.

Letsky, E.A. (1995). Coagulation defects. In: *Medical Disorders in Obstetric Practice*, ed. de Swiet, M., pp. 71–115. Oxford: Blackwell Scientific.

Loke Y.W. & King, A. (2000). Decidual natural-killer-cell interaction with trophoblast:cytolysis or cytokine production? *Biochem. Soc. Trans.*, **28**, 196–8.

Lyall, F., Bulmer, J.N., Kelly, H., Duffie, E. & Robson, S.C. (1999). Human trophoblast invasion and spiral artery transformation: the role of nitric oxide. *Am. J. Pathol.*, **154**, 1105–14.

Magness, R.R. & Rosenfeld, C.R. (1989). Local and systemic estradiol-17β: effects on uterine and systemic vasodilatation. *Am. J. Physiol.*, **256**, E536–42.

Magness, R., Rosenfeld, C.R., Faucher, D.J. & Mitchell, M.D. (1992). Uterine prostaglandin production in ovine pregnancy: effects of angiotensin II and indomethacin. *Am. J. Physiol.*, **263**, H188–97.

Magness, R.R., Shaw, C.E., Phernetton, T.M., Sheng, J. & Bird I.M. (1997). Endothelial vasodilator production by uterine and systemic arteries II. Pregnancy effects on NO synthase expression. *Am. J. Physiol.*, **272**, H1730–40.

Many, A., Hubel, C.A. & Roberts, J.M. (1996). Hyperuricemia and xanthine oxidase in pre-eclampsia, revisited. *Am. J. Obstet. Gynecol.*, **174**, 288–91.

Many, A., Hubel, C.A., Fisher, S.J., Roberts, J.M. & Zhou, Y. (2000). Invasive cytotrophoblasts manifest evidence of oxidative stress in preeclampsia. *Am. J. Pathol.*, **156**, 321–31.

Manyonda, I.T., Slater, D.M., Fenske, C. et al. (1998). A role for noradrenaline in pre-eclampsia: towards a unifying hypothesis for the pathophysiology. *Br. J. Obstet. Gynaecol.*, **105**, 641–8.

McCarthy, A.L., Woolfson, R.G., Raju, S.K. & Poston, Ll. (1993). Abnormal endothelial function of resistance arteries from women with pre-eclampsia. *Am. J. Obstet. Gynecol.*, **168**, 1323–30.

McCarthy, A.L., Taylor, P., Graves, J., Raju, S.K. & Poston, L. (1994). Endothelium dependent relaxation of human resistance arteries in pregnancy. *Am. J. Obstet. Gynecol.*, **171**, 1309–15.

Mendelsohn, M.E. & Karas, R.H. (1999). The protective effects of estrogen on the cardiovascular system. *N. Engl. J. Med.*, **340**, 1801–11.

Mulvany, M.J. & Halpern, W. (1977). Contractile properties of small arterial resistance vessels in spontaneously hypertensive and normotensive rats. *Circ. Res.*, **41**, 19–26.

Myatt,L., Rosenfeld, R.B., Eis, A.L. et al. (1996). Nitrotyrosine residues in placenta: evidence of peroxynitrite formation and action. *Hypertension*, **28**, 488–93.

Nappo, F., De Rosa, N., Marfella, R. et al. (1999). Impairment of endothelial functions and reversal by antioxidant vitamins. *J.A.M.A.*, **281**, 2113–18.

Nelson, S.H., Steinsland, O.S., Suresh, M.S. & Lee, N.M. (1998). Pregnancy augments nitric oxide-dependent dilator response to acetylcholine in the human uterine artery. *Hum. Reprod.*, **13**, 1361–7.

Nisell, H., Hjerndhal, P. & Linde, B. (1985). Cardiovascular responses to circulating catecholamines in normal pregnancy and in pregnancy-induced hypertension. *Clin. Physiol.*, **5**, 479–93.

Nobunaga, T., Tokugawa, Y., Hashimoto, K. et al. (1996). Plasma nitric oxide levels in pregnant patients with preeclampsia and essential hypertension. *Gynecol. Obstet. Invest.*, **41**, 189–93.

O'Hagan, K.P. & Casey, S.M. (1998). Arterial baroreflex during pregnancy and renal sympathetic nerve activity during parturition in rabbits. *Am. J. Physiol.*, **274**, H1635–42.

Pan, Z.-R., Lindheimer, M.D., Bailin, J. & Barron, W.M. (1990). Regulation of blood pressure in pregnancy: pressor system blockade and stimulation. *Am. J. Physiol.*, **258**, H1559–72.

Pascoal, I.F. & Umans, J.G. (1996). Effect of pregnancy on mechanisms of relaxation in human omental microvessels. *Hypertension*, **28**, 183–7.

Pascoal, I.F., Lindheimer, M.D., Nalbantian-Brandt, C. & Umans, J.G. (1998). Preeclampsia selectively impairs endothelium-dependent relaxation and leads to oscillatory activity in small omental arteries. *J. Clin. Invest.*, **101**, 464–70.

Phippard, A.F., Horvath, J.S., Glynn, E.M. et al. (1986). Circulatory adaptation to pregnancy: serial studies of haemodynamics, blood volume, renin and aldosterone in the baboon (*Papio hamadryas*). *J. Hypertens.*, **4**, 773–9.

Pijnenborg, R., Anthony, J., Davey, D.A. et al. (1991). Placental bed spiral arteries in the hypertensive disorders of pregnancy. *Br. J. Obstet. Gynaecol.*, **98**, 648–55.

Poranen, A.K., Ekbland, U., Uotila, P. & Ahotupa, M. (1996). Lipid peroxidation and antioxidants in normal and preeclamptic pregnancies. *Placenta*, **17**, 401–5.

Poston, L., McCarthy, A.L. & Ritter, J.M. (1995). Control of vascular resistance in maternal and fetoplacental vascular beds. *Rev. Pharmacol. Ther.*, **65**, 215–39.

Potter, J.M. & Nestel, P.J. (1979). The hyperlipidaemia of pregnancy in normal and complicated pregnancies. *Am. J. Obstet. Gynecol.*, **133**, 165–70.

Raijmakers, M.T., Zusterzeel, P.L., Steegers, E.A., Demacker, P.N. & Peters, W.H. (2000). Plasma thiol status in pre-eclampsia. *Obstet. Gynecol.*, **95**, 180–4.

Ray, J.G. & Laskin, C.A. (1999). Folic acid and homocysteine metabolic defects and the risk of placental abruption, pre-eclampsia and spontaneous pregnancy loss. *Placenta*, **20**; 519–29.

Redman, C.W.G., Sacks, G.P. & Sargent, I.L. (1999). Pre-eclampsia: an excessive maternal inflammatory response to pregnancy. *Am. J. Obstet. Gynecol.*, **180**, 499–606.

Reister, F., Frank, H.G., Heyl, W. et al. (1999). The distrubution of macrophages in spiral arteries of the placental bed in pre-eclampsia differs from that in healthy patients. *Placenta*, **20**, 229–33.

Roberts, J.M. & Hubel, C.A. (1999). Is oxidative stress the link in the two-stage model of pre-eclampsia? *Lancet*, **354**, 788–9.

Robertson, W.B., Brosens, I. & Dixon, H.G. (1976). The pathological response of the vessels of the placental bed to hypertensive pregnancy. *J. Pathol. Bacteriol.*, **93**, 581–92.

Robertson, W.B., Khong, T.Y., Brosens, I. et al. (1986). The placental bed biopsy: review from three European centers. *Am. J. Obstet. Gynecol.*, **155**, 401–12.

Robinson, L.J., Weremowicz, S., Morton, C.C. & Michel, T. (1994). Isolation and chromosomal localization of the human eNOS gene. *Genomics*, **19**, 350–7.

Robson, S.C., Hunter, S., Boys, R.J. & Dunlop, W. (1989). Serial study of factors influencing changes in cardiac output during human pregnancy. *Am. J. Physiol.*, **356**, H1060–5.

Roggensack, A.M., Zhang, Y. & Davidge, S.T. (1999). Evidence for peroxynitrite formation in the vasculature of women with preeclampsia. *Hypertension*, **33**, 83–9.

Russell, K.R., Haynes, M.P., Sinha, D., Clerisme, E. & Bender, J.R. (2000a). Human vascular endothelial cells contain membrane binding sites for estradiol, which mediate rapid intracellular signalling. *Proc. Natl Acad. Sci. U.S.A.*, **97**, 5930–5.

Russell, K.S., Haynes, M.P., Caulin-Glaser, T. et al. (2000b). Estrogen stimulates heat shock protein 90 binding to endothelial nitric oxide synthase in human vascular endothelial cells. Effects on calcium sensitivity and NO release. *J. Biol. Chem.*, **275**, 5026–30.

Sacks, G.P., Studena, K., Sargent, I.L. & Redman, C.W. (1998). Normal pregnancy and pre-eclampsia both produce inflammatory changes in peripheral blood leukocytes akin to those of sepsis. *Am. J. Obstet. Gynecol.*, **179**, 80–6.

Sattar, N., Gaw, A., Packard, C.J. & Greer, I.A. (1996). Potential pathogenic roles of aberrant lipoprotein and fatty acid metabolism in preeclampsia. *Br. J. Obstet. Gynecol.*, **103**, 614–20.

Schiff, E., Friedman, S.A., Stampfer, M. et al. (1996). Dietary consumption and plasma concentrations of vitamin E in pregnancies complicated by preeclampsia. *Am. J. Obstet. Gynecol.*, **175**, 1024–8.

Schobel, H.P. Fischer, T., Heuszer, K., Geiger, H. & Schmeider, R.E. (1996). Pre-eclampsia – a state of sympathetic overactivity. *N. Engl. J. Med.*, **335**, 1480–5.

Seligman, S.P., Buyon, J.P., Clancy, R.M., Young, B.K. & Abramson, S.B. (1994). The role of nitric oxide in the pathogenesis of preeclampsia. *Am. J. Obstet. Gynecol.*, **171**, 944–8.

Shaamash, A.H., Elsnosy, E.D., Makhlouf, A.M. et al. (2000). Maternal and fetal serum nitric oxide (NO) concentrations in normal pregnancy, pre-eclampsia and eclampsia. *Int. J. Obstet. Gynecol.*, **68**, 207–14.

Sheehan, H.L. (1950). Renal morphology in pre-eclampsia. *Kidney Int.*, **18**, 241–52.

Silver, R.K., Kupfermine, M.J., Russell, T.L. et al. (1996). Evaluation of nitric oxide as a mediator of severe preeclampsia. *Am. J. Obstet. Gynecol.*, **175**, 1013–17.

Sladek, S.M., Magness, R.R. & Conrad, K.P. (1997). Nitric oxide and pregnancy. *Am. J. Physiol.*, **272**, R441–63.

Smarason, A.K., Sargent, I.L., Starkey, P.M. & Redman, C.W.G. (1993). The effect of placental syncytiotrophoblast microvillous membranes from normal and pre-eclamptic women on the growth of endothelial cells in vitro. *Br. J. Obstet. Gynaecol.*, **100**, 943–9.

Smarason, A.K., Allman, K.G., Young, D. & Redman, C.W.G. (1997). Elevated levels of serum nitrate, a stable end product of nitric oxide, in women with pre-eclampsia. *Br. J. Obstet. Gynaecol.*, **104**, 538–43.

Sorensen, J.D., Secher, N.J. & Jespersen, J. (1995). Perturbed (procoagulant) endothelium and deviations within the fibrinolytic system during the third trimester of normal pregnancy. *Acta Obstet. Gynecol. Scand.*, **74**, 257–61.

Sorensen, T.K., Easterling, T.R., Carlson, K.L., Brateng, D.A. & Benedetti, T.J. (1992). The maternal hemodynamic effect of indomethacin in normal pregnancy. *Obstet. Gynecol.*, **79**, 661–3.

Staff, A.C., Halvorsen, B., Ranheijm, T. & Henriksen, T. (1999). Elevated level of free 8-iso-prostaglandin F_2 alpha in the decidua basalis of women with pre-eclampsia. *Am. J. Obstet. Gynecol.*, **181**, 1211–15.

Staff, A.C., Ranheim, T., Henriksen, T. & Halvorsen, B. (2000). 8-iso-prostaglandin $F_{2\alpha}$ reduces trophoblast invasion and matrix metalloproteinase activity. *Hypertension*, **35**, 1307–13.

Starzyk, K.A., Salafia, C.M., Pezzullo, J.C. et al. (1997). Quantitative differences in arterial morphometry define the placental bed in preeclampsia. *Hum. Pathol.*, **28**, 353–8.

Stratta, P., Canavese, C., Porcu, M. et al. (1994). Vitamin E supplementation in preeclampsia. *Gynecol. Obstet. Invest.*, **37**, 246–9.

Suzuki, Y., Kajikuri, J., Suzomori, K. & Itoh, T. (2000). Mechanisms underlying the reduced endothelium-dependent relaxation in human omental resistance artery in pre-eclampsia. *J. Physiol.*, **527**, 163–74.

Taylor, R.N. & Roberts, J.M. (1999). Endothelial cell dysfunction. In: *Chesley's Hypertensive Disorders in Pregnancy*, ed. Lindheimer, M.D., Roberts, J.M. & Cunningham, G. Connecticut: Appleton & Lang.

Uotila, J.T., Tuimala, R.J. & Aarnio, T.M. (1993). Findings on lipid peroxidation and anti-oxidant function in hypertensive complications of pregnancy. *Br. J. Obstet. Gynaecol.*, **100**, 270–6.

Van Buren, G.A., Yang, D. & Clarke, K.E. (1992). Estrogen-induced uterine vasodilation is antagonised by L-nitroarginine methyl ester, an inhibitor of nitric oxide synthesis. *Am. J. Obstet. Gynecol.*, **167**, 828–33.

Veille, J., Li, P., Eisenach, J.C., Massman, A.G. & Figueroa, J.P. (1996). Effects of estrogen on nitric oxide synthase biosynthesis and vascular relaxant activity in sheep uterine and renal arteries in vitro. *Am. J. Obstet. Gynecol.*, **174**, 1043–9.

Veille, J.C., Gorusch, L., Weeks, W. & Zaccaro, D. (1998). Hyperemic response of the brachial artery during the second half of pregnancy. *J. Soc. Gynecol. Invest.*, **5**, 38–43.

Visser, W. & Wallenburg, H.C. (1991). Central hemodynamic observations in untreated preeclamptic patients. *Hypertension*, **17**, 1072–7.

von Dadelszen, P., Hurst, G. & Redman, C.W. (1999). Supernatants from co-cultured endothelial cells and syncytiotrophoblast microvillous membranes activate peripheral blood leukocytes in vitro. *Hum. Reprod.*, **14**, 919–24.

Walsh, S.W., Vaughan, J.E., Wang, Y. & Roberts L.J. (2000). Placental isoprostane is significantly increased in pre-eclampsia *FASEB J.*, **14**, 1289–96.

Wang, Y. & Walsh, S.W. (1996). Antioxidant activities and mRNA expression of superoxide dismutase, catalase, and glutathione peroxidase in normal and preeclamptic placentas. *J. Soc. Gynecol. Invest.*, **3**, 179–84.

Ward, K. & Lindheimer, M.D. (1999). Genetic factors. In: *Chesley's Hypertensive Disorders in Pregnancy*, ed. Lindheimer, M.D., Roberts, J.M. & Cunningham, G, pp. 453–86. Connecticut, USA: Appleton & Lang.

Weiner, C.P., Knowles, R.G. & Moncada, S. (1994). Induction of nitric oxide synthases early in pregnancy. *Am. J. Obstet. Gynecol.*, **171**, 838–43.

Williams, D.J., Vallance, P.J.T., Neild, G.H., Spencer, J.A.D. & Imms, F.J. (1997). Nitric oxide mediated vasodilatation in human pregnancy. *Am. J. Physiol.*, **272**, H748–52.

Xu, D., Martin, P., St John, J. et al. (1996). Upregulation of endothelial and constitutive nitric oxide synthase in pregnant rats. *Am. J. Physiol.*, **271**, R1739–45.

Yallampalli, C. & Garfield, R.E. (1993). Inhibition of nitric oxide synthesis in rats during pregnancy produces signs similar to those of pre-eclampsia. *Am. J. Obstet. Gynecol.*, **169**, 1316–20.

Yang, C.C., Chao, T.C., Kuo, T.B., Yin, C.S. & Chen, H.I. (2000). Pre-eclamptic pregnancy is associated with increased sympathetic and decreased parasympathetic control of HR. *Am. J. Physiol.*, **278**, H1269–73.

Zhou, Y., Damsky, C.H. & Fisher, S.J. (1997). Preeclampsia is associated with failure of human cytotrophoblasts to mimic a vascular adhesion phenotype. One cause of defective endovascular invasion in this syndrome? *J. Clin. Invest.*, **99**, 2152–64.

Index

Note: page numbers in *italics* refer to figures and tables